Essentials of Pharmacology
for Nurses

Essentials of Pharmacology for Nurses

Fourth Edition

Paul Barber and Deborah Robertson

Mc Graw Hill

Open University Press

Open University Press
McGraw-Hill Education
8th Floor, 338 Euston Road
London
England
NW1 3BH

email: enquiries@openup.co.uk
world wide web: www.openup.co.uk

and Two Penn Plaza, New York, NY 10121-2289, USA

First edition published 2020

Commissioning Editor: Sam Crowe
Editorial Assistant: Beth Summers
Content Product Manager: Ali Davis

A catalogue record of this book is available from the British Library

ISBN-13: 978-0-33-524844-5
ISBN-10: 0-33-524844-6
eISBN: 978-0-33-524845-2

Library of Congress Cataloging-in-Publication Data
CIP data applied for

Typeset by Transforma Pvt. Ltd., Chennai, India

Praise for this book

Overall, this book is an excellent resource for healthcare students that will support their learning throughout their training and beyond. It covers fundamental concepts of how the major classes of medications exert their therapeutic effect, but also how side effects and adverse reactions can occur. Chapters on legal aspects of medication administration and drug calculations enhance this usefulness of this book – all of which are supported by example questions, calculations and clinical 'tips'. This book has been fully updated to reflect the 2018 NMC standards and as such provides a one-stop shop for any students studying safe administration of medications.

Dr Andy Powell, Physiology Lead for Nursing, Birmingham City University

The outlay of the chapters is easily navigated and the level of the knowledge that the book starts at is at a basic level enough for any student nurse from year 1-3 to start with and builds in complexity. They are in lovely bite-size chunks that are easy to read and easily understood. The 10 MCQ's at the end of a chapter are a very useful method of chapter consolidation and the case studies further reinforce learning.

Georgina Cox, Senior Lecturer in Adult Health, Middlesex University

Brief table of contents

Detailed table of contents

About the authors

Paul Barber (MSc Practitioner Research, BSc (Hons) Nursing, Dip N (Lond), Cert Ed, RNT, SRN, RMN) commenced his nursing career in 1974 as a cadet nurse. He completed both his Registered Mental Nurse and State Registered Nurse training. Paul spent his early career in surgery, high dependency, and accident and emergency, and then progressed to become manager of a small surgical unit. Paul commenced a teaching career in October 1988 and has held a variety of positions in education from senior lecturer to head of an educational centre. Paul has now retired from full-time teaching as a senior lecturer.

Deborah Robertson joined the School of Health & Society at the University of Salford in March 2018. Prior to that she was in nurse education in the Faculty of Health and Social Care at the University of Chester (starting in 2004). Deborah is an RGN but also holds a BSc (Hons) and PhD in Pharmacology. She teaches on the Non-Medical Prescribing Course where she uses her expertise in pharmacology. Deborah also inputs heavily into the pre-registration nursing curriculum and teaching around anatomy, physiology, pharmacology and medicines management as well as being involved in postgraduate research and education.

Acknowledgements

The authors would like to acknowledge the contributions of Dr. Alexander Robertson, General Practitioner, to some of the clinical therapeutic aspects of Chapters 4–13.

List of abbreviations

5-HT	5-hydroxytryptamine	DVT	deep vein thrombosis
AAA	abdominal aortic aneurysm	EMLA	eutectic mixture of local anaesthetics
ABCDE	airway, breathing, circulation, disability, exposure	EPSE	extra-pyramidal side-effect
ACE	angiotensin-converting enzyme	g	gram
ACS	acute coronary syndromes	GABA	gamma-aminobutyric acid
ADE	adverse drug event	GABA$_A$	GABA receptor subtype A
ADHD	attention deficit hyperactivity disorder	GI	gastrointestinal
ADR	adverse drug reaction	GP	general practitioner
AED	anti-epileptic drug	GTN	glyceryl trinitrate
AF	atrial fibrillation	HIV	human immunodeficiency virus
AIDS	acquired immunodeficiency syndrome	H-receptor	histamine receptor
ARB	angiotensin II receptor blocker	IDDM	insulin-dependent diabetes mellitus
BBB	blood–brain barrier	IM	intramuscular
BHF	British Heart Foundation	INR	international normalized ratio
BNF	British National Formulary	IV	intravenous
BP	blood pressure	kg	kilogram
BZD	benzodiazepine	LABA	long-acting beta 2 agonist
CCB	calcium channel blocker	LAMA	long-acting muscarinic antagonist
CDAO	controlled drug accountable officer	LD	learning disability
CD/LD	carbidopa/levodopa	MAO-B	monoamine oxidase B
CHD	coronary heart disease	MAOI	monoamine oxidase inhibitor
CMP	clinical management plan	mcg	microgram
COPD	chronic obstructive pulmonary disease	MDI	metered dose inhaler
COX	cyclo-oxygenase	mg	milligram
CR	controlled release	mg/kg/day	milligrams per kilogram per day
CSF	cerebrospinal fluid	MHRA	Medicines and Healthcare Products Regulatory Agency
CSM	Committee on Safety of Medicines	MI	Myocardial infarction
CTZ	chemoreceptor trigger zone	mL	millilitre
DA	dopamine	NA	noradrenaline
DH	Department of Health	NARI	noradrenaline reuptake inhibitor
DKA	diabetic ketoacidosis	NG	nasogastric
DM	diabetes mellitus	NHS	National Health Service
DMARD	disease-modifying anti-rheumatoid drug	NICE	National Institute for Health and Care Excellence
DNA	deoxyribonucleic acid	NIDDM	non-insulin-dependent diabetes mellitus
DOAC	direct acting anticoagulant	NMC	Nursing and Midwifery Council
		NPSA	National Patient Safety Agency

NRM	nucleus raphe magnus	RIMA	reversible inhibitor of monoamine oxidase-A
NSAID	non-steroidal anti-inflammatory drug	RNA	ribonucleic acid
NSTEMI	non-ST-segment elevation myocardial infarction	SC	subcutaneous
OCD	obsessive-compulsive disorder	SI	International System of Units
OTC	over the counter	SNRI	serotonin–norepinephrine re-uptake inhibitor
PABA	para-amino benzoate/para-aminobenzoic acid	SSRI	selective serotonin re-uptake inhibitor
PAG	periaqueductal grey	STI	sexually transmitted infection
PDE	phosphodiesterase	STEMI	ST-segment elevation myocardial infarction
PEG	percutaneous endoscopic gastrostomy	TB	tuberculosis
PEP	post-exposure prophylaxis	TCA	tricyclic antidepressant
PGD	Patient Group Direction	TTR	time in the therapeutic range
PPI	proton pump inhibitor	TXA	thromboxane
PrEP	pre-exposure prophylaxis	VTE	venous thromboembolism
prn	*pro re nata*	WHO	World Health Organization
PTSD	post-traumatic stress disorder		

Introduction

This book is aimed largely at nurses in training, but given the level of detail in many areas, qualified nurses will find it useful throughout their careers. It is important to understand that nurses need pharmacology education. This has been clearly outlined in the Pre-Registration Nursing Education Standards set out by the Nursing and Midwifery Council (NMC) in 2018. Nurses require pharmacology education so that they can inform patients about any medications prescribed, the need for those medications and the consequences of both taking and not taking them. The relevant sections of the Standards are outlined in the introductory chapters of the book, but it is important to remember that pharmacological knowledge standards apply throughout this text. Where there are specific standards relating to specific areas of education, these are introduced in the relevant chapters. You should remember that as a student or as a qualified nurse, your adherence to the Code (NMC 2015) includes medicines management.

Learning about medicines is a fundamental part of the nurse's role, whatever the field of nursing you decide to choose as a career pathway. This book is written to engage you in the subjects of pharmacology and calculation of drugs and for you to be able to apply these principles in your practice. First, you will notice that not all drugs are listed. This book is an essentials text and its aim is to introduce you to the most common areas of nursing practice regarding medications. It will focus on some of the major drug groups to outline the importance of your pharmacological knowledge without overwhelming you. Each of the chapters that discusses major drug groups has been enhanced by the inclusion of relevant aspects of physiology to help you understand drug action.

There is some application of drug calculation in all relevant chapters. Some calculations are simple (as they would be in practice) and some are more complicated due to the nature of the drugs. We wanted the calculations to reflect each of the chapter's contents and give you a sense of what might be expected in practice. Very detailed and complex calculations are not included here, as these are covered in other texts, some of which you will find in the recommended reading section at the end of each chapter.

A further feature of the book is the inclusion of case studies. At the end of each chapter there are a number of scenarios, covering relevant fields of practice.

Where possible we have also tried to focus the pharmacology on nursing practice. You will notice that in each chapter there are several boxes entitled 'Clinical tip'. These are designed to increase your understanding of the importance of pharmacology within nursing. They should also assist you in reflecting on your everyday practice in medicines management.

Finally, we have included 10 multiple-choice questions at the end of most chapters. All the questions are based on information included in the chapter, so there are no trick questions. We thought the idea of evaluating what you have gained in knowledge from reading each chapter was important and we hope you enjoy getting them all right! We know how important it is to students to evaluate their learning as they proceed.

References

Nursing and Midwifery Council (NMC) (2015) *The Code: Professional Standards of Practice and Behaviour for Nurses, Midwives and Nursing Associates*. London: NMC. Updated 2018.

Nursing and Midwifery Council (NMC) (2018) *Standards of Proficiency for Registered Nurses*. London: NMC.

Pharmacodynamics and pharmacokinetics

1

Chapter contents

Learning objectives

After studying this chapter, you should be able to:

- Understand what is meant by pharmacokinetics and pharmacodynamics.
- Describe aspects of absorption, distribution, metabolism and excretion of a drug.
- List the principal routes of drug administration.
- Name the phases in hepatic metabolism.
- Describe what is meant by the term 'cell receptor'.
- Understand the concept of receptor occupancy.
- Outline how drugs affect the body.
- Give three examples of different cell receptors.
- Outline what is meant by 'ion channel'.
- Describe the term 'first pass metabolism'.
- Understand at a basic level the term 'affinity'.

Introduction

Part of the nurse's role, alongside the pharmacist, is to ensure that medicines are administered appropriately. The Nursing and Midwifery Council's Standards for Pre- Registration Nursing Programmes published in May 2018 state that education must

> *ensure that field-specific content in relation to the law, safeguarding, consent, pharmacology and medicines administration and optimisation is included for entry to the register in one or more fields of nursing practice*

This is backed up by the Standards of Proficiency for Registered Nurses:

> Platform 3: Assessing needs and planning care
> *3.2 demonstrate and apply knowledge of body systems and homeostasis, human anatomy and physiology, biology, genomics, pharmacology and social and behavioural sciences when undertaking full and accurate person-centred nursing assessments and developing appropriate care plans*
> *3.3 demonstrate and apply knowledge of all commonly encountered mental, physical, behavioural and cognitive health conditions, medication usage and treatments when undertaking full and accurate assessments of nursing care needs and when developing, prioritising and reviewing person-centred care plans*

and

> Platform 4: Providing and evaluating care
> *4.5 demonstrate the knowledge and skills required to support people with commonly encountered physical health conditions, their medication usage and treatments, and act as a role model for others in providing high quality nursing interventions when meeting people's needs*
> *4.14 understand the principles of safe and effective administration and optimisation of medicines in accordance with local and national policies and demonstrate proficiency and*

accuracy when calculating dosages of prescribed medicines
> *4.15 demonstrate knowledge of pharmacology and the ability to recognise the effects of medicines, allergies, drug sensitivities, side effects, contraindications, incompatibilities, adverse reactions, prescribing errors and the impact of polypharmacy and over the counter medication usage*
> *4.16 demonstrate knowledge of how prescriptions can be generated, the role of generic, unlicensed, and off-label prescribing and an understanding of the potential risks associated with these approaches to prescribing*
> *4.17 apply knowledge of pharmacology to the care of people, demonstrating the ability to progress to a prescribing qualification following registration*

That is why it is essential that the nurse has a good knowledge and understanding of pharmacology and the relevant calculations in terms of patient care. Pharmacology is the study of drugs (chemicals) and their interactions with the body. The term is derived from the Greek *pharmakon*, which can mean both 'remedy' and 'poison'. In modern medical practice, drugs are being used more and more to treat and manage disease, so it is vital that nurses understand the basic mechanisms of drug action and reaction.

The aim of this chapter is to introduce the basic principles of pharmacology in relation to nursing practice. The chapter will give you an appreciation of *pharmacodynamics* and *pharmacokinetics*. It will identify the main targets for drug action and allow you to develop an understanding of drug absorption, distribution, metabolism and excretion.

Put quite simply:

- *pharmacodynamics* is the effect that drugs have on the body; while
- *pharmacokinetics* is the study of the way in which drugs move through the body during absorption, distribution, metabolism and excretion.

For drugs to produce their effects, they must interact with the body. This can happen in many ways and depends on the properties of the drug and will be discussed later in this chapter. Pharmacokinetics influences decisions over the route of administration. The processes that occur after drug administration can be broken down into four distinct areas (known as ADME):

A	Absorption of the drug
D	Distribution of the drug molecules
M	Metabolism of the parent drug
E	Excretion or elimination of the drug and its metabolites

Absorption

Before a drug can begin to exert any effect on the body, it has to be absorbed into the body systems. Of the many factors that can affect the absorption process, the most important is the route of administration (see Box 1.1). Many patients require the administration of their medication to be tailored to their particular medical condition or the medication that they have been prescribed. It is thus important that nurses understand the implications attached to choosing the route of administration of drugs based on their absorption, as it can impact on the patient's ability or desire to take their medication.

Box 1.1   Principal routes of drug administration

Route	Advantages	Disadvantages
Enteral routes		
Oral	Convenient, non-sterile, good absorption for most drugs	Gastrointestinal (GI) irritation, potential for interactions, first pass destruction, inactivated by acids, variable absorption
Sublingual/buccal	Avoids first pass (see p. 8), avoids gastric acid	Few preparations suitable
Rectal	Avoids first pass, avoids gastric acid	Less dignified for the patient
Parenteral (refers to IV, IM and SC) routes		
Intravenous (IV)	Rapid action, complete availability	Increased drug levels to heart, must be sterile, risk of sepsis and embolism
Intramuscular (IM)	Rapid absorption	Painful, risk of tissue damage
Subcutaneous (SC)	Good for slower absorption	Absorption variable
Inhaled (lungs)	Large absorption area, good for topical use	Few disadvantages

Other routes include intra-arterial, intrasternal, intrathecal, intra-articular, intraperitoneal, intraventricular, nasal, bronchial, vaginal, skin and conjunctiva

The other factors that can affect the rate and reliability of drug absorption fall into two categories: physiological and physico-chemical. *Physiological* factors relate to human physiological functions:

- **Blood flow to absorbing site.** The better the blood supply to the area, the greater the rate of absorption. Therefore, if a person has a good circulation they will have the ability to absorb the drug well.
- **Total surface area for absorption.** The greater the surface area, the greater the rate of absorption. The intestine has a very large surface area, making it an ideal target for drug absorption. This is why most drugs are given orally when possible.
- **Time of arrival and contact time at absorption site.** The longer the drug is in contact with the absorbing surface, the greater the rate of absorption. Therefore, if a person is suffering from diarrhoea, the chances of a drug given orally being absorbed completely are lowered and other means of administration must be considered.

Physico-chemical factors relate to the chemical make-up of the drug in relation to human physiological functions:

- **Solubility.** How soluble is the drug in body fluids? As the body consists of a large amount of water, drugs can dissolve readily. However, certain drugs do not dissolve into small enough particles to ensure their rapid absorption.
- **Chemical stability.** Will it break down readily?
- **Lipid to water partition coefficient.** Is the drug more fat soluble than water soluble? This is an important thing to consider. As our cells are made up of a phospho-lipid layer, any drug that can dissolve well in lipids will pass through the tissues far more rapidly. Examples of drugs that are highly lipid soluble are anaesthetic agents and benzodiazepines.
- **Degree of ionization.** Some drugs are both weak acids and weak bases (alkalis). These

drugs tend to disassociate when administered. This means that some of the drug remains active and some is inactive. Often this depends on the pH of the solution (i.e. its acidity or alkalinity) in which the drug is being dissolved. For example, a weak acid does not disassociate as much if dissolved in an acid environment. This means that the drug can cross membranes in a more active form than if it had been dissolved in a neutral or base solution.

Clinical tip

It is very important that the patient takes the medicine as directed by the prescriber to obtain the best therapeutic value from it. As a nurse, therefore, you need to understand the mechanics of absorption so that you can explain to the patient why it is important that a drug is taken in the correct way.

Distribution

Once a drug has been administered and absorbed, it must be distributed to its site of action. For some drugs that site is known, and such drugs are available to give locally or topically. All other drugs need to be distributed throughout the body.

There are four main elements to this:

1. **Distribution into body fluids.** These are mainly plasma, interstitial fluid and intracellular fluid. Molecular targets for drugs are found in these areas.

2. **Uptake into body tissues/organs.** Specific tissues take up some drugs – for example, iodine and thyroid gland.

3. **Extent of plasma protein binding.** Plasma proteins such as albumin can bind drug molecules. This varies widely among drugs. Drugs bound to plasma proteins are pharmacologically inert; only free drugs are active.

Some drugs do not bind (e.g. caffeine) whereas others are highly bound (e.g. warfarin, which is 99% bound to plasma proteins). Some drugs can displace others from their binding sites on the plasma proteins – for example, phenylbutazone can displace warfarin from plasma proteins. This is an important consideration for drugs that have this effect.

4 **Passage through barriers.** The two main examples are the placenta and the blood–brain barrier (BBB). Drugs must be highly lipid soluble to pass across these barriers. If not, they may not be able to reach their site of action.

Phase	Process
Phase I metabolism	Oxidation
	Reduction
	Hydrolysis
Phase II metabolism	Conjugation

Table 1.1 Metabolic phases and processes

drug itself is pharmacologically inactive until it is metabolized by the liver to its active form. A good example is codeine, which is metabolized to morphine by the body. The metabolite is more polar (i.e. chemically charged) than the parent drug and therefore is more readily excreted by the kidney. Drug metabolism can influence strength of dose and frequency of dosing. Drugs that are metabolized quickly have a short duration of action and need to be administered more often (two to four times daily). Drugs that are metabolized slowly have a longer duration of action and may only need to be given on a once-daily basis.

Hepatic metabolism

The terms shown in Table 1.1 are different chemical reactions that change the properties of drugs to facilitate their removal from the body by excretion. Most drugs undergo phase I oxidation followed by phase II conjugation.

Clinical tip

As a nurse in practice it is important you have knowledge about drugs such as warfarin so that you can be aware of the symptoms which the patient may display if they become toxic with the drug.

The factors that affect drug distribution are taken into consideration by drug companies when developing and formulating medications. While these factors are of interest, the nurse's main role in monitoring drug distribution is to monitor the onset of the effect of, or the response to, the medication. If analgesia is given and the patient reports reduced or relieved pain, the drug has been distributed to its target site.

Biotransformation

The biotransformation of drugs, which is the process of turning the parent drug into different compounds called metabolites, occurs mainly in the liver (hence the term *hepatic metabolism*). Drug metabolites may have greater, lesser or similar pharmacological activity compared with the parent drug. It may also have a different activity. Some drugs are called *pro-drugs* – that is, the

Clinical tip

It is important as a nurse to recognize that babies, particularly those less than 6 months old, do not have a mature liver and therefore drugs must be given with great caution. Exercise caution also when giving drugs to patients who have diseases that have an impact on liver function – for example, congestive heart failure – as their ability to metabolize a given drug will be greatly impaired.

Excretion

Once a drug has had its desired effect, it needs to be excreted by the body. The principles of excretion include renal elimination and clearance, secretion into bile for faecal elimination and entero-hepatic recirculation. As previously outlined, some drug metabolites can also have pharmacological effects. If these compounds were not to be eliminated, they would accumulate in the bloodstream and could cause toxic and unwanted effects.

The main means of renal elimination is by active glomerular filtration. This is where ionized drugs are actively secreted into the proximal tubule. These ionized compounds are actively excreted by the kidney and are 'pushed' out into urine. A more passive form of drug compound movement occurs in the distal tubule of the kidney. Here there is passive reabsorption and excretion of drug molecules and metabolites according to a concentration gradient. Molecules move from a high concentration to a lower concentration by diffusion. This applies to un-ionized compounds (drugs without charge) and prevents the entire dose of a drug being excreted at once. This helps to maintain circulating plasma levels to allow the drug effect to continue until the next dose is taken.

Clinical tip

People who have renal impairment may require alterations in dose to achieve a therapeutic level. Older patients also need special consideration, as kidney performance declines in the elderly, resulting in a lower glomerular filtration rate.

Excretion into bile is another way of eliminating drug molecules and metabolites. The liver produces bile, which is secreted into the bowel (and some is stored in the gall bladder) and can contain drug metabolites. These are secreted from the liver into bile and into the gut for faecal

elimination. As in renal excretion, not all of the drug and its metabolites are eliminated at once. Some drugs undergo entero-hepatic recirculation. This is where some of the drug is reabsorbed from the gut, back into the bloodstream and presented to the liver for further metabolism. This can help to maintain circulating levels of active molecules to prolong a drug's effect until the next dose. One example of a drug that undergoes this form of elimination is the combined oral contraceptive pill.

General and molecular aspects of pharmacodynamics

It is important that nurses involved in medicines management are aware of the sites of action for many commonly used drugs. Drugs exert their effects at molecular (chemical) targets, of which there are many. Some of the most common are detailed below.

Receptors

The plasma membrane of a human cell is selectively permeable, in that it helps control what moves in and out of the cell. The cell membrane consists of a thin structured bilayer of phospholipids and protein molecules. The surfaces of plasma membranes are generally studded with proteins that perform different functions, such as the reception of nutrients. In biochemistry, these protein molecules are referred to as *receptors*. Molecules that bind to these receptors are called *ligands*. Examples of ligands are neurotransmitters, hormones and drugs.

Many drugs exert their effect through interaction with receptors. Examples include:

- ligand-gated ion channels (ionotropic receptors) such as the $GABA_A$ receptor and the $5\text{-}HT_3$ receptor;
- G-protein coupled receptors such as adrenoceptors and prostaglandin receptors;
- kinase-linked receptors such as the insulin receptor and the receptor for growth hormone;
- nuclear receptors such as the thyroid receptor and oestrogens.

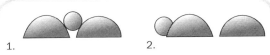

In 1. we see a drug blocking the permeation of the actual ion channel itself.

In 2. we see a drug binding to the channel but not sitting within the channel itself.

Figure 1.1   Drug binding at ion channels

Ion channels

Ion channels, such as those for sodium, calcium and potassium, provide receptors which drugs can interact with. Drug actions at ion channels can take two forms (see Figure 1.1). The first form are known as *channel blockers*, whereby the drug blocks permeation of the channel; the second form are *channel modulators*, whereby the drug binds to a receptor site within the ion channel and modulates permeation of the channel. This can happen by the drug altering the channel's response to its normal mediator.

Enzymes

Enzymes are biological catalysts that increase the rate of chemical reactions in the body. They are integral to many normal physiological functions. Many drugs target enzymes to prevent them from carrying out their normal function – for example, ibuprofen acts on cyclooxygenase enzymes, acting to reduce inflammation. In this example, the substrate arachidonic acid is acted upon by the cyclooxygenase enzyme to produce prostaglandins. Targeting this enzyme with a drug such as ibuprofen reduces the production of the inflammatory agent.

Transport systems

These are also known as carrier molecule interactions. In some transmitter systems, there is normal physiological recycling of the transmitters, such as serotonin. After the release of serotonin from a neurone, it is taken back up by that same neurone using a serotonin-selective re-uptake system. The drug fluoxetine blocks the uptake transporter for serotonin as its mode of action. This results in an increased level of serotonin in the neuronal synapse. This mechanism has an onward effect that facilitates an increase in mood and makes fluoxetine and drugs like it good antidepressants.

Drug action

The time to the onset of drug action involves delivery of the drug to its site of action. This is largely controlled by the:

- route of administration;
- rate of absorption;
- manner of distribution.

These are important considerations, as often we want the drug to have its effect within a certain time frame. We can speed up the time to the onset of drug action in many ways. If the drug is administered orally, we can use liquid or dispersible formulations instead of regular tablets. If drug action is needed more quickly, we can use the intramuscular (IM) or intravenous (IV) route as necessary. For example, if a patient requires pain relief following myocardial infarction, they would be given intravenous morphine rather than an oral preparation.

It is also possible to delay drug onset or prolong the effect by using enteric-coated or slow release preparations orally, or by using the transdermal or subcutaneous (SC) route. For example, people suffering with chronic pain from conditions such as rheumatoid arthritis may be given analgesia in the form of a transdermal patch. This is much preferred by the patient, as it decreases the amount of oral analgesia required.

The duration of drug effect relates to the time it takes for the drug to be removed from its site of action. This is largely controlled by the:

- rate of hepatic metabolism;
- rate of renal excretion.

It is important to know how long a drug will remain effective. Drug companies undertake extensive studies to determine this information. They use the data they obtain to decide upon dosing schedules. It is vital that nurses know the normal dosing schedules for the drugs they are administering (this can easily be found in the British National Formulary, or BNF) so that the correct regimen is implemented. Drugs need to be given more than once to have continued effect. Some drugs need to be given daily, while others need to be given two, three or four times per day to maintain their effective action.

First pass metabolism

Some drugs undergo destruction by *first pass metabolism*. When absorbed through the stomach after oral administration, a drug enters blood vessels that lead directly to the liver. We call this the *portal circulation*. This means that drugs which are largely destroyed by liver enzyme systems will not enter the general systemic circulation. An example of such a drug is glyceryl trinitrate (GTN), which is metabolized completely by the liver at this stage. Therefore, you will find GTN being given via routes other than orally.

The concept of affinity

Drugs have what is termed an *affinity* for their receptors, or chemical targets. This is a measure of how well a drug can bind to its chemical target. The tighter the bond, the better the drug action. Some drugs have a higher affinity for their chemical targets than others. Those with a higher affinity will bind first, in preference to any other drug molecule present. Some drugs have a higher affinity for their targets than even the normal physiological molecule. This can be very useful in drug action, especially where the normal molecule is abundant and is the cause of the problem or symptom the patient is experiencing. Higher affinity means that even small amounts of the drug will bind preferentially.

Agonistic and antagonistic drug action

Drugs can either be *agonists* or *antagonists* at their target sites. This is best explained using receptors as an example (see Figure 1.2). When agonists or antagonists bind to receptors, they are said to *occupy* the receptor site. The amount of drug occupying the receptor site relates to the

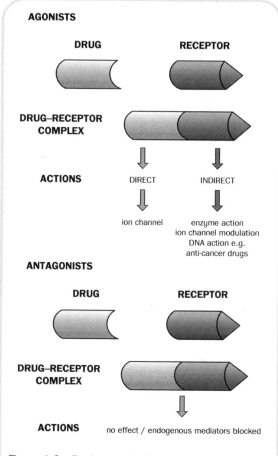

Figure 1.2 Basic receptor theory

magnitude of response to the drug itself. In simple terms, the more of an agonist drug occupying a receptor, the greater the response.

Agonists are drugs that bind to their targets and form a drug–receptor complex. Agonists activate the receptors to produce a response (known as *full agonists*) and have what is termed *positive efficacy*. Antagonists are drugs that bind to their targets and form a drug–receptor complex, but without causing activation or response. They can block the receptor to its endogenous activator, thereby blocking normal function. They have what is termed *zero efficacy*. Receptor occupancy by antagonists is important if the drug is a competitive antagonist, i.e. it competes for occupancy with another drug or with the receptor's normal mediator. The amount of drug occupying will determine any response.

This is a simplistic view of the concepts of agonism and antagonism, as the response of a drug at its chemical target is graded. For agonists we have:

- **Partial agonists:** drugs that bind to their targets and activate them to produce less of a response than we would expect from a full agonist. They have what is termed *partial efficacy*. Taking opioid drugs as an example, morphine is a full agonist but buprenorphine is a partial agonist.
- **Inverse agonists:** drugs that bind to their targets and can reduce the normal activity of that chemical target. They have what is termed *negative efficacy*. Naltrexone is an example of a drug with inverse agonist properties.

For antagonists we have:

- **Competitive antagonists:** drugs that bind to the chemical targets and prevent activation by the normal target agent. Naloxone is a competitive antagonist at opioid receptors and can reverse adverse effects in opioid overdose.
- **Non-competitive antagonists:** drugs that do not necessarily bind to the chemical target but at a point in the chain of events block target activation. Ketamine is a non-competitive antagonist.

Drug specificity

Very few drugs are specific for their intended targets within the body. A prescriber will give a drug with a specific action in mind, for example salbutamol. Salbutamol is a beta2 adrenoceptor agonist.

This means it has its main action at beta2 adrenoceptors in the bronchi. This gives us its desired effect as a bronchodilator, which eases breathing in asthma. However, the action of salbutamol is not that specific and can act on other beta2 adrenoceptors in the body as well as on beta1 adrenoceptors, especially if given in high doses leading to increased receptor occupancy. This is the reason for some of the side-effects of drugs. In the case of salbutamol, action at other beta adrenoceptors can lead to palpitations, while increased occupancy at non-bronchial beta adrenoceptors can cause tremor.

The concepts in this chapter relate to the NMC Standards of Proficiency for Registered Nurses (NMC 2018):

Platform 4: Providing and evaluating care
4.15 demonstrate knowledge of pharmacology and the ability to recognise the effects of medicines, allergies, drug sensitivities, side effects, contraindications, incompatibilities, adverse reactions, prescribing errors and the impact of polypharmacy and over the counter medication usage

and

Platform 3: Assessing needs and planning care
3.2 demonstrate and apply knowledge of body systems and homeostasis, human anatomy and physiology, biology, genomics, pharmacology and social and behavioural sciences when undertaking full and accurate person-centred nursing assessments and developing appropriate care plans

Case studies

① Mrs Asamoah is a 72-year-old woman who has been admitted to the medical unit following a general deterioration in her mobility and ability to carry out most of the activities of living independently. She has suffered from rheumatoid arthritis for many years and takes co-codamol with moderate effect. On admission she looks pale and lethargic and is complaining of pain in her knees and hands. She informs you that she has also been taking atenolol 50 milligrams (mg) daily for the past 5 years.

Following a discussion with her daughter, you learn that she has recently commenced a course of trimethoprim to treat a urinary tract infection but has been reluctant to take it as she claims that she has too many tablets to take and has difficulty swallowing them. What information from Mrs Asamoah's assessment could you now obtain which would help you identify factors influencing the absorption and distribution of the medication she is taking?

② Mr Mambety is a 42-year-old man who is recovering from emergency gastric surgery. He has a history of heavy drinking and cigarette smoking. His post-operative pain is being controlled by a patient-controlled analgesic device and he is beginning to mobilize with assistance. What factors are likely to influence Mr Mambety's ability to metabolize and excrete any drugs he is prescribed during his post-operative recovery?

③ Ben Brown is aged 45 and has Down's syndrome. He currently takes regular Gaviscon as he suffers from indigestion. He has developed a respiratory infection and is to be commenced on erythromycin 250mg four times per day. Erythromycin comes with cautionary labels 5, 9 and 25. Label 5 warns that the erythromycin should not be taken within 2 hours (before or after) antacid preparations and label 9 dictates that the doses be split evenly throughout the day. Label 25 states the drugs should be swallowed whole.

Thinking about the principles of absorption, what do you need to find about from Ben regarding his Gaviscon taking, and what advice and education would you give to Ben to ensure that he takes the medications appropriately?

Key learning points

Introduction

▶ Pharmacology is the study of drugs.
▶ Pharmacodynamics is the effect that drugs have on the body.
▶ Pharmacokinetics is the effect the body has on the drugs.
▶ Pharmacokinetics includes absorption, distribution, metabolism and excretion of drugs.

Absorption

▶ The main factor relating to absorption of drugs is the route of administration.
▶ Physiological considerations in absorption are blood flow, total surface area, time of arrival of the drug and time of drug at absorption site.
▶ Other considerations for absorption are solubility, chemical stability and how soluble the drug is in lipids.

Distribution

▶ Drugs are distributed into major body fluids (e.g. plasma).
▶ Specific tissues may take up certain drugs (e.g. iodine is taken up by the thyroid gland).
▶ Drug distribution is affected by the extent that the drug binds to plasma proteins.
▶ Drug distribution is affected by barriers (e.g. the placenta and the BBB).

Biotransformation

▶ This is the process of metabolizing drugs in the body.
▶ It occurs mainly in the liver and is therefore often called hepatic metabolism.
▶ Some drugs are activated by this hepatic metabolism – these are called pro-drugs.
▶ Drug metabolism is split into two phases in the liver.
▶ An example of phase I metabolism is oxidation.
▶ An example of phase II metabolism is conjugation.

Excretion

▶ Excretion includes renal elimination and faecal elimination.
▶ The main method of renal elimination is by active glomerular filtration.
▶ Drugs can also be eliminated by passive methods in the distal tubules.
▶ Drugs can be eliminated from the body in bile and so removed in the faeces.

General and molecular aspects

▶ Drugs exert their effects at molecular (chemical) targets (e.g. adrenaline receptors).
▶ Drugs can also act by stopping or partially stopping important ions entering the cell (e.g. calcium channel blockers).
▶ Drugs can interfere with enzymes that are produced by the body.
▶ Drugs can work on the transport of chemicals into and out of cells.

Drug action

▶ Drug action relies on the route of administration, rate of absorption and manner of distribution.
▶ The duration of drug effect involves how quickly it is removed from the body.
▶ Some drugs when absorbed from the stomach enter the portal circulation and pass through the liver. This is called the first pass effect.
▶ Drug action can also be affected by drug affinity.
▶ The greater the affinity, the better the drug action.

Agonistic and antagonistic drug action

▶ Agonists activate receptors to produce a response.
▶ Antagonists bind with receptors but do not activate them or cause a response. They can actually block the activation of receptors.
▶ Partial agonists produce a response. However, this is less than would be expected from a full agonistic drug.

▶ Inverse agonists are drugs that can reduce the normal activity of the cell.
▶ Competitive antagonists are drugs that prevent activation of the cell by their normal agent.
▶ Non-competitive antagonists are drugs that may block the receptor but not in a permanent way.

Multiple-choice questions

Try answering these multiple-choice questions to test what you have learned from reading this chapter. You can check your answers at the end of the book.

1. **A drug that binds to a cell receptor and affects a response is called ...**

a) An agonist
b) An antagonist
c) A receptor blocker
d) A channel blocker

2. **Most drugs and metabolites are excreted by ...**

a) The kidneys
b) The lungs
c) Bile
d) Saliva

3. **The four processes in pharmacokinetics are ...**

a) Stomach, liver, kidney and lungs
b) Receptors, ion channels, transport systems and enzymes
c) Administration, absorption, metabolism and elimination
d) Absorption, distribution, metabolism and excretion

4. **Pharmacodynamics is defined as ...**

a) The effect our body has on drugs
b) The action of the liver on drug molecules
c) The effect a drug has on our bodies
d) The movement of a drug around the body

5. **The main method of renal elimination of a drug is by ...**

a) Passive distal excretion
b) Active glomerular filtration
c) Selective reabsorption
d) Active secretion into the collecting duct

⟶

←

6. **How many phases of hepatic metabolism are there?**

a) 1
b) 2
c) 4
d) 10

7. **What route should drugs subject to complete destruction by first pass metabolism *not* be given by?**

a) Intravenous
b) Intramuscular
c) Sublingual
d) Oral

8. **Which of the following is a plasma protein?**

a) Prostacyclin
b) Albumin
c) Protamine
d) Meatamine

9. **A pro-drug is ...**

a) A drug given to promote growth
b) A drug given in its active form
c) A drug given to prevent metabolism of another drug
d) A drug given in its inactive form, requiring metabolism

10. **An antagonist can be ...**

a) Competitive and non-competitive
b) Competitive and complementary
c) Competitive and comparative
d) Competitive and conjugated

Recommended further reading

Beckwith, S. and Franklin, P. (2011) *Oxford Handbook of Prescribing for Nurses and Allied Health Professionals*, 2nd edition. Oxford: Oxford University Press.

Brenner, G.M. and Stevens, C.W. (2017) *Pharmacology*, 5th edition. Philadelphia, PA: Elsevier.

Downie, G., Mackenzie, J. and Williams, A. (2007) *Pharmacology and Medicines Management for Nurses*, 4th edition. Edinburgh: Churchill Livingstone.

Greenstein, B. and Gould, D. (2008) *Trounce's Clinical Pharmacology for Nurses*, 18th edition. New York: Churchill Livingstone.

Karch, A.M. (2017) *Focus on Nursing Pharmacology*, 7th edition. Philadelphia, PA: Lippincott Williams & Wilkins.

Nursing and Midwifery Council (NMC) (2018) *Standards of Proficiency for Registered Nurses*. London: NMC.

Simonson, T., Aarbakke, J., Kay, I., Coleman, I., Sinnott, P. and Lyssa, R. (2006) *Illustrated Pharmacology for Nurses*. London: Hodder Arnold.

Willihnganz, M. and Clayton, B.D. (2016) *Basic Pharmacology for Nurses*, 17th edition. St Louis, MO: Mosby Elsevier.

Adverse drug reactions and interactions

2

Learning objectives

After studying this chapter, you should be able to:

- Convey the importance of recognizing adverse drug reactions and interactions.
- Describe why drug interactions occur during absorption, distribution, metabolism and excretion of drugs.
- Explain what is meant by the terms 'enzyme inducer' and 'inhibitor'.
- Define the term 'adverse drug reaction'.
- Outline what is meant by 'ion channel'.
- Describe the term 'first pass metabolism'.
- Understand at a basic level the term 'affinity'.
- Give two examples of different drug reactions.
- Define pharmacovigilance.
- Outline the use of the yellow card system.

- Be aware of anaphylaxis.
- List three common drugs that are frequently implicated in drug reactions.
- Discuss the steps taken in minimizing drug interactions in patient care.
- Describe why elderly people and children are at a higher risk of drug interaction than other age groups.

Introduction

The aim of this chapter is to introduce you to the concepts of adverse drug reactions and drug interactions and side-effects. According to Veeren and Weiss (2016), emergency hospital admissions due to adverse drug reactions (ADRs) are an increasing problem in the National Health Service (NHS). The likelihood of drug interactions and adverse reactions is increased in patients on more than one medicine, and highest in those who take more than four medications (polypharmacy). The incidence is also increased in elderly patients. As many elderly people are on several medicines, they as a group are often at higher risk of interactions and adverse reactions.

Main mechanisms of drug interactions

Drug interactions can be:

- pharmacokinetic; and/or
- pharmacodynamic.

Pharmacokinetic interactions can occur in any of the four pharmacokinetic processes:

- absorption;
- distribution;
- metabolism;
- excretion.

Absorption

The most common absorption interactions occur when medicines are taken by the oral route. Many drugs require precise conditions for optimal absorption in the stomach and upper gastrointestinal (GI) tract. Anything which disrupts these conditions can affect drug absorption. Examples include:

- Taking medication with or after a meal: the presence of food in the stomach can delay drug absorption. Sometimes we use this to our advantage, but some drugs need to be taken on an empty stomach.
- Taking medication at the same time as an antacid preparation. Antacids such as Gaviscon coat the stomach and delay drug absorption, thus taking them at the same time as some drugs must be avoided.
- Crushing or splitting tablets. Some tablets need to travel intact through the stomach before being absorbed optimally in the small intestine, or have a coating that delays their absorption. Crushing or splitting tablets may change the rate of absorption of these drugs.

Clinical tip

Do not crush or tamper with tablets or capsules: many are specially designed to be absorbed in a specific manner in a specific time frame. If in doubt how a medicine should be taken, consult your pharmacist.

Always follow any instructions given with oral medicines to ensure their optimal absorption.

Distribution

Some drugs are bound to plasma proteins during their distribution through body fluids. The efficiency of a drug can be affected by the degree to which it binds to proteins within the blood plasma. The less a drug binds to a plasma protein, the more efficient it is in diffusing and crossing cell membranes. An example of a common blood protein that drugs can bind to is albumin. Due to protein binding of a drug, the drug exists in two forms, namely protein bound and unbound (free), the unbound form being the active component of the drug. The bound portion remains inactive unless displaced from the protein. Any medications that may displace other medicines from plasma proteins could change the level of free drug in the plasma. Drugs associated with this sort of interaction are usually listed as incompatible in Appendix 1 of the British National Formulary (BNF).

Clinical tip

When working in the clinical setting it is important to be thinking of the age of the person you are dealing with. For example, neonates, infants and older people have a reduced amount of plasma proteins, therefore doses of drugs in these patients should reflect physiological differences.

Metabolism

Some drugs can interfere with the effectiveness of drug metabolizing enzymes in the liver. These drugs can have one of two effects:

1. **Enzyme inducer:** this is where the drug increases the effectiveness of the enzymes and metabolizes more quickly. This means that the effectiveness of other drugs and their duration of action may be reduced.

2. **Enzyme inhibitor:** this is where the drug decreases the effectiveness of the enzymes and metabolizes more slowly. This means that the effectiveness of other drugs and their duration of action may be increased.

Drugs that modify metabolizing enzymes should be given with caution to patients on other medicines,

and the effects should be monitored. Having the pharmacist on the ward on a daily basis, monitoring prescriptions while liaising with both the medical and nursing staff, is of great importance in identifying any such problems.

Clinical tip

When nursing neonates and infants, you will notice that certain drugs are given at a reduced dose. This is because of the immature liver's poorer ability to metabolize drugs.

Excretion

Relatively few drugs have a dramatic effect on drug excretion. Non-steroidal anti-inflammatory drugs (NSAIDs) can affect the kidney tubule and modify the excretion and reabsorption of some drugs. *Pharmacodynamic* interactions are more common and fall into two categories.

1. **Additive effects of drugs with similar actions.** For example, giving an angiotensin-converting enzyme (ACE) inhibitor (e.g. Lisinopril) with a diuretic (e.g. bendroflumethiazide) may lead to an adverse fall in blood pressure.

2. **Competing effects of drugs with opposite actions.** For example, giving a beta blocker drug for hypertension (e.g. propranolol) to an asthmatic patient may render their beta agonist drug (e.g. salbutamol) ineffective in managing their asthma symptoms.

Clinical tip

As a nurse you should keep accurate fluid balance records because patients' renal function needs to be optimal to avoid toxicity. Often, the first indicator of renal insufficiency is a change in urinary output.

Adverse drug reactions

An adverse drug reaction (ADR) (sometimes called an adverse drug event, or ADE) is a negative event that follows the prescription and administration of a medication, but is different from a side-effect. This is because some side-effects can be beneficial. The study of ADRs is called *pharmacovigilance.*

The World Health Organization's (WHO) definition of an adverse drug reaction is 'a response to a drug which is noxious and unintended, and which occurs at doses normally used in man for the prophylaxis, diagnosis or therapy of disease or for the modification of a physiological function' (WHO 1972: 9). Adverse drug reactions can be classified according to their cause:

- Type A: augmented effects – an exaggeration of the drug's normal pharmacological action.
- Type B: bizarre effects – unexpected.
- Type C: chronic effects – occur with long-term use.
- Type D: delayed effects – occur some time after ceasing taking the medication.
- Type E: end-of-treatment effects.
- Type F: failure of therapy.

The most common types of ADR are augmented and bizarre.

Type A: augmented

This is where the reaction is an augmentation of the drug's pharmacology. This means we can often predict these reactions from our knowledge of the pharmacodynamic properties of a drug. For example, a patient on an antihypertensive drug may develop dizziness and fainting because of too large a fall in blood pressure. Patients on NSAIDs can develop gastric irritation due to the drug's action on protective gastric mucous. These types of reactions are mainly dose dependent: the higher the dose, the greater the likelihood of an adverse reaction. They are the most common ADRs but are associated with low morbidity and mortality.

Type B: bizarre

This is where the reaction is wholly unexpected and could not be predicted from the pharmacodynamic properties of the drug. Examples include anaphylaxis to a particular drug, and a red pinprick rash with penicillin. These types of reactions are not dose dependent and can occur even at low starting doses. They are rarer than Type A but are associated with higher morbidity and mortality.

Clinical significance of drug reactions

The clinical significance of a drug reaction depends on many factors and can determine how health care professionals respond to such a reaction.

Some patients can tolerate side-effects or ADRs of medications if the benefit of the drug outweighs the inconvenience. When side-effects cannot be tolerated, this may be classed as a Type A ADR.

Type A ADR

If a patient reports an ADR, there are a variety of responses. The prescriber should be informed immediately so that appropriate action can be taken. This might include:

- stopping the medication altogether;
- reducing the dose of the drug;
- switching to an alternative drug.

The ADR should always be recorded in the patient's notes. Poor management of ADRs can lead to problems with patients adhering to their medication regimens, so this is an area that should be taken very seriously.

Type B ADR

Type B ADRs are more serious than Type A and require prompt detection and rapid action. The drug suspected of causing the adverse reaction should be withheld and the prescriber informed immediately. Any resuscitative measures should be undertaken at once to prevent serious complications. The drug should be stopped, and an alternative found where necessary. This type of ADR should always be recorded in the patient's notes and be easily visible to any future prescriber.

All Type B and many Type A ADRs should be reported to the Medicines and Healthcare Products Regulatory Agency (MHRA) via the yellow card found in the back of the BNF or online. This allows pharmacovigilance and allows a fuller profile of the drug to be built up.

Pharmacovigilance

Pharmacovigilance relates to the detection, assessment, understanding and prevention of adverse drug effects. The word derives from the Greek *pharmakon*, 'drug' and the Latin *vigilare*, 'to keep awake or alert, to keep watch'. In daily practice, we are mostly concerned with the side-effects of medicines that may be intolerable to our patients or cause them to experience adverse effects as described above. Pharmacovigilance involves collecting, monitoring, researching, assessing and evaluating information from health care providers and patients on the adverse effects of medications with a view to:

- identifying new information about medicines to inform prescribing practice;
- preventing harm to patients.

Very helpful information on pharmacovigilance is provided by the MHRA (n.d.).

The yellow card system

The yellow card system is vital in helping the MHRA monitor the safety of all the medicines and vaccines available. Before a medicine is granted a licence so that it can be made available in the UK, it must pass strict tests and checks to ensure that it is acceptably safe and effective. All effective medicines, however, can cause side-effects (or ADRs, see above), which can range from minor to very serious. Even if there is only a *suspicion* that a medicine or combination of medicines has caused a side-effect, patients and health professionals should send the MHRA a yellow card. Yellow card reports on suspected side-effects are evaluated, together with other sources of information such as clinical trial data, medical literature or data from international medicines regulators, to pinpoint previously unidentified safety issues. The MHRA will act, whenever necessary, to ensure that medicines are used in a way that minimizes risk, while maximizing patient benefit. More

information on the yellow card scheme is provided by the MHRA (2015).

> **Clinical tip**
>
> You must learn to actively listen to the patient and become observant. Look at the prescription chart to see if the person has been prescribed any new medication. Remember: always report any signs or symptoms to the nurse in charge.

Major groups of drugs involved in adverse drug reactions

Some drugs are more likely to result in ADRs than others. This means that their prescribing and administration should be closely monitored. They include:

- antibiotics;
- antipsychotics;
- NSAIDs;
- drugs with a narrow therapeutic index (e.g. warfarin and digoxin);
- lithium;
- diuretics;
- benzodiazepines; and
- newly licensed medicines.

Many of these medications have limited alternatives that are as effective for some patients, which means that a reaction may be inevitable.

Steps to minimize the effects of adverse drug reactions

Several steps can be taken to minimize or prevent ADRs:

- Drugs should only be prescribed for a good indication, particularly during pregnancy.
- A check should be made of all previous medications taken.
- Any previous reactions to medicines should be assessed.

19

■ Any non-drug allergies should be identified, including food allergies/sensitivities or topical allergies (e.g. sticking plasters).

■ Other drug use should be verified, including over the counter (OTC) medications, herbal remedies and any illicit or recreational drugs taken.

■ Age should always be taken into consideration (e.g. is the patient elderly or a young child?).

■ Check for any hepatic and/or renal disease.

■ Always maintain yellow card reporting to uphold pharmacovigilance.

■ Prescribing should be in accordance with any established protocols.

■ Clear instructions regarding medication administration should always be provided to the patient.

■ Familiar drugs should be prescribed where possible, as side-effect profiles are better known.

■ Always inform the patient of possible side-effects to help them identify ADRs.

Nurses have an important role in ADR monitoring. They are well placed to spot ADRs, as they are often the people administering the medication to the patient and patients may find it easier to talk to nurses about their medicines during the drug round than to the prescribing doctor. If you suspect a reaction, you must follow local policies and procedures for its reporting and management.

Anaphylaxis

Anaphylaxis is an *acute multi-system severe type I hypersensitivity allergic reaction*. The term derives from the Greek words *ana*, 'against' and *phylaxis*, 'protection'. Anaphylactic shock or true anaphylaxis is associated with systemic vasodilation that results in low blood pressure. It is also associated with severe bronchoconstriction to the point where the individual finds it increasingly difficult to breathe. Anaphylaxis can present with many different symptoms, which usually develop quickly over a few minutes. The most common systems affected include the skin, the respiratory system, the gastrointestinal system, the heart and vasculature, and the central nervous system. Anaphylaxis can occur in response to any allergen. Common triggers include insect bites or stings, foods, medications

and latex. The most common medicines to trigger anaphylaxis are antibiotics, aspirin, ibuprofen and other analgesics.

Treatment

The Resuscitation Council in the UK issues guidelines for the treatment and management of anaphylaxis (Resuscitation Council 2008). The key points are:

Treatment of an anaphylactic reaction should be based on general life support principles:

■ use the airway, breathing, circulation, disability, exposure (ABCDE) approach to recognize and treat problems;

■ call for help early;

■ treat the greatest threat to life first;

■ initial treatments should not be delayed by the lack of a complete history or definite diagnosis.

Patients having an anaphylactic reaction in any setting should expect the following as a minimum:

■ recognition that they are seriously unwell;

■ an early call for help;

■ initial assessment and treatments based on an ABCDE approach;

■ adrenaline therapy if indicated;

■ investigation and follow-up by an allergy specialist.

For the full guidance, see the Resuscitation Council website.

Age-related adverse drug reactions

As previously noted, the elderly and the very young should be closely monitored when prescribed medications that are associated with a high incidence of drug reactions or side-effects. The elderly often have changes in sensitivity to drugs because of:

■ a reduction in drug binding sites;

■ impaired organ function (liver/kidneys);

■ altered metabolizing enzyme systems in the liver.

All of the above can lead to potentiation of drug action, which in turn can result in further side-effects. These are normal manifestations of the ageing process.

By looking at the four processes of pharmacokinetics, it becomes clear why this needs to be considered:

Absorption

Absorption of drugs, especially via the oral route, can be affected by many age-related changes, including:

- reduced acid secretion resulting in higher pH;
- reduced gut motility;
- reduced muscle mass;
- reduced surface area of absorption sites;
- reduced blood flow to absorption sites.

Although overall drug absorption is not changed significantly for most elderly patients, as nurses we need to consider the best route of administration to optimize absorption.

Distribution

In the elderly, the distribution of drugs from their absorbing site can be affected by many factors. For example, albumin, the main protein of human plasma and a major binder of drugs, may be reduced by as much as one-fifth of normal adult values in the elderly. Furthermore, elderly individuals may be on a variety of medications that could displace other drugs from plasma protein binding sites, thus increasing the risk of raised plasma levels of some drugs in the elderly.

The elderly also experience changes in body composition, which can affect distribution. An increase in percentage body fat and a decrease in total body water are the main contributing factors. The increase in body fat means some lipid soluble drugs are more readily distributed and stored.

Metabolism

The liver of elders is smaller than that of the typical adult liver, as its mass decreases with age. This leads to a concomitant decrease in the amount of liver metabolizing enzymes, thereby reducing the capacity to metabolize drugs. Compound this with reduced hepatic blood flow and we can see that the overall effectiveness of the liver as a detoxifying organ is reduced. However, the clinical significance of these changes are difficult to judge, as they vary considerably from person to person.

Excretion

By the age of 65, the human kidney is almost a third less efficient. This is due to a reduction in renal clearance, a decrease in glomerular filtration, and often a reduced circulating blood volume, which may partly be due to a decreased fluid intake. Drugs and their metabolites, if not cleared by the kidney, can build up and become toxic quickly in the elderly, and this is often the reason for reduced drug doses after the age of 65 to try to prevent toxic build-up.

Medicine-related problems are more likely to be associated with older people who:

- take four or more medicines (polypharmacy);
- take digoxin, warfarin, NSAIDs, diuretics or benzodiazepines;
- have recently been discharged from hospital;
- have a low level of social support;
- have poor hearing, vision or dexterity;
- experience confusion, disorientation or depression.

It is also important to consider the effects of comorbidities in the elderly population from two perspectives:

1. the concomitant conditions themselves, and
2. the medications used to treat the concomitant conditions.

Some medical conditions can be cautions or contraindications for some drug therapy. An appropriate medical history should be taken from each elderly patient to establish the presence of any comorbid conditions. Then, using the BNF together with clinical knowledge, you should be able to highlight any concerns regarding the introduction

---

Box 2.1 Pharmacokinetic features in children and adolescents

Absorption (children and adolescents)	Distribution (children under 6)
■ Delayed gastric emptying ■ Slower GI transit (longer contact) ■ Thinner skin ■ Use of rectal administration	■ Plasma protein levels lower immediately after birth, especially in premature babies ■ Presence of bilirubin can affect binding to plasma proteins ■ More body water for drug distribution
Metabolism (children under 3 months)	**Excretion (children under 6 months)**
■ Liver maturity happens quickly after birth in term babies, usually by 4 weeks ■ Conjugation of bilirubin occurs ■ Increased clearance after 4 weeks due to relative liver mass and hepatic blood flow being higher	■ Glomerular filtration is 40% of adult level at birth ■ Tubular secretion processes poorly developed ■ Renal maturity slower than liver, reaching full maturity only after 6 months in the term infant

---

of a new medication. It is important that nurses are aware of all patients' medical conditions when reviewing drug charts and medications.

Whereas it is often the case that a variety of medications could be prescribed for a single condition, the scope is much more limited in patients with comorbid conditions. Thus careful drug choice and good drug administration and patient monitoring is essential for the comorbid patient.

Children cannot simply be viewed as small adults when it comes to medication. They respond differently to drugs for many reasons, most of which can be related to pharmacokinetics (see Chapter 1; see also Box 2.1).

Absorption

This can be a major factor in drug problems with children under the age of 12. Delayed gastric emptying results in drugs taken orally remaining in the stomach for longer, which can in turn delay the absorption of drugs from the small intestine. Children have a longer GI transit time, which means drugs are in contact with their absorbing sites for longer. Also, young children have trouble swallowing tablets and often cannot tolerate liquid medicines well.

> **Clinical tip**
>
> Drugs are sometimes administered rectally in small children. If drugs are given by the transdermal route, the fact children have thinner skin means that they absorb the drug more quickly by this route.

Distribution

Plasma protein levels are lower immediately after birth, especially in premature babies. This means that the availability of proteins for drug binding is limited compared with adults. This can be a problem with drugs that are extensively bound to plasma proteins. If plasma protein levels are reduced there are fewer sites to bind, which increases the available drug, hence effectively increasing the dose, which can lead to Type A reactions.

Metabolism

Children metabolize drugs differently to adults, especially in the first few weeks of life. This can lead to higher levels of an active drug being present for longer and produces a risk of Type A reactions. The liver takes time to mature over the first few weeks and months of life, and as the liver contains the enzymes necessary for drug metabolism, the immature liver is an important consideration in drug prescribing. It is important to remember that as a proportion of body size, the mass of the liver is larger in children than it is in adults.

Excretion

A child's kidney is not fully developed at birth and is unable to process drug molecules efficiently. This leads to a delay in the excretion of drug molecules, allowing them to circulate for longer, again with the risk of Type A reactions.

All of the above mean that children require lower doses of medicines than adults, not simply because they are smaller, but also because their organ systems are not fully developed. The doses of drugs can be increased at 6 months and slowly raised to adult values for many drugs by the age of 12, when organ maturity is achieved.

Drug–drug interactions

Drug–drug interactions fall into two categories: pharmacokinetic and pharmacodynamic. A *pharmacokinetic* drug interaction occurs when one drug alters the absorption, protein binding, metabolism or excretion of another, resulting in altered bioavailability of the drug and thus its pharmacological effect. For example, the presence of magnesium in many antacid medications reduces the absorption of iron preparations if taken orally and at the same time. Concomitant administration should be avoided.

A major worry regarding pharmacokinetic interactions is when one occurs in the liver at the level of the liver enzyme systems. Some drugs can induce or inhibit liver drug metabolizing enzymes, leading to a change in how other drugs are metabolized by those same enzymes. Common interactions of this sort include:

- **Enzyme induction**, which can be caused, for example, by carbamazepine, rifampicin, phenobarbital, phenytoin, tobacco (increase in theophylline when stop smoking) or alcohol.
- **Enzyme inhibition**, which can be caused, for example, by cimetidine, erythromycin, antidepressants or sodium valproate.

A *pharmacodynamic* interaction occurs with drugs that have similar or antagonistic effects. For example, morphine, which acts as an agonist at opioid receptors, can be antagonized using naloxone, an antagonist at the same receptor site. Their effects can cancel one another out. However, this is desirable in the event of morphine overdose, when naloxone is used as an antidote. Thus such an interaction can sometimes be beneficial.

When two drugs have a similar pharmacodynamic effect, the effect can be magnified if the two drugs are given together. For instance, there is a risk of bleeding if aspirin is given to a patient who is already taking warfarin. This is an unwanted interaction, as the outcome could be detrimental.

Consult Appendix 1 of the BNF for drug–drug interactions, where you will find a comprehensive list of drugs and the drugs they interact with. The interactions are categorized as pharmacokinetic, pharmacodynamic or unknown, as well as mild, moderate or severe. It is often also important to check the interaction status of herbal or alternative medicines, such as St. John's Wort, and even some foodstuffs, such as grapefruit juice, as these also exert an effect on liver enzymes.

The concepts in this chapter relate to the NMC Standards of Proficiency for Registered Nurses (NMC 2018):

Platform 4: Providing and evaluating care
4.15 demonstrate knowledge of pharmacology and the ability to recognise the effects of medicines, allergies, drug sensitivities, side effects, contraindications, incompatibilities, adverse reactions, prescribing errors and the impact of polypharmacy and over the counter medication usage

and

Platform 3: Assessing needs and planning care
3.2 demonstrate and apply knowledge of body
systems and homeostasis, human anatomy and
physiology, biology, genomics, pharmacology

and social and behavioural sciences when
undertaking full and accurate person-centred
nursing assessments and developing appropriate
care plans

Case studies

① Marek Brodzki is a 19-year-old man who has been newly commenced on antibiotics for a post-operative wound infection. You are helping him to dress when you notice a red pin-prick rash all over his upper body. You suspect this has been caused by the antibiotics. What are your responsibilities in this matter and what course of action should be taken regarding:

- the antibiotics?
- recording of the incident?
- prevention of recurrence?

② Sue Kent is an elderly woman on many different medicines to manage her complex health needs. One of her medicines is ibuprofen for her knee pain. She is also on warfarin for her atrial fibrillation. Using the BNF, identify any possible interactions between these drugs and whether suitable alternatives or further prescribing may be necessary.

③ Ethel Bassett is a 77-year-old obese female with type 2 diabetes, high blood pressure, heart failure, moderately severe kidney disease, high cholesterol, heartburn, severe knee arthritis, burning neuropathy in her feet, glaucoma, depression and insomnia. She is being treated with a range of medicines. With reference to this lady, explain the interaction between normal ageing and responses to drug therapy in older people.

④ Safiso is 18 months old and has been admitted to hospital following a simple febrile seizure. She has red ears and throat and has a probable viral upper respiratory tract infection. Her parents are very anxious and worried that she will have another fit and want her to have medicine to control her temperature. With reference to this child, explain how the age of the child is important when considering the concept of pharmacokinetics to drug therapy in the young person.

Key learning points

Introduction

▶ Hospital admissions thought to be associated with adverse drug reactions are increasing in the UK.
▶ The risk of adverse drug reactions increases with the number of drugs being taken.
▶ The elderly are a higher risk group.

←

Main mechanisms of drug interactions

▶ The presence of food in the stomach can delay absorption.
▶ Taking medication at the same time as an antacid preparation can affect drug absorption.
▶ Crushing or splitting of tablets can affect how they are absorbed by the body.
▶ Some drugs can bind to plasma proteins, therefore affecting their distribution in the body.
▶ Some drugs increase the effectiveness of enzymes in the liver to break down other drugs more quickly – these are called enzyme inducers.
▶ Some drugs decrease the activity of enzymes in the liver, thus affecting the duration of action of certain drugs – these are called enzyme inhibitors.
▶ Very few drugs have dramatic effects on drug excretion.
▶ Non-steroidal anti-inflammatory drugs may affect excretion and reabsorption of certain drugs.

Adverse drug reactions

▶ An ADR is a negative event that follows prescription and administration of a medication.
▶ The most common types of ADR are augmented and bizarre.
▶ An augmented ADR is often a predictable reaction. These types of reaction are mainly dose dependent.
▶ A bizarre ADR is wholly unexpected and could not be predicted from the properties of the drug (e.g. anaphylaxis). These reactions are not dose dependent and are less common than augmented ADRs.

Clinical significance of drug reactions

▶ When side-effects cannot be tolerated, there is a Type A ADR.
▶ When a Type A ADR is reported, a drug may be withdrawn, the dose reduced or an alternative drug prescribed.
▶ All ADRs should be reported in the patient's documentation.
▶ Poor management of ADRs can lead to poor adherence to medication regimes.
▶ Type B ADRs require prompt detection and rapid action. The drug should be immediately stopped, and an alternative found.
▶ All Type B and many Type A ADRs should be reported via the yellow card found in the BNF.
▶ Some drugs are more likely to cause ADRs than others (e.g. warfarin).
▶ Steps to minimize the effects of drug interactions should be taken (e.g. check all previous medications).

Age-related adverse drug reactions

▶ The elderly and children are at greater risk of drug reactions.
▶ The elderly are often more sensitive to drugs, take more than four medicines and have less social support.
▶ Children respond differently to drugs for many reasons, most of which can be related to differences in the absorption, distribution, metabolism and excretion of drugs compared with adults.

→

Drug–drug interactions

▶ Many drugs can interact with other medications the patient is taking.

▶ It is essential to consult Appendix 1 of the BNF to assess the risk of drug–drug interactions.

▶ Drug interactions can be pharmacokinetic or pharmacodynamic.

Multiple-choice questions

Try answering these multiple-choice questions to test what you have learned from reading this chapter. You can check your answers at the end of the book.

1.   **What does ADR stand for?**

a)   A drug response
b)   Adverse drug reaction
c)   A dangerous reaction
d)   Avoidable drug response

2.   **What are the two main types of ADR?**

a)   Accidental and bizarre
b)   Accelerated and bad
c)   Augmented and bizarre
d)   Absolute and beneficial

3.   **Drug interactions can be ...**

a)   Predictable and non-predictable
b)   Pharmacokinetic and pharmacodynamic
c)   Found in polypharmacy
d)   All of the above are true

4.   **The elderly are ...**

a)   Not affected by ADRs
b)   All on four or more medicines
c)   Unable to tolerate side-effects
d)   More susceptible to drug interactions

5.   **Children react to drug therapy differently to adults because ...**

a)   They have an immature liver and kidneys
b)   They are smaller

←

c) They may not be able to tolerate more than one drug

d) All of the above are true

6. **The side-effects of drugs …**

a) Can always be predicted

b) Can always be avoided

c) Can sometimes become ADRs

d) Only happen at high doses

7. **Pharmacodynamic interactions can occur when …**

a) Two drugs are given at the same time of day

b) Two drugs are given for the same condition

c) The action of one drug competes with the action of another

d) One drug blocks the absorption of another

8. **Which of the following is an *adverse* reaction?**

a) Sedation with a sleeping tablet

b) Reduced blood pressure with an antihypertensive drug

c) Nausea with an emetic drug

d) Rash with an antibiotic drug

9. **A drug given to prevent an adverse effect is called …**

a) A pro-drug

b) A prophylactic drug

c) A drug given to prevent metabolism of another drug

d) A placebo

10. **Anaphylaxis is an example of …**

a) A Type B ADR

b) A predictable drug side-effect

c) Polypharmacy

d) A Type A ADR

Recommended further reading

Brenner, G.M. and Stevens, C.W. (2017) *Pharmacology*, 5th edition. Philadelphia, PA: Elsevier.

Downie, G., Mackenzie, J. and Williams, A. (2007) *Pharmacology and Medicines Management for Nurses*, 4th edition. Edinburgh: Churchill Livingstone.

Greenstein, B. and Gould, D. (2008) *Trounce's Clinical Pharmacology for Nurses*, 18th edition. New York: Churchill Livingstone.

Karch, A.M. (2017) *Focus on Nursing Pharmacology*, 7th edition. Philadelphia, PA: Lippincott Williams & Wilkins.

Medicines and Healthcare Products Regulatory Agency (MHRA) (2015) *The Yellow Card Scheme: Guidance for Healthcare Professionals, Patients and the Public*. Last updated 2019. Available at: https://www.gov.uk/guidance/the-yellow-card-scheme-guidance-for-healthcare-professionals.

Medicines and Healthcare Products Regulatory Agency (MHRA) (n.d.) *Services and Information*. Available at: https://www.gov.uk/government/organisations/medicines-and-healthcare-products-regulatory-agency/services-information.

Nursing and Midwifery Council (NMC) (2018) *Standards of Proficiency for Registered Nurses*. London: NMC.

Resuscitation Council UK (2008) *Emergency Treatment of Anaphylactic Reactions: Guidelines for Healthcare Providers*. London: Resuscitation Council UK. Last updated 2012. Available at: https://www.resus.org.uk/anaphylaxis/emergency-treatment-of-anaphylactic-reactions/.

Simonson, T., Aarbakke, J., Kay, I., Coleman, I., Sinnott, P. and Lyssa, R. (2006) *Illustrated Pharmacology for Nurses*. London: Hodder Arnold.

Veeren, J.C. and Weiss, M. (2016) Trends in emergency hospital admissions in England due to adverse drug reactions: 2008–2015, *Journal of Pharmaceutical Health Services Research*, 8: 5–11.

World Health Organization (WHO) (1972) *International Drug Monitoring: The Role of National Centres*, Technical Report No. 498. Geneva: WHO.

Drug calculations and numeracy skills

3

Chapter contents

Learning objectives

After studying this chapter, you should be able to:

■ Understand the importance of numeracy skills in nursing.
■ Be aware of the International System (SI) of units of number and be able to convert from one unit to another.
■ Be able to perform basic mathematics tasks of addition, subtraction, multiplication and addition.
■ Use basic mathematics to calculate simple drug dosages.

Introduction

An important part of the nurse's role is to ensure that dosages of medicines are calculated and administered appropriately. That is why it is essential that the nurse has a good knowledge and understanding of basic mathematical and arithmetic skills in relation to drug calculation. The NMC Standards of Proficiency for Registered Nurses (NMC 2018) state:

> Platform 4: Providing and evaluating care
> *4.14 understand the principles of safe and effective administration and optimisation of medicines in accordance with local and national policies and demonstrate proficiency and accuracy when calculating dosages of pre-scribed medicines*

The aim of this chapter is to introduce the basic principles of numeracy and the specifics of calculating drug dosages to help you can gain the knowledge and skills to meet the NMC standard. We will cover basic arithmetic principles and use worked examples to illustrate each area to help develop your knowledge and understanding. Where appropriate we will refer you to other texts or sources of information to augment your skills.

An introduction to number

It is important that you are familiar with the structure of numbers and how they are expressed in written form. Going back to basics and starting from simple principles will help you develop your knowledge as we explore the area of drug calculation.

Number format and the way numbers are written and expressed are important. We are all familiar with numbers but how many of us think about their written format and what it means when we perform calculations?

Number order

The order in which digits are placed within a written number tells us the value of those digits. Single digits are represented by the numbers 0 to 9. They form the basis of all the numbers that are possible. See Box 3.1 for how numbers are ordered to form numbers.

So if we take some numbers at random, we can work out the value of each digit within those numbers:

> 17 contains the digits 1 (tens column) and 7 (units column)
> 183 contains the digits 1 (hundreds column), 8 (tens column) and 3 (units column)
> 4567 contains the digits 4 (thousands column), 5 (hundreds column), 6 (tens column) and 7 (units column)

The same principles can be applied to numbers that contain digits after the decimal point, as shown in Box 3.2. So again, if we look at some numbers at random, we can work out the value of each digit within those numbers too:

> 1.2 contains the digits 1 (units column) and 2 (tenths column)
> 2.75 contains the digits 2 (units column), 7 (tenths column) and 5 (hundredths column)
> 3.825 contains the digits 3 (units column), 8 (tenths column), 2 (hundredths column) and 5 (thousandths column)

Box 3.1 Order of numbers

Hundreds of thousands	Tens of thousands	Thousands	Hundreds	Tens	Units
100000–999999	10000–99999	1000–9999	1000–999	10–99	0–9

Box 3.2 Order of numbers after the decimal point

Units	Decimal point	Tenths	Hundredths	Thousandths
1	.	1	1	1

Box 3.3 Mathematical symbols and notation

Mathematical symbol(s)	What it means	When to use
+	Plus or add	Calculations requiring addition
−	Minus or subtract	Calculations requiring subtraction
× or *	Multiply or times	Calculations requiring multiplication
÷ or /	Divide	Calculations requiring division
=	Equals	All calculations

Take some numbers you see in everyday practice. Reflect on what position each digit takes within each number and how you think of that number. Consider the following things about number order:

- It helps us decide how big or small a number is.
- It helps us decide how numbers relate to one another.
- It helps us structure our working to ensure we carry out calculations properly.

We will apply the principle of number order when we begin to carry out simple calculations. But before we get to grips with drug calculations, let's remind ourselves of basic arithmetic skills and how to manipulate numbers.

Basic arithmetic skills

These basic skills form the foundation of all drug calculations and are thus a good place to begin. The processes involved are addition, subtraction,

multiplication and division. We need to know what these mean and understand related mathematical symbols and notation before we can start to put these processes into practice.

Take a look at Box 3.3. You need to be familiar with all the symbols there and their meanings before moving on, so look carefully at each one and ensure you can pair the correct process with its accompanying mathematical symbol.

Now let us look at these processes one by one.

Addition

Addition is the process of taking two or more numbers and combining them to make a new number. It is a simple process but often used to work out how many tablets a patient needs to take at any one time. For example:

Jane is on medication A for her heart and takes 1 tablet in the morning.
She is also on a medication B for her blood pressure for which she needs to take 2 tablets in the morning.

Finally, she is on medication C for pain for which she takes 2 tablets in the morning.

How many tablets does she take first thing?

Let's break this down into a sum:

A is 1

B is 2

C is 2

Now let's add them all together and use the mathematical symbols:

$$1 + 2 + 2 = 5$$

Thus Jane takes five tablets every morning.

Addition of number is a process for which the order of the digits needs to be considered before starting the process. Here is a simple example to show you how to add different numbers together.

In the number 51 we have 5 (tens) and 1 (units). If we want to add the number 22, we have to ensure that we add the tens together and then the units together. We would therefore place them in the following way:

$$51$$
$$\underline{22 +}$$
$$\underline{73}$$

We can see that the 5 and the 2 combine to form 7 (tens column) and the 1 and the 2 combine to form 3 (units column), giving us the new number of 73.

The same principles apply to larger numbers and we must ensure that units, tens, hundreds and so on are all in the correct place before carrying out the addition process.

Try the following to test your addition skills (the answers can be found at the end of the chapter):

$$11 + 27 =$$
$$23 + 45 =$$
$$101 + 273 =$$
$$450 + 339 =$$
$$1022 + 2174 =$$

Subtraction

Subtraction is the process of taking one or more numbers from a starting number to make a new

number. Again, this is a simple process that is often used to work out how long a bottle of medication will last.

John has a 100mL bottle of medication. He knows he need to take 10mL per day and he has already had 4 days' worth from it, so has used 40mL. He is going away for 7 days and knows he needs 70mL to last him the entire period he is away. He needs to calculate how much is left in his current bottle.

He started with 100mL and has used 40mL. Let's turn that into a calculation and use the mathematical symbols:

$$100 - 40 = 60mL$$

It is clear that John does not have enough medication for his trip and must obtain more.

As with addition, it is important that we consider the order of the digits in the number before commencing the process. Here is a simple example to show you how to subtract different numbers from one another:

In the number 59 we have 5 (tens) and 9 (units). If we want to subtract the number 22, we must ensure that we pair the tens together and then the units together. We would therefore place them in the following way:

$$59$$
$$\underline{22 -}$$
$$\underline{37}$$

Try the following to test your subtraction skills (the answers can be found at the end of the chapter):

$$19 - 17 =$$
$$53 - 41 =$$
$$177 - 73 =$$
$$458 - 334 =$$
$$1726 - 1114 =$$

Multiplication

Multiplication is the process of taking one or more numbers and combining them to make a new number called a product. Many of you will have learned simple multiplication (or times) tables at school. This gives us a good grounding in multiplication of small numbers and helps us to work

×	1	2	3	4	5	6	7	8	9	10
1	1	2	3	4	5	6	7	8	9	10
2	2	4	6	8	10	12	14	16	18	20
3	3	6	9	12	15	18	21	24	27	30
4	4	8	12	16	20	24	28	32	36	40
5	5	10	15	20	25	30	35	40	45	50
6	6	12	18	24	30	36	42	48	54	60
7	7	14	21	28	35	42	49	56	63	70
8	8	16	24	32	40	48	56	64	72	80
9	9	18	27	36	45	54	63	72	81	90
10	10	20	30	40	50	60	70	80	90	100

Table 3.1 Number multiplication table

out how to do this as number size increases. As we often give drugs many 'times' a day, we can use multiplication to calculate the total amount of medicine a person needs in a day.

For example, Francine needs her medication 4 times per day. On each occasion she needs to take 2 tablets. How many does she take in a day?

$$4 \times 2 = 8 \text{ tablets per day}$$

Knowledge of our 2 or 4 times table will have helped with this. It is worthwhile revising your tables to familiarize yourself with simple multiplication. Tables are aplenty on the internet, including that on the Maths is Fun website (2015). Or they can be bought in book form from many retailers. Use the number table in Table 3.1 to find the above answer.

When multiplying larger numbers, it is important that we consider the order of the digits in the number before commencing the process. Here is a simple example to show you how to multiply larger numbers:

In the number 55 we have 5 (tens) and 5 (units). If we want to multiply by the number 4, we must ensure that we place the tens and then the units correctly. We would therefore place them in the following way:

$$55$$
$$44 \times$$
$$\underline{220}$$

This allows us to multiply the units by 4 ($4 \times 5 = 20$);
then the tens by 4 ($4 \times 50 = 200$);
to give an answer of 220.

Try the following to test your multiplication skills (the answers can be found at the end of the chapter):

$$3 \times 4 =$$
$$9 \times 7 =$$
$$10 \times 3 =$$
$$20 \times 4 =$$
$$6 \times 15 =$$

Division

This is the opposite of multiplication where we take one number and divide it by another to create a new number. If we know the total amount of a drug a patient has to receive over one day, we can use division to calculate how much should be given for each individual dose, noting that the drug must not be administered all at once.

For example, Sam requires 100mg of medication to be given today, but that100mg has to be split into 4 equal doses. How many milligrams should each dose contain?

$$100 / 4 = 25\text{mg per dose}$$

When dividing numbers, it is important that we consider the order of the digits in the number before commencing the process. Here is a simple example to show you how to divide one number by another:

In the number 66 we have 6 (tens) and 6 (units). If we want to divide by the number 3, we must ensure that we place the tens and then the units correctly. We would therefore place them in the following way:

$$\frac{66}{3\,/} $$
$$\underline{22}$$

This allows us to divide the units by 3 (6 / 3 = 2); then the tens by 3 (60 / 3 = 20); to give an answer of 22.

Try the following to test your division skills (the answers can be found at the end of the chapter):

$$12 / 4 =$$
$$150 / 3 =$$
$$500 / 2 =$$
$$20 / 4 =$$
$$600 / 5 =$$

Calculator skills

Of course, for all the basic mathematical skills above most of us would use a calculator to derive our answer. Being able to use a calculator is an essential skill in numerical practice. You should use a calculator you are familiar with and be aware of all its functions and how to use them. It should be used primarily to check calculations – do not rely solely on a calculator, as there is no substitute for your own numerical ability.

Practise using your calculator for the four basic processes above by addressing the same questions provided in each section. Did you arrive at the same answers as when you worked them out yourself?

Basic introduction to units and conversions

Before performing many drug calculations, you will need to convert the numbers you use in the calculation so that they all appear in the same units. You should be familiar with the units in Box 3.4, as they are the most common used in drug calculation.

To convert from a smaller unit (e.g. gram) to a larger unit (e.g. kilogram), divide by 1000, thus:

$$5000g \div 1000 = 5kg$$

To convert from a larger unit (e.g. gram) to a smaller unit (e.g. milligram), multiply by 1000, thus:

$$5g \times 1000 = 5000mg$$

It is important to be comfortable with unit conversions before progressing to using a drug calculation formula. Practise some conversions before you move on.

Basic formula

There is more than one way to do a drug calculation, but the simplest and most widely used method is the basic formula shown here:

$$\frac{D \times Q}{H} = X$$

where:

$$D = \text{desired dose}$$

Box 3.4 Equivalencies of weight

Unit	Symbol	Equivalent	Symbol
1 kilogram	kg	1000 grams	g
1 gram	g	1000 milligrams	mg
1 milligram	mg	1000 micrograms	mcg
1 microgram	mcg	1000 nanograms	ng

H = strength available

Q = quantity or unit of measure (for tablets Q = 1, for liquids Q can vary)

X = dose to be determined / amount to be given

The steps when using the basic formula method are as follows:

- First, memorize the formula.
- Remember to convert all the units to the same system and size.
- Place all the unit information into the correct positions within the basic formula.
- Calculate your answer.
- Label all answers (e.g. tablets, capsules, millilitres).

Here are some examples:

Example 1

The doctor orders a dose of 0.05mg to be given orally.

You have 25 microgram tablets.

How many tablets should you give?

$$\frac{50}{25} \times 1 = X$$

$$\frac{2}{1} \times 1 = 2$$

$$X = 2 \text{ tablets}$$

Example 2

The patient requires 400mg of liquid to be given orally.

You have 250mg in 5mL of solution.

What volume of drug should you give?

$$\frac{400}{250} \times 5 = X$$

$$\frac{8}{5} \times 5 = 8$$

$$X = 8\text{mL}$$

Example 3

The patient needs 240mg of drug D by injection.

You have 150mg in 5mL of solution.

How many mL will you administer?

The dose has to be given at a rate of 1mL every 30 seconds: how long will each dose last?

$$\frac{240}{150} \times 5 = X$$

$$\frac{24}{15} \times 5 = 8\text{mL to be given}$$

1mL every 30 seconds = 2mL every minute:

$$\frac{8}{2} = 4 \text{ minutes}$$

Making numeracy into drug calculation

So far, we have considered basic processes, unit conversion and the basic formula for calculation. These can help in many of the worked examples above, but there are other areas of drug calculation we need to explore in more depth.

Solid dose calculations

Many of the drug calculations you will perform will be solid dose calculations, as tablets and capsules are used for a high proportion of prescribed medications. Let us apply the basic formula to each of the drug prescriptions for solid dose medication below to help cement your understanding of these types of calculation. Remember that, when using the basic formula equation for solid dose drugs, Q will always = 1.

Example 1

Your patient needs 150mg of Drug A.

50mg tablets are available.

How many tablets will you give?

$D = 150$

$H = 50$

$Q = 1$

So our calculation should look like this:

$$150 / 50 \times 1 = 3 \text{ tablets}$$

Can you see how that works? Here are some more.

Example 2

Your patient needs 375mg of Drug B.

75mg tablets are available.

How many tablets will you give?

$D = 375$

$H = 75$

$Q = 1$

So our calculation should look like this:

$$375 / 75 \times 1 = 5 \text{ tablets}$$

Example 3

Your patient needs 37.5mg of Drug C.

12.5mg tablets are available.

How many tablets will you give?

$D = 37.5$

$H = 12.5$

$Q = 1$

So our calculation should look like this:

$$37.5 / 12.5 \times 1 = 3 \text{ tablets}$$

Example 4

Your patient needs 400mg of Drug D.

200mg tablets are available.

How many tablets will you give?

$D = 400$

$H = 200$

$Q = 1$

So our calculation should look like this:

$$400 / 200 \times 1 = 2 \text{ tablets}$$

Example 5

Your patient needs 0.5mg of drug E.

250mg tablets are available.

How many tablets will you give?

First, we need to make a unit conversion so:

$$0.5 \times 1000 = 500 \text{mg}$$

$D = 500$

$H = 250$

$Q = 1$

So our calculation should look like this:

$$500 / 250 \times 1 = 2 \text{ tablets}$$

We hope these examples have helped you to understand the processes involved in solid dose calculation.

Liquid dose calculations

Many medications are available in liquid form, either as oral or injectable liquids. The principles are the same for each. Let us apply the basic formula to each of the drug prescriptions for liquid dose medication below to help cement your understanding of these types of calculation. Remember that, when using the basic formula equation for liquid dose drugs, Q will vary.

Example 1

Your patient needs 125mg of Drug A by subcutaneous (SC) injection.

50mg in 1mL of liquid for SC injection is available.

How many mL will you administer?

$D = 125$

$H = 50$

$Q = 1$

So our calculation should look like this:

$$125 / 50 \times 1 = 2.5 \text{mL}$$

Can you see how that works? Here are some others:

Example 2

Your patient needs 150mg of Drug B orally.

125mg in 5mL of syrup is available.

How many mL will you administer?

$D = 150$

$H = 125$

$Q = 5$

So our calculation should look like this:

$$150 / 125 \times 5 = 6 \text{mL}$$

Can you see how Q changed from 1 to 5 for this calculation?

Example 3

Your patient needs 25mg of Drug C by intravenous (IV) injection.

10mg in 1mL of liquid for IV injection is available.

How many mL will you administer?

$D = 25$

$H = 10$

$Q = 1$

So our calculation should look like this:

$$25 / 10 \times 1 = 2.5\text{mL}$$

Example 4
Your patient needs 240mg of Drug D by intramuscular (IM) injection.
150mg in 5mL of liquid for IM injection is available.
How many mL will you administer?

$D = 240$
$H = 150$
$Q = 5$

So our calculation should look like this:

$$240 / 150 \times 5 = 8\text{mL}$$

Example 5
Your patient needs 150mg of Drug E orally.
250mg in 10mL of liquid is available.
How many mL will you administer?

$D = 150$
$H = 250$
$Q = 10$

So our calculation should look like this:
$150 / 250 \times 10 = 6\text{mL}$

We hope these examples have helped you to understand the processes involved in liquid dose calculation.

Bolus doses and drug calculations of time
Sometimes a bolus dose, or a one-off dose, will have been prescribed. It is often the case that a bolus dose cannot be given in an instant, such as when swallowing a tablet, but must be infused over a period of time. Here is an example to illustrate this point:

Example 1
Your patient requires a bolus dose of 2g of medication.
500mg in 5mL solution is available for injection.
The drug can be given at a rate of 1mL every minute.
First, to calculate our dose we need to make a unit conversion:

$2 \times 1000 = 2000\text{mg}$
$2000 / 500 \times 5 = 20\text{mL}$
So we know we need to give 20mL, and we can do so at a rate of 1mL every minute:
$20 \times 1 = 20$ minutes to give the dose

That was quite simple so let's look at some others:

Example 2
Your patient requires a bolus dose of 1.2g of medication.
300mg in 5mL solution is available for injection.
The drug can be given at a rate of 1mL every 30 seconds.
First, to calculate our dose we need to make a unit conversion:

$$1.2 \times 1000 = 1200\text{mg}$$
$$1200 / 300 \times 5 = 20\text{mL}$$

So we know we need to give 20mL, and we can do so at a rate of 1mL every 30 seconds:

$$20 \times 30 = 600 \text{ seconds}$$

To convert to minutes, we need to divide by 60, thus:

$$600 / 60 = 10 \text{ minutes to give the dose}$$

Example 3
Your patient requires a bolus dose of 3.6g of medication.
600mg in 2mL solution is available for injection.
The drug can be given at a rate of 1mL every 15 seconds.
First, to calculate our dose we need to make a unit conversion:

$$3.6 \times 1000 = 3600\text{mg}$$
$$3600 / 600 \times 2 = 12\text{mL}$$

So we know we need to give 12mL, and we can do so at a rate of 1mL every 15 seconds.

$$12 \times 15 = 180 \text{ seconds}$$

To convert to minutes, we need to divide by 60, thus:

$$180 / 60 = 3 \text{ minutes to give the dose}$$

We hope these examples have helped you to understand the processes involved in bolus dose calculations over time.

Drug calculations by weight

Some medications require us to calculate the dose based on a patient's weight. These drugs are prescribed on a mg per kg basis and therefore we must obtain the patient's weight in kilograms. Many of these calculations are for medication for children and it is essential we get the doses correct, as errors can lead to overdose and complications. Here is an example to illustrate the point:

Example 1
Your patient requires their medicine at a dose of 60mg/kg/day (milligrams per kilogram per day). The patient weighs 12kg.
So the calculation will look like this:

$$60 \times 12 = 720\text{mg per day}$$

This might be a one-off dose or it may be required to be split. Let's say we want to give it in 4 divided doses, thus:

$$720 / 4 = 180\text{mg per dose}$$

Can you see how that worked? Here are some others:

Example 2
Your patient requires their medicine at a dose of 30mg/kg/day.

The patient weighs 15kg.
The dose must be given in 3 divided doses.
So the calculation will look like this:

$$30 \times 15 = 450\text{mg per day}$$
$$450 / 3 = 150\text{mg per dose}$$

When a dose calculation by weight needs to be made for a child, a liquid dose calculation might also need to be made. Here are all the steps involved:

Example 3
Your patient requires their medicine at a dose of 50mg/kg/day.
The child weighs 20kg.
The drug must be given in 4 divided doses.
You have a liquid available that is 125mg in 5mL.
So the calculation will look like this:

$50 \times 20 = 1000\text{mg per day}$
$1000 / 4 = 250\text{mg per dose}$
$250 / 125 \times 5 = 10\text{mL per dose}$

We hope that you are now clear about making weight calculations.

You should now be in a position to attempt the practice calculation questions at the end of this and the other chapters in the book. Have a look at the case studies below where drug calculations would be needed for the proper delivery of medication.

Case studies

① James Jones is 4 years old and has a fever. His doctor has prescribed paracetamol to help reduce his temperature and wants it given at a dose of 60mg per kg per day, but it must be divided into 4 doses and not given all at once. James has been weighed on admission and he is 16kg. Work out how much paracetamol he can have per day and how much he can have if this must be divided into 4 doses.

With this chapter in mind, outline which mathematical processes you would have to use and which drug calculations you would need to perform. Reflect on the importance of getting this calculation correct.

② Helen Taylor is admitted for surgery and requires a bolus dose of antibiotic before theatre. She is prescribed 300mg of Ciprofloxacin by intravenous infusion over 60 minutes. The dose must be prepared, and you have a 200mL bottle containing 2mg per mL. How many mL from the bottle is required to give 300mg and how much will be left in the bottle? If this dose is to be given as prescribed, at what rate does it need to be delivered over 60 minutes?

With this chapter in mind, outline which mathematical processes you would have to use and which drug calculations you would need to perform. Reflect on the importance of getting this calculation correct.

Key learning points

▶ Numeracy is integral to safe nursing practice.
▶ The ability to use basic principles such as addition, subtraction, multiplication and division is paramount in health care.
▶ The ability to convert between units of mass lays the foundations for drug calculations.
▶ The ability to calculate doses in solid and liquid form is essential, as is the ability to calculate drug administration over time and by weight.

Answers to questions in this chapter

Addition

$$11 + 27 = 38$$
$$23 + 45 = 68$$
$$101 + 273 = 374$$
$$450 + 339 = 789$$
$$1022 + 2174 = 3196$$

Subtraction

$$19 - 17 = 2$$
$$53 - 41 = 12$$
$$177 - 73 = 104$$
$$458 - 334 = 124$$
$$1726 - 1114 = 612$$

Multiplication

$$3 \times 4 = 12$$
$$9 \times 7 = 63$$
$$10 \times 3 = 30$$
$$20 \times 4 = 80$$
$$6 \times 15 = 90$$

Division

$$12 / 4 = 3$$
$$150 / 3 = 50$$
$$500 / 2 = 250$$
$$20 / 4 = 5$$
$$600 / 5 = 120$$

Calculations

1. How many micrograms are in 2mg?

2. How many grams are in 600mg?

3. How many milligrams are in 1.2g?

4. How many micrograms are in 5mg?

5. A doctor has prescribed 0.25mg of digoxin. You have 125 microgram tablets in stock. How many should you give?

6. How many 25mg tablets should be administered for a prescribed dose of 0.05g?

7. How many mL should be administered if your patient requires 250mg and you have 100mg in 5mL solution?

8. How many mL should be administered if your patient requires 1.5g and you have 500mg in 5mL strength liquid?

9. How long will it take to deliver a bolus dose of 1g of your drug if you have 250mg in 5mL solution which can run over 1mL every 30 seconds?

10. How much medication should you administer to your patient if they require their drug at a dose of 50mg/kg/dose and they weigh 15kg?

Recommended further reading

Downie, G., Mackenzie, J. and Williams, A. (2007) *Pharmacology and Medicines Management for Nurses*, 4th edition. Edinburgh: Churchill Livingstone.

Lapham, R. (2015) *Drug Calculations for Nurses: A Step-by-Step Approach*, 4th edition. London: Arnold.

Maths is Fun (2015) *Learn Your Multiplication Tables*. Available at: https://www.mathsisfun.com/tables.html.

Nursing and Midwifery Council (NMC) (2018) *Standards of Proficiency for Registered Nurses*. London: NMC.

Shihab, P. (2014) *Numeracy in Nursing and Healthcare: Calculations and Practice*, 2nd edition. London: Routledge.

Starkings, S. and Krause, L. (2018) *Passing Calculations Tests in Nursing*, 4th edition. London: Sage.

Local anaesthetics and analgesics

4

Chapter contents

Learning objectives

After studying this chapter, you should be able to:

- Understand how a nerve impulse is initiated and transmitted.
- Describe pain reception, transmission and interpretation.
- Outline the body's analgesic system.
- Discuss the mode of action of local anaesthetic agents.
- Identify the major ways local anaesthetic agents are administered.
- List unwanted effects of local anaesthetic agents.

- ■ Name at least two major drugs from the non-steroidal anti-inflammatory and opioid classifications of analgesics.
- ■ Compare the mode of action of non-steroidal anti-inflammatory and opioid analgesics.
- ■ Demonstrate knowledge of the unwanted effects of non-steroidal anti-inflammatory and opioid classifications of analgesics.
- ■ State the major opioid antagonist used in clinical practice.
- ■ Define the term 'adjuvant drug'.
- ■ Outline the use of novel analgesics in neuropathic pain
- ■ Correctly solve several drug calculations about local anaesthetics and analgesic drugs.

Introduction

Pain is a sensation that lets us know about damage to our tissues. It is one of our normal defence mechanisms and is important to our survival. Therefore, when we consider modifying the experience of pain, it is important to remember that, although distressing and unpleasant, pain has a role to play in protecting us. It is possible to suffer severe pain without any obvious tissue damage or injury, such as trigeminal neuralgia (severe burning or stabbing pain in the face arising from one of the nerves carrying sensation). On the other hand, pain may become a dominant feature in a person's life long after tissues have healed, such as phantom limb pain. It is also possible that tissue damage in one part of the body can lead to pain being perceived in another part of the body, something that is called *referred pain*.

Pain is therefore a difficult concept to define. As it becomes more chronic in nature (i.e. more than 6 months in duration), it begins to affect all activities of daily living, not just from a physical but also from a psychological and sociological perspective. The nurse has a unique role to play in minimizing pain for patients. To carry out this role effectively, nurses need to have some understanding of the drugs used in pain relief. The NMC Standards of Proficiency for Registered Nurses (NMC 2018) state:

Platform 4: Providing and evaluating care
4.8 demonstrate the knowledge and skills required to identify and initiate appropriate interventions to support people with commonly

encountered symptoms including anxiety, confusion, discomfort and pain

We first need to remind ourselves of the basic principles of the initiation and conduction of nerve impulses and the body's pain pathways and analgesic system.

Neurones

Neurones are specialized cells in the nervous system whose function is to transmit messages. A neurone has branch-like processes called dendrites that convey incoming messages (action potentials) towards the cell body (see Figure 4.1). The cell body houses the nucleus and therefore is the metabolic centre. Structures known as *axons*, which terminate in *axon terminals*, conduct impulses away from the cell body. Housed in the axon terminals are hundreds of small sacs (vesicles), which contain *neurotransmitters*. The nerve impulse therefore travels from the dendrites along the axon and finishes at the axon terminal where the impulse stimulates the release of the neurotransmitter.

Several neurones are covered with a substance called myelin, formed by supporting cells called Schwann cells, which wrap themselves around the axon. The myelin covering acts as an insulator for the nerve and affects the speed at which messages can travel along individual neurones.

Neurones carrying messages from the internal organs and skin into the central nervous system are called *sensory (afferent) neurones*. Conversely, neurones carrying messages out of the central

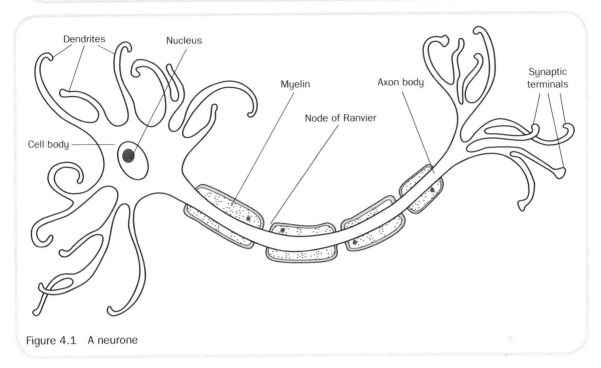

Figure 4.1   A neurone

nervous system to the muscles, glands and internal organs are called *motor (efferent) neurones*.

The nerve impulse

At rest, the inside of a neurone has a negative charge compared to the outside, which is positive. This is because the inside of a neurone carries a lot of negatively charged particles called *anions*. Anions are large particles that have difficulty moving through the wall of the neurone. In contrast, the outside of the neurone contains lots of positively charged particles called *cations*. The major cation in our discussion here is sodium.

To trigger the sensation of pain, the inside of the neurone must become positively charged. A nociceptive stimulus can cause chemicals to be released by damaged tissue (examples of these include bradykinin, histamine, serotonin, potassium and other proteolytic enzymes), which in turn can bring about a change in the neuronal membrane, allowing sodium to pass into the neurone. As the sodium enters, the membrane becomes even more permeable to sodium. This continues until the inside of the neurone is positively charged in

relation to the outside. This build-up of positively charged sodium is termed *depolarization*.

At the synapse, where one neurone meets another, neurotransmitters must be released to stimulate the next neurone to continue to pass the message onwards. This process is important when considering analgesics and how they work. Once the neurone has converted to a positive environment, calcium channels in the membrane open, so allowing calcium to enter. The influx of calcium attracts small sacs called synaptic vesicles, which are full of neurotransmitters, towards the synapse. When these vesicles reach the synapse, they fuse with the neurone membrane and release the neurotransmitter into the synapse itself (see Figure 4.2).

The neurotransmitters that are important in the pain pathway are substance P, neurokinin A and B, and glutamate. Once the neurotransmitter attaches itself to receptors on the other side of the synapse, this neurone then becomes permeable to sodium and the process continues (see Figure 4.3).

Having discussed the initiation and transmission of a nerve impulse, we need now to consider the body's pain pathways.

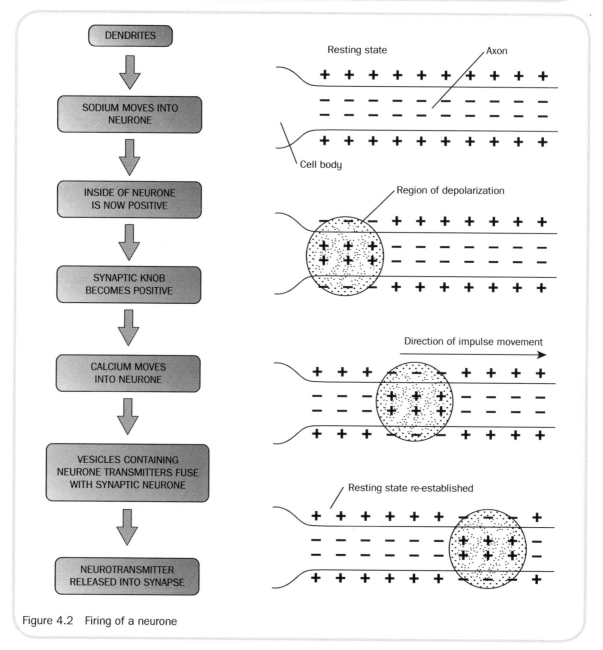

Figure 4.2 Firing of a neurone

Pain reception

Pain is received via specialist receptors called *nociceptors*, which are free nerve endings that lie in the tissues. They are most plentiful in the skin; as you move deeper into the tissues of the body, they become fewer in number. Nociceptors can be stimulated by mechanical, thermal and chemical means and have a high threshold. This means that only stimuli indicating some degree of tissue damage are perceived as pain. Nociceptors are *non-adapting*, which means they are stimulated at the same level of intensity each time the threshold level is reached. In other words, you do not raise the threshold at which the nociceptors are stimulated

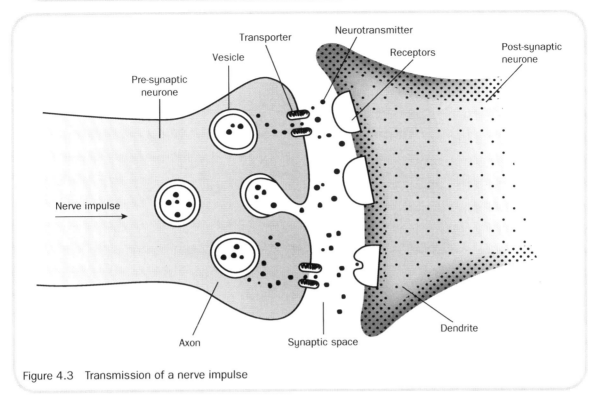

Figure 4.3   Transmission of a nerve impulse

just because the pain is constant. This is an important aspect to our survival.

In addition to noxious stimuli like heat and pressure, nociceptors can become sensitive to a variety of chemicals that are present after local tissue injury. These substances include potassium, serotonin, bradykinin, histamine and prostaglandins. Prostaglandins are normally produced by the body to ensure the smooth running of our internal environment (homeostasis). They are especially important in the case of certain medicines, such as NSAIDs.

Painful stimuli are received by the nociceptors and then transmitted by two different types of nerve fibres: A-delta fibres and C fibres. *A-delta fibres* are myelinated fibres, small in diameter, which are stimulated by mechanical means. A myelinated nerve is one covered by a fatty insulating substance called myelin. As the fibres are myelinated, they convey impulses very quickly. Stimulation of these fibres leads to sharp prickling pain that the person can easily localize. *C fibres* are

also fibres of small diameter but are unmyelinated and so convey impulses more slowly, resulting in a 'burning' or 'aching' pain that is harder to pinpoint. It will tend to be more general in nature, and a good example is abdominal pain.

Both A-delta and C fibres synapse with the next neurone in the pathway in the dorsal horn of the spinal cord. It is in this area of the dorsal horn (i.e. the substantia gelatinosa) that Melzack and Wall (1965) proposed a gate-controlled entry for the sensation of pain into the central nervous system. If the gate is opened a person will perceive pain, whereas if the gate is closed they will not.

The sensation of pain is then carried by what are referred to as the *spinothalamic tracks*, which carry impulses from the spinal cord up to the thalamus. One track carries information from the A-delta fibres and the other from the C fibres. These tracks once again synapse in the thalamus and the impulses are conveyed to several areas, including the sensory cortex, where they are interpreted as pain (see Figures 4.4 and 4.5).

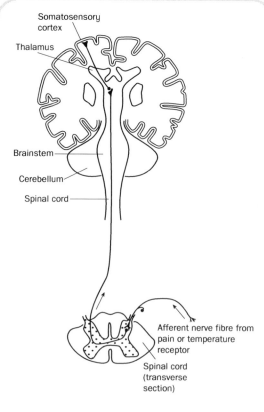

Figure 4.4 Spinothalamic tracks

The body's analgesic system

As with other sensory systems in the body, the pain pathway has a descending mechanism (see Figure 4.6). This mechanism constitutes the body's attempt to modify the pain we interpret. In other words, it is our inbuilt analgesic system.

This analgesic system commences at an area of the brain called the periaqueductal grey (PAG). This is a tiny part of grey matter that lies in the mid-brain. It receives input from several brain areas, among them the hypothalamus, cortex and thalamus. The PAG is thought to be the mechanism by which the gate to pain can be closed. It would certainly explain in physiological terms why psychological approaches to pain management are successful.

The PAG connects to an area in the medulla called the nucleus raphe magnus (NRM). This in turn sends fibres down the spinal cord and they interact at the dorsal horn. Therefore, higher brain centres have the infrastructure to open or close the gate to pain in the substantia gelatinosa.

Substance P is a neurotransmitter that has been implicated in the transmission of pain, but there are also several peptides that have been implicated

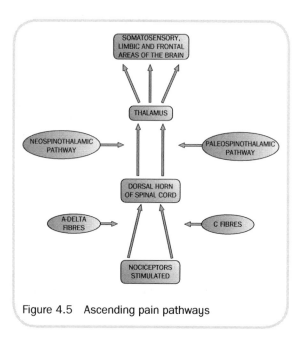

Figure 4.5 Ascending pain pathways

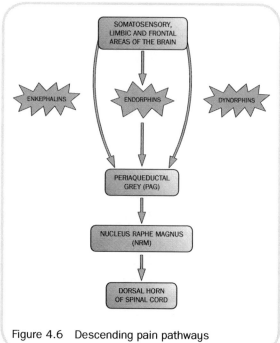

Figure 4.6 Descending pain pathways

in the brain's analgesic system. The three families of these peptides are *endorphins, dynorphins* and *enkephalins*. The discovery of these proteins has been very valuable in our understanding of why opiate drugs, including morphine, have such a unique effect on the body.

Types of pain

Nociceptive (tissue) pain

Nociceptive pain results from tissue damage. Intact pain pathways report this damage via their neurones, and pain is experienced. Nociceptive pain can be further subdivided into *somatic* and *visceral* (gut) pain. It can be experienced as sharp, dull or aching pain. There may be radiation of the pain, especially visceral pain, but it will not be in a direct nerve distribution. For example, gall bladder pain can radiate to the tip of the left shoulder blade. Nociceptive pain generally responds to NSAIDs and opioids, both of which will be addressed later in this chapter. Conditions associated with inflammation, bone pain and joint disease are particularly responsive to NSAIDs.

Neuropathic (nerve) pain

Neuropathic pain may occur when there is either damage to or dysfunction of nerves in the peripheral or central nervous system. This results in faulty signals being sent to the brain and experienced as pain. Neuropathic pain can be either peripheral (outside the central nervous system) or central (spinal cord and brain) in origin. Examples of neuropathic pain include diabetic neuropathy, trigeminal neuralgia, postherpetic zoster pain (peripheral pains) and thalamic pain syndrome (a central pain). Neuropathic pain frequently exists alongside nociceptive pain. Examples include trauma that damages tissue and nerves, burns (that burn skin as well as nerve endings) and external nerve compression. Examples of the latter include tumours that press on (compress) nerves and the pain of sciatica, caused by herniated intervertebral discs pressing on nerves.

Patients often describe neuropathic pain as a 'burning sensation'. They may also describe it as feeling like an electric shock or lightning bolt.

Sometimes, stimuli that usually do not cause pain, such as light touch, may elicit a painful response. A light stroke of the cheek that results in the sudden pain of trigeminal neuralgia is an example of this type of pain. Sometimes patients do not describe the sensation as being 'painful' but rather as feeling unpleasantly strange or 'tingly', rather like an arm feels when it wakes up from 'going to sleep'. This is called a dysesthesia. Diabetic neuropathy commonly results in this type of sensation.

Neuropathic pain in the peripheral nervous system frequently follows a nerve distribution. This distribution may follow a particular nerve, as in sciatic pain or trigeminal neuralgia, or may represent the distribution of terminal nerve endings, as in the 'stocking-glove' distribution of peripheral neuropathies. Neuropathic pain is relatively resistant to NSAIDs and opioids, although they may be helpful in certain cases. The other major classes of medications useful for neuropathic pain, tricyclic antidepressants and gabapentin, will be discussed later.

Acute and chronic pain

Pain can also be classified in terms of how long a person has experienced it for. A short duration would be classed as acute pain whereas a longer duration would be classified as chronic pain.

Acute pain

Acute pain is of recent onset and of limited duration. Sufferers often describe it as being sharp or stabbing in nature, at times like an electric shock. This is a warning to the body that something is not right and that damage to cells may be occurring. Examples of conditions that might lead to acute pain are:

■ bone fracture;
■ after having surgery;
■ following first degree burns;
■ lacerations to the skin;
■ giving birth;
■ dental surgery.

Acute pain can be measured on a scale. It can be a generally mild pain that soon disappears, or it might go to the other end of the scale where a person describes it as excruciating and such pain might last for a few weeks or months. However, in most cases acute pain lasts no more 6 months. If it continues for more than 6 months, it would likely be classified as chronic pain. Furthermore, acute pain usually disappears when the underlying cause of the pain has been treated or healing has taken place.

A pain scale can help nurses to determine the severity of a patient's pain, and the subsequent effectiveness of analgesia administered. Adults are frequently asked to quantify their pain numerically, on a scale of 1–10. Using this scale, 0 equates to no pain while 10 represents the worst possible pain imaginable. Numerical scores are not so useful with children, however; instead, nurses can use the FACES scale (Wong and Baker 2001), where the child can point to the facial expression that best relates to how they feel.

Chronic pain

If the person continues to experience pain for more than 6 months, the pain will have become chronic in nature. Also, in some individuals the pain may persist despite their injury having healed. Pain signals may remain active in the nervous system for months or even years. Chronic pain also leads to other physiological effects in the body, so that the person might also complain of tense muscles, a lack of energy, limited mobility and changes in appetite.

Individuals may have an emotional component to their pain when it becomes chronic in nature. It is not unusual for the person to become depressed, angry or anxious, even fearful of re-injury. Such strong emotional responses to the pain may also hinder their ability to return to normal work or leisure activities. Chronic pain, therefore, is a a very complex phenomenon to treat. Examples of common chronic pain complaints include:

- a longstanding headache;
- lower back pain;
- pain due to cancers;
- pain suffered by people with arthritis;
- pain resulting from damage to nerves, for example trigeminal neuralgia.

Chronic pain might have begun as acute pain, perhaps due to an initial trauma, injury or infection. However, some people suffer chronic pain in the absence of a past injury or physiological evidence of body damage. Indeed, as in arthritis or phantom pain, there might be no known cure for the disease and any interventions we make will be palliative rather than curative.

Local anaesthetics

Local anaesthetics are analgesic drugs designed to be used clinically to produce a reversible loss of sensation in a part of the body. Generally, there are two classes of local anaesthetic: *ester agents* such as cocaine, procaine and amethocaine, and *amides* such as lidocaine, prilocaine and bupivacaine. The difference between the two classes relates to biochemistry:

- Esters are more unstable in solution than amides and are broken down relatively quickly by enzymes in the plasma. One of the products produced when this group of drugs is broken down is a compound known as para-amino benzoate acid (PABA). These drugs have been associated with allergic responses and hypersensitivity reactions, so caution should be exercised.
- The amides display fewer of the above problems. It is more common in practice for drugs of this class to be used.

Mode of action

Local anaesthetics block the sodium channels in the neuronal membrane. If sodium cannot cross the semi-permeable membrane, then the inside of the neurone cannot become depolarized, i.e. the environment remains negative rather than becoming positively charged. Local anaesthetics tend to block conduction more effectively in nerve fibres of small diameter, thus making them perfect for the A-delta and C fibres described earlier. Thus, pain is blocked more effectively than other sensations, such as touch. Also, this makes it possible to provide a good level of analgesia with limited loss of motor function. This will be observed, for example, following an epidural anaesthetic during labour.

One of the problems encountered when giving a local anaesthetic is that many of them cause the surrounding vessels to dilate. This can lead to rapid absorption of the drug, reducing its effect. For this reason, a vasoconstrictor is sometimes added to increase potency and prolong action. Vasoconstrictors also decrease the likelihood of systemic side-effects, making local anaesthetics safer. The most common drug added to local anaesthetics is adrenaline.

The effect of vasoconstrictors on the potency and duration of action of local anaesthetics varies according to the drug being given and the site at which it is being used.

> ### Clinical tip
>
> Solutions containing adrenaline should never be used for infiltration around the penis or in finger or toe blocks, as the constrictive effects could lead to severe ischaemia and necrosis in the small vessels in these parts of the body.

Topical anaesthesia

Local anaesthetics are produced that are effective for the skin, eyes, ears, nose and mouth (e.g. prilocaine and lidocaine). When used topically, the onset of action is around 5–10 minutes, the drug action lasting between 30 and 60 minutes. This method of application numbs a small area of skin so is ideal for relieving pain from sunburn, minor burns and insect bites. Topical application can also be administered to the surface of the eye allowing certain operative procedures to take place. It must be remembered that significant amounts of these drugs can be absorbed, especially if applied to very vascular areas.

Infiltration anaesthesia

This technique is used to provide anaesthesia for minor surgical procedures such as dental work. Lidocaine and prilocaine are again frequently used with the patient feeling pressure but no pain. The

> ### Clinical tip
>
> If you work in paediatric practice, you will come across EMLA or Ametop cream. This is a cream eutectic mixture of local anaesthetics, usually used to provide surface anaesthesia of the skin in children prior to insertion of a cannula. EMLA cream is a mixture of equal proportions of lidocaine and prilocaine. The medicine should be applied to the skin under an occlusive dressing and should be left for 60 minutes before the procedure takes place.

onset of action is very rapid, while the duration of action depends on the drug being used. Prilocaine has the shortest period of action (15–30 minutes), while lidocaine provides a moderate length of anaesthesia (60 minutes). Bupivacaine has the longest duration of action, at around 200 minutes but has a slow onset of up to 30 minutes. Often the effects of the local anaesthetic continue after the procedure is concluded, so providing extra pain relief. As discussed earlier, the addition of adrenaline will increase the quality and duration of these anaesthetics.

Nerve blockade (conduction anaesthesia)

As the name implies, in conduction anaesthesia the nerves relating to the area being operated upon are blocked with a local anaesthetic. The blockade may be minor (e.g. intercostals) or deep (e.g. brachial plexus). Drugs such as lidocaine are used for minor blocks and have an onset of 5–10 minutes and duration of 1–2 hours. In a major blockade, the onset can be more variable so communication with the patient is paramount. The local anaesthetic in this case takes a little longer to act (10–15 minutes), but has a longer duration of action, at around 3–4 hours. Bupivacaine can be effective for up to 10 hours. The main advantage of this approach is that a relatively small amount of the drug can be administered to achieve a wide area of anaesthesia. This can be of benefit, for example, in the case of a neck of femur fracture in a patient who is not suitable for general anaesthetic, and is called a femoral block. Nerve blockade can also be used in conjunction with a general anaesthetic to reduce the number of drugs used in the procedure and any resulting side-effects.

Extradural, epidural and caudal anaesthesia

For each of these procedures, the local anaesthetic is injected between the dura (the outside covering of the brain and spinal cord) and the periosteum of the bones lining the spinal cord. Either lidocaine or bupivacaine is used with this technique. The advantage of an epidural approach is that a carefully placed needle can achieve a pain-free band from about the mid-chest to the mid-thighs but at the same time allow the legs to maintain their normal strength. A further local anaesthetic can be administered into a reservoir connected to a fine tube placed in the patient's lower back.

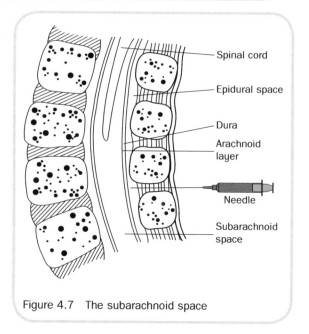

Figure 4.7 The subarachnoid space

distal forearm fractures. First, the limb is elevated to encourage drainage of blood. A blood pressure cuff would have been applied prior to the procedure and this is now inflated to above the arterial pressure by 100mmHg to a maximum of 300mmHg.

The local anaesthetic (prilocaine at 0.5% strength, prepared according to patient weight) is then injected into a previously cannulated vessel. The anaesthetic agent infiltrates the tissues below the level of the blood pressure cuff. The onset of action is almost immediate, giving excellent anaesthesia for any procedure lasting up to a maximum of 45 minutes (RCEM 2017).

Clinical tip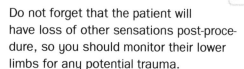

Do not forget that the patient will have loss of other sensations post-procedure, so you should monitor their lower limbs for any potential trauma.

Spinal anaesthesia

This is a specialized procedure which anaesthetizes the lower half of the body and does not maintain leg strength: the patient will be unable to move their legs. The local anaesthetic in this case is administered directly into the cerebrospinal fluid. The drug is rapidly taken up, which leads to a faster onset and requires a smaller dose. Care must be taken if using this route of administration with a pregnant woman, as the volume of the subarachnoid space (see Figure 4.7) is diminished, and therefore a reduced dose is required.

Clinical tip

Systemic blood levels of prilocaine are not significant at a dose of 3mg/kg, providing the cuff is not deflated for a period of 15 minutes following initial injection.

Intravenous local anaesthesia

This is sometimes referred to as a *Biers block* and is usually used to assist doctors to manipulate

Unwanted effects of local anaesthetics

Local anaesthetics are relatively safe if they are administered in an appropriate dosage and given

Box 4.1   Administration of local anaesthetics

Topical	Applied directly to the skin, eyes, ears, nose or mouth
Infiltration anaesthesia	Applied by penetration of surrounding tissue area
Nerve blockade	Applied as close to neurone supplying pain sensation to an area of the body as possible
Epidural	Applied to space between the dura and skull
Spinal	Applied directly into the subarachnoid space
Intravenous	Applied directly into the vein of a limb

into the correct anatomical area. It is especially important to avoid unwanted effects of this group of drugs on the central nervous system and the cardiovascular system.

These drugs have a profound effect on the central nervous system due to their mode of action on cell membranes. Initial mild symptoms may include a feeling of dizziness, leading to sensory disturbances. Severe central nervous system responses to local anaesthetics include major convulsions, followed by acute central nervous system depression as indicated by respiratory arrest and coma.

The cardiovascular effects tend to be associated with myocardial depression and vasodilation. The myocardium loses its ability to contract effectively and coupled with the dilation of vessels, leads to a rapid and life-threatening fall in blood pressure.

Clinical tip

Health care professionals must always be alert to the possibility of accidental injection of local anaesthetics into veins and arteries.

A true allergic reaction to a local anaesthetic agent is rare. Some people are sensitive to what are called *parabens* (preservatives in local anaesthetics). The preservative, methylparaben or propylparaben,

may act as the allergen. The symptoms that occur following a possible allergic reaction to a local anaesthetic agent must be distinguished from toxic reactions due to over-dosage (unintended intravenous injection) and reactions occurring as a side-effect of adrenaline (used as an additive).

In the rare event that a patient is sensitive to a local anaesthetic, skin tests should be undertaken using preparations without parabens. In addition, adrenaline-containing preparations are avoided, as they mask a positive skin test.

The analgesic ladder

Before discussing further analgesics, it is useful to consider whether a framework exists to help in planning the pharmacological pathway for a patient in severe or chronic pain. The World Health Organization (WHO 1966) offers what is commonly known as the *analgesic ladder*. This is a step-by-step escalation of a variety of analgesics depending upon the severity of pain experienced and is administered in standard doses at regular intervals. Step 1 commences with the use of paracetamol and NSAIDs such as ibuprofen. If the pain continues the patient moves on to Step 2. This step involves giving the patient a weak opioid such as codeine. If the pain is still not controlled, the final step in the ladder is to administer a strong opioid such as morphine. Progress up the ladder frequently involves using analgesic drugs in combination (see Figure 4.8). This ladder was originally derived to help manage cancer pain but has been widely adopted to treat many types of severe or enduring pain.

Non-steroidal anti-inflammatory drugs

Non-steroidal anti-inflammatory drugs (NSAIDs) are a group of drugs commonly given to patients who complain of mild to moderate pain. These drugs are also known to lower body temperature (they are *antipyretic*) and have anti-inflammatory properties (see Chapter 6). Earlier we discussed tissue injury and how prostaglandin release is implicated in this. When cells are damaged, they release a substance called *arachidonic acid*. This in turn is utilized in two metabolic pathways, one of these being the cyclooxygenase pathway which

creates several products, among them prostaglandins (we will revisit these pathways in Chapter 6). Prostaglandins are responsible for making the nociceptors more sensitive. As a result, when pain-producing products, such as bradykinins, are released, greater pain is felt by the individual.

NSAIDs are thought to decrease the amount of prostaglandin produced by blocking the cyclooxygenase pathway. Hence this group of drugs is effective for a range of conditions, such as pain from arthritis, toothache, periods and even cancer. The blockage of the pathway is useful in terms of the amount of pain we feel; however, it also produces side-effects.

Prostaglandins contribute to our natural balance (homeostasis) and have important roles to play within the body. The prostaglandin I-2 is responsible for ensuring the mucous lining of our digestive tract remains effective. Prostaglandin E-2 has a role to play in the kidneys, where it helps to maintain the correct pressure for the kidneys to filter water and waste products (see Figure 4.9) Therefore, interference with prostaglandin production has a price and this is shown in the gastrointestinal and renal side-effects of using this group of drugs. It is important to also note that some patients with cardiovascular conditions may not be suitable for NSAID use and careful consideration of the cautions and contraindications in the BNF is necessary by the prescriber.

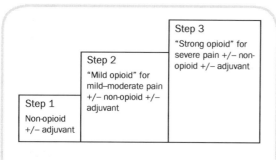

Figure 4.8   The analgesic ladder adapted from WHO (1966)

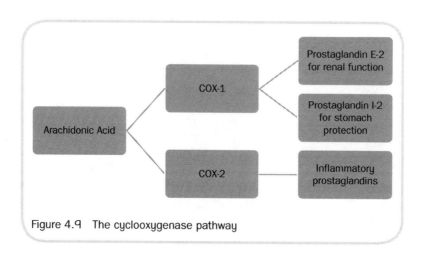

Figure 4.9   The cyclooxygenase pathway

Aspirin

Aspirin was the first drug to be discovered in this category. It has a long history, going back to the fifth century BC and the Greek physician Hippocrates, who wrote about the pain-relieving effects of willow bark (from which salicylic acid is derived). The discovery of aspirin, however, is attributed to the German chemist Felix Hoffmann in 1897, who was working under the direction of Arthur Eichengrün at Bayer pharmaceuticals (Sneader 2000). Aspirin is a weak acid and so is absorbed better in an acid environment such as the stomach, although the small intestine absorbs the greatest amount of the drug due to its large surface area.

For adults, doses of 300mg to 900mg are generally given four times a day. The correct dose of aspirin depends on the condition being treated. For mild-to-moderate pain, it is usually given at a dose of 300mg to 600mg four times a day. Due to its gastrointestinal side-effects, it is best given with or after food in an enteric coated form, which discourages breakdown in the stomach and small intestine.

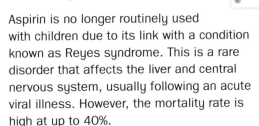

Clinical tip

Aspirin is no longer routinely used with children due to its link with a condition known as Reyes syndrome. This is a rare disorder that affects the liver and central nervous system, usually following an acute viral illness. However, the mortality rate is high at up to 40%.

Other contraindications are also associated with aspirin. The drug should be avoided in patients with known allergies to ibuprofen and naproxen, or with kidney disease, peptic ulcers or gastritis. Patients with a tendency to bleeding disorders (e.g. haemophilia) should also avoid this drug. Taking aspirin with other drugs, such as warfarin (see Chapter 7 on anticoagulants) is also known to increase the chances of gastrointestinal bleeding. Asthmatic patients should be alerted to the possibility of it causing a severe reaction. It is estimated that 4–10% of patients who suffer from asthma are at risk of having a severe reaction to the drug (Hamad et al. 2004). Aspirin also has several other side-effects that are dealt with in more detail later.

Ibuprofen

Ibuprofen is another drug that blocks cyclooxygenase, the enzyme that makes prostaglandins, resulting in lower levels of these in the body. Ibuprofen is prescribed for mild-to-moderate pain, caused by many and diverse conditions. The usual dose for minor aches and pains, including painful periods and a high temperature, is 200mg to 400mg three to four times per day.

As with other drugs in this class, ibuprofen can be enteric coated and should be taken with or just following food. The drug is known to have many interactions. If taken with lithium (a mood stabilizer), it may lead to increased levels of lithium due to its influence on lithium excretion by the kidneys. It should also be avoided during pregnancy, as no adequate studies have been completed on its safety in pregnant women.

The side-effects of ibuprofen are similar to those of other drugs in this category, such as rash, abdominal pain, nausea, diarrhoea and heartburn (dyspepsia). Renal function is also affected, so ibuprofen should be used cautiously in patients who already have a degree of renal impairment or congestive cardiac failure.

Naproxen

Naproxen is another NSAID that is used on a regular basis. It is frequently prescribed to patients who have pain and inflammation due to rheumatic disease and is often the drug of choice for musculoskeletal pain in the joints, muscles and tendons. It is also used to treat dysmenorrhoea and gout.

Naproxen comes in tablet form, either a gastro-resistant tablet or an effervescent tablet, and is also available as an oral suspension.

Naproxen tablets should be taken with food to reduce stomach irritation (Cautionary label 21 in the BNF). The recommended dose for pain is 500mg to 1g daily in two divided doses. However, the dosing interval depends on the formulation

Clinical tip

Naproxen effervescent tablets are to be dissolved in water before taking. The solution is rapidly absorbed from the gut, so this type of tablet provides pain relief more quickly than the other types. However, the solution is more likely to irritate the stomach lining, because it doesn't have the advantage of the gastro-protective enteric coat. The dispersible tablets are therefore most suitable for short-term use and should not be used for more than 3 months.

used and the condition being treated – the dose for gout, for example, is 750mg initially followed by 250mg every 8 hours for the duration of the attack.

Like other NSAIDs, naproxen is associated with several suspected or probable interactions that affect the action of other drugs. The most common side-effects involve the gastrointestinal system. The drug can cause ulcerations, abdominal burning, pain, cramping, nausea, gastritis and even serious gastrointestinal bleeding and liver toxicity; rash, kidney impairment, ringing in the ears and light-headedness are also known to occur. NSAIDs reduce the flow of blood to the kidneys and impair their function. This impairment is most likely to occur in patients who already have reduced kidney function or congestive heart failure, and use of NSAIDs in these patients should be considered with caution. Individuals with asthma are more likely to experience allergic reactions to NSAIDs.

As with ibuprofen, naproxen may increase circulating levels of lithium by reducing the excretion of lithium by the kidneys. Increased levels of lithium may lead to lithium toxicity. This is particularly important to bear in mind if the patient is being treated with lithium for other problems. Naproxen may also lower a patient's blood pressure, reducing the effects of blood pressure medications. This may occur because prostaglandins play a role in the regulation of blood pressure. Individuals taking oral anticoagulants such as warfarin should avoid NSAIDs because they also affect the clotting cascade by their actions on prostaglandins, which in turn could increase the patient's international normalized ratio (INR) (see Chapter 7).

Paracetamol

Paracetamol relieves pain and fever in adults and children and is probably the most widely used medicine in fulfilling this role. It can be prescribed by a doctor or pharmacist, but generally it is bought as an over the counter (OTC) medicine. Although the drug was first discovered in 1893, it was not used commercially until the 1950s. Much remains unknown about its mechanism of action.

Paracetamol does not appear to have any significant action on either of the cyclooxygenase pathways. This helps to explain why it is free from the gastrointestinal side-effects typical of NSAIDs. A third previously unknown pathway is initiated by an enzyme found in the brain and spinal cord. This enzyme is specifically affected by paracetamol and it is this effect that explains its effectiveness in relieving pain and reducing fever without GI side-effects.

Clinical tip

Sometimes, stomach ulceration and bleeding can occur without any abdominal pain. Black tarry stools (melaena), weakness and dizziness upon standing may be the only signs of internal bleeding. So listen to the patient and monitor them for these signs and symptoms.

Clinical tip

The recommended adult dose for paracetamol is 1000mg every 4–6 hours, and no more than eight tablets in a 24-hour period. If this dose is adhered to, there are few if any toxic effects. There are no groups of people who should not take paracetamol and interactions with other medicines are rare.

Paracetamol is quickly absorbed by the body and its peak serum levels occur within approximately 30 minutes to 2 hours after ingestion. Elimination is also rapid: paracetamol has a half-life of about 2 hours. It is vital that the recommended dose be adhered to, because a substantial overdose of paracetamol is likely to result in liver damage and requires immediate treatment. When paracetamol is broken down by the liver, it produces an active by-product. To neutralize this by-product, the liver attaches a substance known as glutathione to it. In overdose, the rate of the by-product increases far more rapidly than the liver can manufacture glutathione. Eventually the liver stores are exhausted and the reactive by-product starts to damage the liver tissue itself.

Treatment of overdose requires skilled hospital management. An antidote called *N*-acetylcysteine is available and is given intravenously. This restores the liver's capacity to produce glutathione and, therefore, protects against damage to the liver. It is important that the antidote is administered quickly, and it is best given within 12 hours of ingestion. However, it has been shown that the antidote has beneficial effects even as much as 48 hours post-ingestion.

Clinical tip

It is worth remembering that paracetamol is often combined with decongestant ingredients in cold and flu remedies and with other analgesics such as codeine in the preparation known as co-codamol. Therefore, this should be considered by the patient if taking the full dose so that accidental overdose is avoided. The size of retail packs is also intended to reduce the risk of overdose. Pharmacies are limited to a maximum of 32 tablets per pack, while shops are limited to packs of 16. Although multiple packs can be purchased, if more than 100 tablets are needed, a doctor's prescription will be necessary.

Opioid analgesics

These drugs are given for moderate-to-severe pain (see the WHO analgesic ladder in Figure 4.8). Opioid drugs are a class of natural, synthetic and semi-synthetic agents and are used for their analgesic, anti-tussive (stop you coughing) and anti-diarrhoeal properties. This class of drugs is derived from the opium poppy, whose properties have been known for centuries. They are subject to the Misuse of Drugs Act 1971.

Clinical tip

You may find several terms that are used interchangeably when describing drugs in this category: 'narcotic', 'opiate' and 'opioid'. You will also see them referred to as 'weak', 'strong', 'natural', 'semi-synthetic' and 'synthetic'.

All opioids exert their effect through binding with specific receptors called opioid receptors located in the central nervous system (brain and spinal cord) or peripherally in the GI tract. There are four types designated by the Greek letters μ (mu), κ (kappa), σ (sigma) and δ (delta). Different opioid analgesics bind in different ways with a variety of these receptors, thus explaining why such a range of effects and side-effects can occur.

Opioid drugs are agonistic in nature, i.e. they mimic our own endorphins, bringing about a similar analgesic reaction. There are numerous opioid analgesic preparations, some natural (e.g. morphine and codeine) and some synthetic (e.g. diamorphine, methadone, fentanyl and meperidine). We will focus on morphine as a strong agonistic opioid, fentanyl as a synthetic opioid and codeine as a moderate agonist or weak opioid.

Morphine

Opioid drugs are thought to have several mechanisms of action. You will recall that at the beginning of this chapter we discussed the importance of calcium channels opening to allow the transmission of a nerve signal across a synapse. Morphine is thought to block these channels from opening so that the pain signal breaks down. It is also thought that morphine opens potassium channels in neurones, so making the inside more negative, a condition known as *hyperpolarization*. This makes the firing of a pain neurone more difficult.

The most important effects of morphine, and many of the opioids related to it, occur on the central nervous system and the GI tract and include:

- **Analgesia.** This term refers to the loss or relief of pain but without the loss of consciousness. Morphine is useful in both acute and chronic types of pain. It not only raises the level at which pain is initiated (higher threshold) but also alters the brain's perception of the pain. The person is still aware of the pain but does not recognize it as an unpleasant sensation.
- **Euphoria.** When a person takes morphine, it makes them feel a powerful sense of contentment and well-being, often described as a 'rush'. This is a very positive effect, as pain often leads to anxiety and agitation. Patients who are prescribed the drug for acute pain tend to be euphoric, whereas this effect may diminish or disappear in patients with chronic long-standing pain.
- **Respiratory depression.** This is caused by the respiratory centre in the brainstem becoming less sensitive to the respiratory drive of carbon dioxide. It is one of the more worrying side-effects that you need to be aware of, particularly as it can occur with therapeutic doses. It is the most common cause of death in acute opioid poisoning.
- **Depression of the cough reflex.** This does not match the analgesic or respiratory depressive effects of morphine. Therefore, weaker opiates, such as codeine, can be used in antitussive preparations.
- **Nausea and vomiting.** This occurs in up to 40% of people prescribed morphine when they first start to take the drug. As they become

tolerant of the medicine, this effect is reduced. These side-effects are thought to be brought about by morphine's effects on a particular area of the brain known as the chemoreceptor trigger zone (CTZ).
- **Pupillary constriction.** Pinpoint pupils are caused by morphine. The drug stimulates a pair of cranial nerves called the oculomotor nerves which cause this phenomenon.
- **Effects on the GI tract.** Morphine reduces the rate at which the GI system moves (motility). This leads to constipation, which is often severe and very troublesome for the patient. All patients receiving morphine should be considered for an aperient. Morphine also affects the smooth muscle of the biliary tract, causing a rise in the pressure within this system. It is due to this effect that morphine should be avoided in people suffering from biliary colic due to gallstones: if morphine is given, it might increase the pain rather than lessen it. The general slowing of the gut may affect the absorption of other drugs.

Clinical tip

The appearance of pinpoint pupils is still considered a significant diagnostic feature of opiate overdose as other causes of unconsciousness tend to cause the pupils to dilate.

Despite its side-effects, morphine is still regarded as the gold standard by which other analgesic medications are measured. Absorption of the drug from the GI tract is not particularly good. A significant first pass effect occurs in the liver, meaning a subcutaneous, intramuscular or intravenous injection is usually given.

Repeated doses of morphine cause tolerance, resulting in the need to prescribe a higher dose of the drug to achieve the same effect. Both physical and psychological dependence do occur.

Fentanyl

Fentanyl is a powerful synthetic opiate analgesic similar to but approximately 100 times more potent than morphine, with 100mcg of fentanyl approximately equivalent to 10mg of morphine. It is typically used to treat patients with severe pain, or to manage pain after surgery. It is also used to treat chronic pain in patients who are physically tolerant to opiates.

Fentanyl is a narcotic analgesic that acts predominately at the m-opiate receptor. Apart from analgesia, the fentanyls as a group produce drowsiness and euphoria, the latter being less pronounced than with morphine. The most common side-effects include nausea, dizziness, vomiting, fatigue, headache, constipation, anaemia and peripheral oedema. Tolerance and dependence develop rapidly after repeated use. Characteristic withdrawal symptoms (sweating, anxiety, diarrhoea, bone pain, abdominal cramps, shivers or 'goose flesh') occur when use is stopped.

Serious interactions can occur when fentanyls are mixed with heroin, cocaine, alcohol and other central nervous system depressants such as benzodiazepines. The use of human immunodeficiency virus (HIV) protease inhibitors such as ritonavir has been reported to increase plasma levels and reduce elimination of co-administered fentanyl. As with morphine, overdose results in respiratory depression that is reversible with naloxone.

As it has a wide range of uses for both acute and chronic pain, fentanyl comes in a number of formulations, including intravenous injection, lozenges and transdermal patches. Such skin patches should only be used to control moderate-to-severe chronic (around-the-clock, long-lasting) pain that cannot be controlled by the use of other pain medications in people who are tolerant to narcotic pain medications. Fentanyl patches should not be used to treat mild pain, short-term pain, pain after an operation or medical or dental procedure, or pain that can be controlled by medication that is taken as needed. Patches are usually applied to the skin once every 72 hours. The doctor may start the patient on a low dose and gradually increase this, not more often than once every 3 days at first, and then not more often than once every 6 days.

> **Clinical tip**
>
> The medication in fentanyl patches is contained in a gel that is sealed between layers of the patch. If this gel leaks from the patch, remove it immediately without touching the gel. If you do touch the gel, wash the affected area immediately with large amounts of clean water. Do not use soap, alcohol or other cleansers.

Fentanyl skin patches can be habit forming. The patient should be reminded not to apply more than one patch at a time, or to wear them for longer than the period prescribed. Equally they should not cease to use without consulting their doctor, as there is a danger of symptoms of withdrawal that include restlessness, teary eyes, runny nose, yawning, sweating, chills, hair standing on end, muscle aches, large pupils, irritability, anxiety, backache, pain in the joints, weakness, stomach cramps, difficulty falling asleep or staying asleep, nausea, loss of appetite, vomiting, diarrhoea, a fast heartbeat and rapid breathing.

Codeine

Codeine is a less potent analgesic than morphine and is frequently referred to as a weak opioid. However, it has one advantage over morphine in that it is well absorbed when taken orally, although when increased to higher doses for severe pain the analgesic effect does not increase in parallel. Large amounts of the drug do not provide extra analgesia; therefore, it is only suitable for mild-to-moderate pain. Codeine has a lower potential for dependency making abuse of the drug less likely, although cases have been reported. The drug is a good antitussive at doses that do not produce analgesia, and thus has the potential for use in cough medicines. However, in most non-prescription cough medicines it has been replaced by newer drugs such as dextromethorphan, a synthetic narcotic, which has the same antitussive properties. Codeine is used in drugs that are classed as *analgesic mixtures*. For example, co-codamol tablets contain paracetamol and codeine phosphate in varying ratios (available preparations are codeine 8mg/paracetamol 500mg, codeine 15mg/paracetamol 500mg and codeine 30mg/paracetamol 500mg). Another analgesic mixture that you will come across regularly is co-dydramol, which contains dihydrocodeine 10mg and paracetamol 500mg per tablet.

Tramadol

Tramadol is a strong analgesic painkiller but a moderate strength opioid. It can be used in acute and chronic pain. Like other opioids, it has the potential to become addictive and patients should be monitored for signs of this as well as tolerance (the need for more of the drug to produce the same response), and the lowest possible does to produce the analgesic effect should be administered. Daily does of over 400mg should not be given. Although able to be used in chronic pain, the manufacturer recommends that tramadol should not be administered for longer than absolutely necessary. Dose adjustments (reductions) may be needed in the over-75s and its use is not recommended in children under 12.

When a patient starts taking any opioid, it is very important that you warn them of the possible sedative effects and discuss the dangers of driving or operating heavy machinery. This is a requirement of legislation amending the Road Traffic Act to incorporate The Drug Driving (Specified Limits) (England & Wales) (Amendment) Regulations 2015.

Opioid antagonists

As discussed above, respiratory depression is a side-effect of opiates. Therefore, in opioid overdose, an antidote is necessary. This comes in the form of a drug called naloxone, which attracts strongly to all three opioid receptors. Naloxone blocks the actions of morphine and our own endorphins by occupying the opioid receptors without bringing about any response, so effectively stopping anything else connecting to the receptor. Naloxone therefore quickly reverses the effects of opioid drugs.

Clinical tip

The main clinical use of naloxone is to treat respiratory depression caused by opioid drugs in overdose, whether accidental or intentional. It is usually given intravenously, and its effects are immediate. It has a relatively short half-life, as it is quickly metabolized by the liver. Therefore, when treating a patient, you may see the drug repeatedly used in order to maintain respiratory function.

Drugs for neuropathic pain

Neuropathic pain is caused by damage to nerves and often does not respond to the common painkillers we have discussed so far. Newer drugs, or drugs used for other purposes have been found to be beneficial in managing this type of pain in some patients. Very often these drugs are prescribed to patients with long-term intractable pain who may be under the management of a specialist pain team or in a shared care arrangement between the pain team and their GP.

Amitriptyline

Amitriptyline is a tricyclic antidepressant drug that has been used for many years. As other antidepressants were developed this drug, due to its many side-effects, became less favoured in the treatment of depression (see Chapter 12 for its mechanism of action), although evidence is emerging of its usefulness in treating pain that has a neuropathic component. The BNF section on managing neuropathic pain suggests its use, or its close relative nortriptyline, or the use of anti-epileptic medicines. The use of amitriptyline in this condition is unlicensed but there is a growing body of evidence to support its use as seen in a Cochrane review of 2015 (Moore et al. 2015).

Gabapentin and pregabalin

These two drugs are anti-epileptic medications and are sometimes referred to as gabapentinoids.

The pharmacodynamic mechanism is to block calcium channel mediated neurotransmission but the actual link to the analgesic effect is poorly understood and may be related to activity in the dorsal horn of the spinothalamic tract (Chincholkar 2018). These drugs have been licensed for treatment of peripheral neuropathic pain and their use has increased dramatically over recent years (Morrison et al. 2017). They are of proven benefit to some patients – many patients and prescribers find the side-effects and risk of adverse reactions to outweigh the potential benefits. There is a risk of addiction and concomitant misuse with opioid medication and as such they became controlled drugs, subject to the Misuse of Drugs Act 1971 in 2019.

Case studies

① Dawn Mason, a 40-year-old woman, has undergone major abdominal surgery. The medical staff have decided to change her analgesia from opioids to NSAID medication as she is 4 days post-surgery. A health care assistant approaches you and asks you to explain the mode of action of the different types of analgesia and why the patient is now stepping down from one set of analgesia to another. Discuss this with reference to:

- the mode of action of these two drugs;
- the importance of stepping down post-operative analgesia;
- the maintenance required to achieve a steady plasma concentration of analgesic;
- how you would put this information into terms that the health care assistant will understand.

② Alex Smith is a 9-year-old boy who has sustained a broken arm after falling from his bike. The doctor has prescribed him paracetamol and ibuprofen. The dose he can have for each drug is:

- ibuprofen 200mg every 6–8 hours;
- paracetamol 500mg every 4–6 hours, maximum 2g in 24 hours.

You must explain to Alex and his parents how these drugs work and the importance of regular medication to manage Alex's pain. Discuss this with reference to:

- pharmacodynamics: mode of action of the two drugs;
- pharmacokinetics: the need for regular dosing to achieve a therapeutic plasma concentration;
- how you would put this information in terms that Alex and his parents will understand.

③ Michael Nozic is a 56-year-old male who has a history of osteoarthritis, worsened by hip dysplasia. His pain has become much less tolerable during the past year and his ability to carry out certain activities of living has been reduced drastically. He was admitted for a total hip replacement and has just returned from theatre to your ward. He has had a spinal anaesthetic and sedation during the procedure.

With reference to his spinal anaesthetic, what nursing observations would you make on Mr Nozic during his immediate post-operative care?

④ Ruby Mtumba is a 71-year-old female. She has been referred to the pain team because her pain is becoming more persistent and widespread. She is complaining of pain in her lower back, neck and shoulders. This lady is a widow, but her daughter has moved in to help her, especially as the pain is stopping her carry out daily activities.

→

With reference to the WHO's analgesic ladder (see Figure 4.8), explain how this lady's pain should have been pharmacologically managed.

⑤ Jonti Williams is aged 35 and has neuropathic pain resulting from a slipped disc causing sciatica. Jonti has Down's Syndrome and suffers from focal epileptic seizures. His current anti-epileptic medication is gabapentin 300mg three times daily.

Using the BNF, look at the range of medication that may be prescribed for Jonti's pain, and any potential interactions with his current medication.

Key learning points

Introduction

- ► Pain alerts us to tissue damage.
- ► Pain is a defence mechanism.
- ► We can suffer pain without tissue damage.
- ► Pain is a difficult concept to define.
- ► At rest, the inside of a neurone carries a negative charge.
- ► For the neurone to fire, the inside must become positive.
- ► Sodium moves into the neurone to allow it to become positively charged.
- ► The pre-synaptic neurone allows calcium to enter.
- ► The neurotransmitter allows the post-synaptic neurone to be excited or inhibited.
- ► Pain is received by nociceptors.
- ► Nociceptors are fired by heat, pressure or chemicals.
- ► Nociceptors are non-adapting, high-threshold fibres.
- ► Pain is transmitted by A-delta and C fibres.
- ► A-delta and C fibres synapse in the dorsal horn of the spinal cord.
- ► The pain impulse is interpreted in several areas in the brain.
- ► The analgesic system is a descending one.
- ► It is thought to close the gate to pain stimuli.
- ► Endorphins, dynorphins and enkephalins are important in modifying pain.
- ► Nociceptive pain results from tissue damage.
- ► Neuropathic pain is damage to nerves in the peripheral or central nervous system.
- ► The duration of pain results in it being classified as either acute or chronic.

Local anaesthetics

- ► Produce a reversible loss of sensation.
- ► There are two classes: esters and amides.
- ► Block sodium channels in the neurone.
- ► Usually used as dilute preparations (e.g. lidocaine 1%).

←

- ▶ Can cause vasodilation (so are often given with adrenaline).
- ▶ Can be given topically, via infiltration, as a nerve block, as an epidural, as a spinal anaesthetic or as an intravenous injection.
- ▶ Can cause central nervous and cardiovascular side-effects.

Non-steroidal anti-inflammatory drugs

- ▶ Used for mild-to-moderate pain.
- ▶ Lower body temperature and have anti-inflammatory properties.
- ▶ Block the production of prostaglandins.
- ▶ Block cyclooxygenase pathways.
- ▶ Limit prostaglandin effects on the nociceptors.
- ▶ Have marked gastrointestinal and renal side-effects.
- ▶ Paracetamol damages the liver if the recommended dose is not followed.
- ▶ Paracetamol overdose is treated with *N*-acetylcysteine.

Opioid analgesics

- ▶ Given for moderate-to-severe pain.
- ▶ Work on receptors in the central nervous system.
- ▶ Some drugs are natural compounds, while some are synthetic agents.
- ▶ Block entry of calcium into pre-synaptic neurone.
- ▶ Open potassium channels making it harder for the pain neurone to fire.
- ▶ Main effects are on the central nervous system and gastrointestinal tract.
- ▶ Morphine is the gold standard by which other opioids are measured.
- ▶ Morphine can cause tolerance and dependence.
- ▶ Fentanyl is a powerful synthetic opiate analgesic similar to, but approximately 100 times more potent than, morphine.
- ▶ Fentanyl is used to treat patients with severe pain, or to manage pain after surgery.
- ▶ Fentanyl is also used to treat people with chronic pain who are physically tolerant to opiates.
- ▶ Codeine is a weak opioid.
- ▶ Tramadol is an opioid of moderate strength.
- ▶ Naloxone is given to reverse the effects of morphine.

Drugs for neuropathic pain

- ▶ Amitriptyline is a tricyclic antidepressant useful in managing neuropathic pain.
- ▶ Gabapentin and pregabalin are anti-epileptic drugs useful in managing neuropathic pain. They are controlled drugs.

Calculations

1 Pethidine 100mg in 2mL is available to you. However, the patient has been prescribed 75mg. How much do you give?

2 A patient requires 1000mg of paracetamol in liquid form. The stock you have contains 125mg in 5mL. How many mL would you give?

3 Codeine is available in three strengths as tablets: 5mg, 10mg and 20mg. What is the least number of tablets you can give if the prescription is a dose of 50mg?

4 900mg of gabapentin is required to be given. You have 0.3g capsules. How many would you give?

5 A patient is prescribed an injection of 80mg of pethidine. You have available 100mg in 1mL. How much fluid would you draw up?

6 You have oral amitriptyline 10mg in a 5mL solution. The patient is prescribed 25mg. How much do you administer?

7 The maximum dose of paracetamol is 4g in a 24-hour period. The tablets are 500mg. What is the maximum number of tablets you can give in a 24-hour period?

8 A patient requires 4mg of intramuscular morphine sulphate. You have reconstituted the morphine to make a dose of 10mg in 1mL. How much do you draw up?

9 35mg of codeine is to be given to a patient subcutaneously. You have available 50mg in 1mL. How much do you administer?

10 Fentanyl 75mcg is to be given intravenously. You have fentanyl 0.1mg in 1mL available. How much would you draw up

Multiple-choice questions

Try answering these multiple-choice questions to test what you have learned from reading this chapter. You can check your answers at the end of this book.

1. What is the role of prostaglandins in the reception of pain?

a) They make the nociceptors more sensitive
b) They directly stimulate the nociceptors
c) They stimulate the release of bradykinin
d) They only act on receptors in the central nervous system

2. Local anaesthetic agents work by ...

a) Opening potassium channels
b) Opening sodium channels

←

c) Blocking potassium channels
d) Blocking sodium channels

3. Why are some local anaesthetics given with adrenaline?

a) Adrenaline is needed in order for local anaesthetics to work
b) Adrenaline counteracts the vasodilation caused by local anaesthetics
c) Adrenaline makes local anaesthetics work more quickly
d) Adrenaline helps the local anaesthetic enter the cells

4. NSAIDs work by …

a) Blocking production of bradykinin
b) Making the neurone fire more frequently
c) Stimulating the body's own analgesic system
d) Blocking production of prostaglandins

5. Why is it important to tell a patient who has been prescribed paracetamol to be careful when buying OTC medicines?

a) It could be expensive for them
b) You must only take paracetamol on its own
c) Paracetamol is often combined with cold and flu remedies
d) Paracetamol easily interacts with OTCs

6. Ibuprofen must be taken with caution if the patient is also taking lithium – why?

a) The patient may forget to take the medicine
b) It may increase the lithium level in the blood
c) It will make the lithium inactive
d) Ibuprofen also affects mood

7. One of the mechanisms of opiates is thought to be …

a) Blockage of calcium channels
b) Opening of calcium channels
c) Blockage of sodium channels
d) Opening of sodium channels

8. Which of the following channels are blocked by gabapentin?

a) Sodium
b) Potassium
c) Calcium
d) Chloride

→

9. **Why is it good practice to ensure patients are prescribed an aperient when taking morphine?**

a) Because morphine makes some people vomit
b) The patient will be having a poor diet
c) The patient is not likely to be moving
d) It reduces the rate at which the gastrointestinal system moves

10. **What drug is given to reverse the effects of morphine?**

a) Neomycin
b) Nandrolone
c) Naloxone
d) Neostigmine

Recommended further reading

Barber, P. (ed.) (2013) *Medicine Management for Nurses Case Book.* Maidenhead: Open University Press.

Brenner, G.M. and Stevens, C.W. (2017) *Pharmacology,* 5th edition. Philadelphia, PA: Elsevier.

Chincholkar, M. (2018) Analgesic mechanisms of gabapentinoids and effects in experimental pain models: a narrative review, *British Journal of Anaesthesia,* 120 (6): 1315–34.

Cornock, M. (2005) Pain relief and the law, *Nursing Standard,* 19 (51): 28.

Downie, G., Mackenzie, J. and Williams, A. (2007) *Pharmacology and Medicines Management for Nurses,* 4th edition. Edinburgh: Churchill Livingstone.

Gatford, J.D. and Phillips, N. (2011) *Nursing Calculations,* 8th edition. Edinburgh: Churchill Livingstone Elsevier.

Godfrey, H. (2005) Physiology of pain: understanding pain, Part 1: physiology of pain, *British Journal of Nursing,* 14 (16): 846–52.

Godfrey, H. (2005) Pain management: understanding pain, Part 2: pain management, *British Journal of Nursing,* 14 (17): 904–9.

Greenstein, B. and Gould, D. (2008) *Trounce's Clinical Pharmacology for Nurses,* 18th edition. New York: Churchill Livingstone.

Hamad, A.M., Sutcliffe, A.M. and Knox, A.J. (2004) Aspirin induced asthma: clinical aspects, pathogenesis and management, *Drugs,* 64 (21): 2417–32.

Karch, A.M. (2017) *Focus on Nursing Pharmacology,* 7th edition. Philadelphia, PA: Lippincott Williams & Wilkins.

Lapham, R. (2015) *Drug Calculations for Nurses: A Step-by-Step Approach,* 4th edition. London: Arnold.

Mann, E. and Redwood, S. (2000) Improving pain management: breaking down the invisible barrier, *British Journal of Nursing,* 9 (19): 2067–72.

Melzack, R. and Wall, P.D. (1965) Pain mechanisms: a new theory, *Science,* 150: 971–9.

Moore, R.A., Derry, S., Aldington, D., Cole, P. and Wiffen, P.J. (2015) Amitriptyline for neuropathic pain in adults, *Cochrane Database of Systematic Reviews,* Issue 7. Art. CD008242 (DOI: 10.1002/14651858.CD008242.pub3).

Morrison, E.E., Sandilands, E.A. and Webb, D.J. (2017) Gabapentin and pregabalin: do the benefits outweigh thee harms?, *Journal of the Royal College of Physicians Edinburgh,* 47 (4): 310–13.

National Institute for Health and Care Excellence (NICE) (2007) *Clinical Guideline CG52: Drug Misuse in Over 16s – Opioid Detoxification.* London: NICE.

Nursing and Midwifery Council (NMC) (2018) *Standards of Proficiency for Registered Nurses.* London: NMC.

Royal College of Emergency Medicine (RCEM) (2017) *Intravenous Regional Anaesthesia for Distal Forearm Fracture (Bier's Block).* London: RCEM.

Scottish Intercollegiate Guidelines Network (SIGN) (2013) *SIGN 136: Management of Chronic Pain. A National Clinical Guideline.* Edinburgh: SIGN.

Simonson, T., Aarbakke, J., Kay, I., Coleman, I., Sinnott, P. and Lyssa, R. (2006) *Illustrated Pharmacology for Nurses.* London: Hodder Arnold.

Sneader, W. (2000) The discovery of aspirin: a reappraisal, *British Medical Journal,* 321 (7276): 1591–4.

UK Government (1971) The Misuse of Drugs Act.

UK Government (2015) *The Drug Driving (Specified Limits) (England & Wales) (Amendment) Regulations.* Retrieved from: https://www.legislation.gov.uk/ukdsi/2015/9780111128824.

Wong, D.L. and Baker, C.M. (2001) Smiling faces as an anchor for pain intensity scales, *Pain,* 89 (2/3): 295–300.

World Health Organization (WHO) (1966) *Cancer Pain Relief.* Geneva: WHO.

Antimicrobials

5

Chapter contents

Learning objectives

After studying this chapter, you should be able to:

- Describe a bacterial cell.
- Explain the mode of action of a range of antibiotics used in practice settings.
- Demonstrate an understanding of what unwanted effects antibiotics have on humans.
- Discuss drugs that are used to treat tuberculosis.
- Define what is meant by viral disease.
- Describe the mode of action and side-effects of antiviral medicines.
- Identify the three main causes of fungal infection.
- Explain how antifungal medicines act.
- Demonstrate an understanding of the links between the pharmacology of antimicrobial therapies and the care given by the health practitioner.
- Solve correctly a number of drug calculations with regard to antimicrobial medicines.

Introduction

Part of the nurse's role is to ensure that medicines are administered appropriately. The Nursing and Midwifery Council's Standards for Pre-Registration Nursing programmes published in May 2018 state that education must

> ensure that field-specific content in relation to the law, safeguarding, consent, pharmacology and medicines administration and optimisation is included for entry to the register in one or more fields of nursing practice

This is backed up by the Standards of Proficiency for Registered Nurses as follows:

> Platform 2: Promoting health and preventing ill health
> 2.12 protect health through understanding and applying the principles of infection prevention and control, including communicable disease surveillance and antimicrobial stewardship and resistance

The Global Burden of Disease Study of 2017 shows that communicable (or infectious) disease is still a major cause of death and disability throughout the world. Many micro-organisms live either inside or on the outside of the human body. These can live harmlessly on the host or can cause disease. Other micro-organisms are present in the external environment and are introduced into our bodies when eating and drinking, breathing or on physical contact.

Micro-organisms that live in or on our bodies for the most part have a harmless relationship with us and can be beneficial – for example, bacteria in the GI system break down foodstuffs, allowing us to absorb nutrients. Unfortunately, at times of vulnerability these same organisms can cause infection and damage. Other micro-organisms that are not normally present in the body attempt to invade our tissues, causing damage that can be life-threatening. Any invasion or abnormal growth pattern of micro-organisms which causes our body to defend itself is called an *infection*. A common example would be respiratory infections – the inflammation of the membrane that lines the respiratory tract and associated structures.

Micro-organisms are categorized into four main groups: bacteria, viruses, protozoa and fungi. Other groups such as algae and parasitic infections will not be considered here. Bacteria and fungi are capable of existing independently of their host, i.e. us. Some protozoa and certainly viruses need the mechanisms from our cells in order to replicate and grow.

This chapter is designed to provide an introduction to some of the medicines used in combating infections caused by micro-organisms. These drugs are referred to as *antimicrobials*. The chapter covers antibiotic therapy, antiviral therapy, antiprotozoa therapy and, finally, antifungal therapy. We provide examples of common drugs that you are likely to encounter in your clinical practice.

Bacterial infection

Bacteria are classified into several types based on their shape. When viewed through a microscope, some look like rods and are called *bacilli*. Some have a curved rod shape and are known as *vibrio*. Others are round and are called *cocci*. Still others have a spiral or corkscrew shape and are known as spirilla or *spirochetes*. Bacteria are also categorized by whether they take up a stain called *gram stain*: bacteria that absorb this stain are termed *gram positive*, while those that do not are *gram negative*.

Whether or not a gram stain is taken up depends on the thickness of the cell walls of the bacteria. Gram-negative bacteria have a thin cell wall, whereas the cell wall of gram-positive organisms is much thicker and can absorb the stain.

Bacteria cells are different from those of humans. Bacteria do not have a nucleus and so are called *prokaryotes*. Animal (including human) cells do have a nucleus and are called *eukaryotes*. This and other differences between bacteria and human cells is important, as antibiotics are designed to target these differences, thus combatting the bacteria while leaving our own cells with little or no damage.

On the very outside of a bacterium is a wall made largely from a sugar called peptidoglycan. This is unique to prokaryotic cells. Beneath this wall is a plasma membrane very similar to our own that consists of a sandwich of phospholipids and proteins. Together, the cell wall and plasma membrane are called the *bacterial envelope*.

A bacterium contains cytoplasm which carries similar organelles to our own. However, the genetic material is arranged in one long strand that floats around in the cytoplasm. A prokaryotic cell does not have any mitochondria and energy production is carried out in the plasma membrane (see Figure 5.1).

Antibiotics are described as being *bactericidal* (i.e. they kill bacteria) or *bacteriostatic* (i.e. they prevent the growth and replication of the bacteria so they do not multiply and they die after their natural cycle has elapsed). This gives the body's natural defence mechanisms time to recognize and deal with the infection. The distinction between these two terms is not black and white because in certain conditions a bactericidal antibiotic may only have a bacteriostatic effect and vice versa. Their spectrum of effects can be governed by dosage, outside influences and the health of the patient.

Selective toxicity is the ability of the antimicrobial to harm a pathogen (bacteria) without harming our own cells. Therefore, when discussing selective toxicity in terms of an antibiotic, health care practitioners are referring to the range between the dose necessary to inhibit or destroy the bacteria and the dose at which our own cells become harmed. Thus, an antibiotic that is far more toxic to the bacteria than our cells is said to have a greater selective toxicity.

ANTIBIOTIC ACTIONS

Different antibiotics interfere with bacterial cell processes in different ways and we will explore each in turn.

Interference with folate

Folate is a vitamin required by both bacterial and human cells. Bacteria must make their own folate and cannot absorb it directly from the environment. Humans cannot make their own and must obtain it from their diet or through a supplement if needed.

A group of antibiotics called sulfonamides exploit this unique ability of bacterial cells. Bacteria need a substance called para-aminobenzoic acid (PABA) as a precursor to synthesize the folate they need. Sulfonamides are structural analogues of PABA and act as a competitive antagonist and are taken up by the bacteria as a pseudo-precursor preventing the synthesis of folate. In this way,

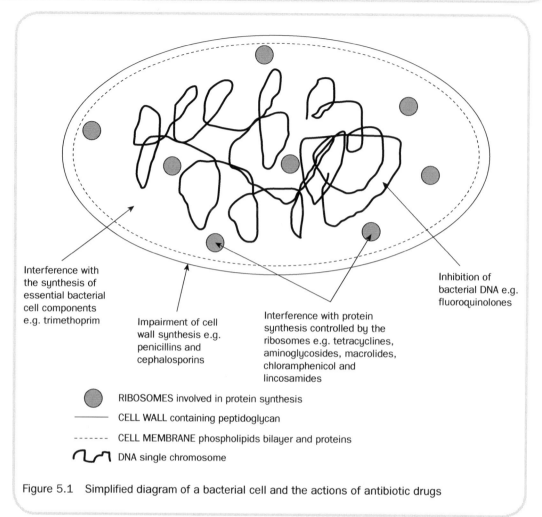

Interference with the synthesis of essential bacterial cell components e.g. trimethoprim

Impairment of cell wall synthesis e.g. penicillins and cephalosporins

Interference with protein synthesis controlled by the ribosomes e.g. tetracyclines, aminoglycosides, macrolides, chloramphenicol and lincosamides

Inhibition of bacterial DNA e.g. fluoroquinolones

⬤ RIBOSOMES involved in protein synthesis

— CELL WALL containing peptidoglycan

----- CELL MEMBRANE phospholipids bilayer and proteins

⌢⌐ DNA single chromosome

Figure 5.1 Simplified diagram of a bacterial cell and the actions of antibiotic drugs

they prevent the cell reproducing and are therefore bacteriostatic in nature.

Trimethoprim

This drug inhibits the enzyme dihydrofolate reductase in the same pathway as the sulfonamide class of drugs but targets a specific part of the pathway. Trimethoprim is given orally as it is well absorbed by the GI system. The drug is usually given to treat urinary and respiratory infections and may be prescribed in combination with sulfamethoxazole as co-trimoxazole. It is the drug of choice in patients with acquired immunodeficiency syndrome (AIDS) with a *Pneumocystis* pneumonia caused by *Pneumocystis jirovecii*, which is associated with a weak immune system.

The side-effects of trimethoprim include nausea, vomiting, certain blood disorders and skin rashes. The drug can also lead to the development of a rare type of anaemia due to its effects on folate.

Beta-lactam antibiotics

Beta-lactam is a chemical structure which is central to many antibiotics. The beta-lactam ring is at the core of the antibiotic structure and is fundamental for its effect on bacterial cell walls. Peptidoglycan makes up to 50% of the cell wall in bacteria, which in some cells is very thick. However, certain antibiotics stop the bacterial cell from making this substance, thus rendering the cell useless. This is how drugs such as the penicillins and cephalosporins work.

Penicillins

The first penicillin was the naturally occurring benzylpenicillin, whose discovery is accredited to the scientist Sir Alexander Fleming in 1928. Benzylpenicillin is poorly absorbed from the GI tract, so can only be administered by injection. Also, because it has been in use for so long, many bacteria have developed enzyme systems to combat its effects. Therefore, various semi-synthetic versions have been prepared by altering the basic biochemistry of the drug. These constitute the penicillin class of drugs which can be given orally or by injection. Examples include piperacillin, flucloxacillin, ampicillin and amoxicillin.

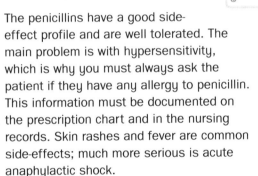

Clinical tip

The penicillins have a good side-effect profile and are well tolerated. The main problem is with hypersensitivity, which is why you must always ask the patient if they have any allergy to penicillin. This information must be documented on the prescription chart and in the nursing records. Skin rashes and fever are common side-effects; much more serious is acute anaphylactic shock.

The penicillins are among the drugs most likely to cause anaphylactic reactions and are thought to be responsible for 20% of drug-related anaphylaxis deaths in Europe and up to 75% of such deaths in the USA (Jethwa 2015). It is sometimes feasible to carry out a skin test for hypersensitivity. However, the results are not always conclusive, and the patient may suffer a severe reaction to only a small amount of the drug. Cefuroxime appears to be a safer alternative but is not completely safe, so care must be taken.

The penicillins can have an adverse effect on the normal bacteria that live in our digestive system.

Sometimes this results in diarrhoea, which can lead to a lack of vitamin K absorption. In addition, infections by micro-organisms not sensitive to penicillin can occur. This can affect the fine balance in the digestive system between good and bad bacteria.

Cephalosporins

This group of drugs is structurally related to the penicillins. Similarly, many semi-synthetic drugs have also been developed. As a result, there is a large range of medicines in this group that can be prescribed for infections.

These drugs work in the same way as the penicillins, in that they affect the production of peptidoglycan in the cell wall of bacteria. They are extremely important owing to the production of enzymes against the biochemical make-up of penicillins, which have made those drugs less effective in preventing infection.

Although some cephalosporins (e.g. cefalexin) may be given orally, most are given via the IV or SC route, including cefuroxime and cefotaxime. After being absorbed, cephalosporins are widely distributed in the tissues of the body. Some, such as cefuroxime, can actually cross the blood–brain barrier (BBB). This drug therefore is useful for infections of the central nervous system. Excretion is mainly by the kidneys but some cephalosporins, including cefoperazone, are eliminated in the bile, which makes them especially useful in treating cholecystitis. Some of these drugs can work on both gram-negative and gram-positive bacteria.

As the side-effects are similar to those of the penicillins, hypersensitivity reactions can occur. Between 0.5 and 6.5% of penicillin-sensitive patients will also be allergic to cephalosporins (NICE 2019), so it is essential to check for any allergies when assessing the patient. Diarrhoea can be a significant side-effect with this group of medicines. If a woman is taking the combined oral contraceptive pill, its effectiveness can be reduced. Thus the patient should be informed of the need to take additional contraceptive protection for the duration of the drug and for 7 days after.

Clavulanic acid

Clavulanic acid is a beta-lactamase inhibitor. Beta-lactamases are enzymes that are produced by some bacteria and are responsible for their resistance to beta-lactam antibiotics like the penicillins (cephalosporins are relatively resistant to beta-lactamase). These antibiotics have a common element in their molecular structure: a four-atom ring known as a beta-lactam. The lactamase enzyme breaks the ring open, deactivating the molecule's antibacterial properties.

Clavulanic acid itself has only weak antimicrobial activity, despite sharing the beta-lactam ring that is characteristic of beta-lactam antibiotics. However, when combined with a penicillin group antibiotic, they have the potential to overcome certain types of antibiotic resistance including resistance in bacteria that secrete beta-lactamase, and which otherwise would inactivate most penicillins. In its most common form, the potassium salt potassium clavulanate is combined with amoxicillin (co-amoxiclav, commercially known as Augmentin). Despite this, some bacterial strains have emerged that are resistant even to such combinations.

The use of clavulanic acid with a penicillin is not risk-free, however, and there has been an associated increased incidence of cholestatic jaundice and acute hepatitis during therapy or shortly after – in particular in men and those over the age of 65. The associated jaundice is usually self-limiting and very rarely fatal (NICE 2019). This is supported by a recommendation that amoxicillin/clavulanic acid preparations be reserved for bacterial infections likely to be caused by amoxicillin-resistant (beta-lactamase-producing) strains, and that treatment should not normally exceed 14 days.

Another beta-lactamase inhibitor, tazobactam, can be given in combination with piperacillin to increase the effectiveness of the penicillin in the face of drug-resistant organisms.

Interference with protein synthesis

Protein synthesis takes place in the ribosomes within cells. However, the ribosomes of human cells are different from those of bacterial cells. This is another difference between cell types that can be exploited by antibiotic therapy.

Tetracyclines

The tetracyclines act by stopping bacterial cells from making essential proteins. The group includes lymecycline, tetracycline, oxytetracycline and minocycline. The spectrum of these medicines is broad, and they are effective against both gram-negative and gram-positive bacteria.

Tetracyclines are usually given by mouth but can be administered by other routes. Absorption is better if they are given on an empty stomach as they can be absorbed erratically, and this is not helped by the presence of food.

> **Clinical tip**
>
> Tetracycline binds to calcium and also to metals such as magnesium, iron and aluminium. This stops its absorption into the body. Therefore, you should advise a patient not to take milk with the tablets. You should also inform them that many OTC antacid remedies contain magnesium and aluminium so should be avoided during treatment. Iron preparations should also be avoided when taking antibiotics from the tetracycline family because they bind with the drug creating a substance that is poorly absorbed from the GI tract.

Gastro-intestinal problems are probably the most common unwanted effect of this group of antibiotics. This is usually due to direct irritation by the medicine and also a decrease in the balance of normal intestinal bacteria (flora). Because they bind calcium, it is possible for tetracycline drugs to be deposited in growing bones and teeth. This can cause staining of teeth, underdevelopment of the teeth (hypoplasia) and bone deformities. For these reasons, tetracyclines should not be given to children under 12, pregnant women or nursing mothers.

Like other antibiotics, many strains of micro-organisms have now developed resistance to the tetracyclines, thus reducing their effectiveness in clinical practice.

Chloramphenicol

Chloramphenicol is similar in action to the tetracycline group. It is also a broad-spectrum antibiotic that can be used against both gram-positive and gram-negative organisms. It is rapidly and completely absorbed when given orally and reaches its maximum effect in the plasma within 2 hours. If necessary, it can be given by other routes, such as topically into the eye for conjunctivitis. The drug has a wide distribution in the tissues of the body, including the cerebrospinal fluid, around the brain and spinal cord.

The main unwanted effect of this drug is that it can cause a severe depression of the bone marrow. This results in a fall in all blood cell elements and a condition called aplastic anaemia. This side-effect is very rare but can occur in low doses in some individuals. This drug is given for certain acute or serious infections (e.g. against gram-negative bacteria which cause meningitis), but is more often used topically for eye and ear infections.

Aminoglycosides

This group of antibiotics includes gentamycin, streptomycin, tobramycin and neomycin and acts by inhibiting bacterial protein synthesis. The aminoglycosides are useful against both gram-negative and gram-positive organisms. However, these drugs are only bactericidal in the presence of oxygen. Therefore, bacteria that thrive in oxygen-poor environments (anaerobes) are only minimally affected. As with other groups of drugs, the resistance of micro-organisms to the aminoglycosides is increasing all the time.

One of the most commonly used drugs in this group is gentamycin. This is given by either the IV or IM route as it is not absorbed by the GI system. The drug has a fairly rapid half-life of 2–3 hours, requiring a dose to be given three times a day. The main problem with this drug is its serious toxic effects. It can have a devastating effect on the

inner ear (ototoxicity). This means that the patient may suffer damage to either their hearing or their ability to balance. The other major side-effect is damage to the kidney tubules (nephrotoxicity), which can be reversed if the drug is stopped.

Due to its side-effects, it is important that gentamycin is kept within a therapeutic range in the plasma and monitoring of blood levels should be done regularly.

Clinical tip

The side-effects of gentamycin mean that gentamycin levels must be monitored by staff. A blood sample is usually taken at specific times – either just prior to administration or 30 minutes afterwards. It is therefore very important that prescribers have this information relayed to them accurately by the monitoring staff member.

Macrolides

Erythromycin was the only drug in this group for many years. However, several new drugs have been developed, including clarithromycin and azithromycin. As with the other antibiotics in this section, the macrolides inhibit protein synthesis in the bacterium.

Erythromycin destroys a similar range of micro-organisms as penicillin and is often the first drug of choice if a patient has a penicillin allergy. The drug is mainly prescribed for gram-positive organisms and spirochetes. It has very limited success with gram-negative organisms.

All drugs in this group can be given orally and they spread throughout most tissues of the body. They do not cross the BBB into the central nervous system and they do not penetrate synovial fluid. The macrolides possess different half-lives, which is why some are given more often in a day than others. They have an unusual action in that they are taken up and concentrated in phagocytic cells – the group of white cells responsible for digesting bacteria. Inside these phagocytic cells there are pockets of cell-destroying enzymes called lysosomes. Macrolides are absorbed into these pockets and therefore considerably enhance the phagocytic killing capacity of these cells.

Unwanted GI problems are the main issue when taking these medicines. If erythromycin is administered intravenously rather than orally, a degree of inflammation and damage to the vessel that the drug is entering (thrombophlebitis) can be expected.

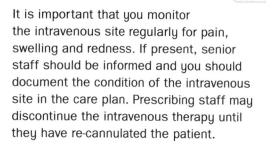

Clinical tip

It is important that you monitor the intravenous site regularly for pain, swelling and redness. If present, senior staff should be informed and you should document the condition of the intravenous site in the care plan. Prescribing staff may discontinue the intravenous therapy until they have re-cannulated the patient.

Lincosamides

The drug of note in this group is clindamycin, whose mechanism of action involves inhibition of protein synthesis in bacteria. It works against a range of organisms, including gram-positive cocci and a range of anaerobic bacteria.

Clindamycin can be given orally or by other routes and becomes well distributed in the body tissues, including bone. Like a number of other antibiotics, it does not have the capacity to cross the BBB. The usual dose is 150–300mg four times a day.

Unwanted effects are mainly GI in nature and the patient may suffer from diarrhoea. In rare cases, this may become life-threatening when they develop a condition called *pseudomembranous colitis*. This is an acute inflammation of the colon caused by toxins released from micro-organisms that are resistant to clindamycin; an example would be infection with a bacterium called *Clostridium difficile*.

Inhibition of bacterial DNA

Deoxyribonucleic acid (DNA) is found in all living cells and carries the organism's genetic information. In bacteria, this information is *supercoiled* and takes up very little space. In order for the bacteria to survive through to replication, this information needs to be copied. To do this, an enzyme called *topoisomerase II* is required to uncoil parts of the supercoiled material. A group of antibiotics called fluoroquinolones affect the ability of the bacteria to use topoisomerase II, thus reducing the ability to replicate.

Fluoroquinolones

The most common antibiotic in this group of drugs is ciprofloxacin, a *broad-spectrum* antibiotic. It is so useful because it is effective against micro-organisms that have become resistant to the penicillins, cephalosporins and aminoglycosides. This drug can be given orally and is well absorbed. It enters many tissues but concentrates in particular in the kidneys, prostate gland and lungs, making it ideal for fighting infection in these areas of the body.

Clinical tip

As with the tetracyclines, the rate of absorption of fluoroquinolones is diminished by metals such as aluminium and magnesium, so they should not be used while taking antacids that contain these elements.

Side-effects are rare, usually mild in nature and disappear rapidly once the drug has been stopped. In the main, GI problems like diarrhoea are reported. Sometimes people also complain of developing a skin rash, headaches and dizziness. One of the main drug interactions with ciprofloxacin occurs when it is given to patients with chronic respiratory conditions who are receiving a drug called theophylline. The ciprofloxacin inhibits enzymes in the liver that are normally responsible for the metabolism of theophylline. This results in a build-up of theophylline in the plasma, eventually reaching toxic proportions.

> ### Clinical tip
>
> Ciprofloxacin should not be given to patients on theophylline. If there is no alternative, the prescriber should closely monitor the levels of theophylline in the blood.

Antibiotic resistance and antimicrobial stewardship

One of the main concerns of modern medicine is *antibiotic resistance*. If an antibiotic is used long enough, or used inappropriately and indiscriminately, bacteria will emerge that are resistant to that antibiotic. The existence of antibiotic-resistant bacteria creates the danger of life-threatening infections that don't respond to antibiotic treatment.

The rise in the occurrence of antimicrobial resistance has prompted guidelines for health care professionals involved in antimicrobial therapy. NICE guideline NG15 (2015) outlines the systems and processes for effective use and stewardship; it would be worth viewing this guideline before reading further.

Causes of antibiotic resistance

The misuse of antibiotics is associated with medicine, agriculture and household products. Common examples include erroneous antibiotic prescriptions for non-bacterial infections and the addition of antibiotics to livestock feed and cleaning agents, which have helped create a reservoir of antibiotic-resistant bacteria.

Irregular combinations of bacteria have sometimes perpetuated drug-resistant microbes. One example was when *Staphylococcus aureus* was shown to develop vancomycin resistance genes through cohabitation with the vancomycin-resistant bacterium, *Enterococcus faecalis*, in the wound of a hospitalized patient. Through mechanisms of genetic exchange between bacterial species, the mere co-existence of these two particular bacteria helped to bring about drug resistance in *S. aureus*.

Enhanced transmission of resistance factors, or the increased efficiency with which resistance genes are exchanged, is another important way that antibiotic resistance is perpetuated. Factors that contribute to enhanced transmission include the survival of patients with chronic disease, an increased number of immunosuppressed individuals, substandard hospital hygiene, more international travel and cuts in health care administration budgets.

Profit also has a role to play in the development of drug resistance. The pharmaceutical industry has increasingly been busy with hugely profitable 'blockbuster' drugs for allergies and depression, and 'lifestyle' drugs for conditions such as baldness and impotence. This has led to a reduction in antibiotic and vaccine research and development.

In many cases, drug-resistant bacteria have been met with antibiotics that are nothing more than replicas of previous drugs. There is an urgent need for new avenues of therapeutic treatment, and a new era of prophylactic (preventative) treatment has now begun.

Drugs used to treat tuberculosis

Tuberculosis (TB) is usually caused by inhalation of *Mycobacterium tuberculosis*. This bacterium has a very tough envelope and can survive for long periods in dry conditions. This coating also protects the organism, making it resistant to destruction by the body's natural defences. The bacterium can invade and survive within our phagocytic cells. The damage to our tissues is usually caused by the body's inflammatory response to the infection rather than the result of any toxin released by the organism. Guidelines for management of TB were issued by NICE in 2016 to include latent and active TB treatments. These guidelines were updated in 2019 to include cautions on the use of fluoroquinolones in TB after reports of disabling side-effects.

Initial infection of the lungs is labelled *primary TB*. The bacteria are engulfed by phagocytic cells in the lungs. These cells attempt to communicate with T-lymphocytes which themselves attempt to resist the infection, but the increase in phagocytic cells at the site of infection is relatively ineffective. Instead, more and more of the phagocytic cells become infected by the bacteria and are carried into the lymphatic system where they eventually reach what is known as the *hilar lymph nodes* within the lungs.

The body manages to 'wall off' these infected phagocytes by creating pockets called *tubercles*. These are balls of infection with a necrotic centre surrounded by infected phagocytic cells wrapped in a capsule of collagen (protein) fibres. These tubercles may remain in the lungs, but the patient suffers no further symptoms of the disease. This is known as *latent TB*. If the person's immune system becomes compromised, the condition is activated again from its dormant state to revert to active TB. Reactivation may take place due to a number of circumstances, including poor nutrition and a lowered immune system.

This reactivation is labelled *secondary TB*. The lung tissue itself now becomes necrotic, creating large cavities. As with the tubercles, these cavities remain encapsulated by connective tissue and may lie dormant or be reactivated once again.

Isoniazid

This drug is specific against mycobacteria and is therefore appropriate for the treatment of TB. It is bacteriostatic when the organisms are not active but becomes bactericidal when they start to divide and multiply. The drug diffuses through cells and crosses the BBB into the cerebrospinal fluid. This is important, as it penetrates well into the tubercles described earlier.

The normal dose for an adult is up to 300mg per day and is usually given as a tablet. Some people break down this drug rapidly in the liver and some do not. The latter tend to have a better therapeutic response, as the drug manages to reach a more constant level in the plasma.

Side-effects are related to the dose given, the most common being skin problems. Patients who metabolize isoniazid more slowly are at greater risk of side-effects if they are dosed too often.

Isoniazid affects enzymes in the liver that break down certain anticonvulsant drugs. Phenytoin, ethosuximide and carbamazepine can all be increased in the plasma if given with isoniazid.

Rifampicin

Rifampicin acts by interfering with ribonucleic acid (RNA) in the bacteria, so affecting protein synthesis within the organism. This antibiotic has a broad range of activities and is effective against both gram-positive and gram-negative organisms. It is the most active agent in the fight against TB to date. It can penetrate the phagocytic cells that have ingested the tubercle bacillus. Once inside, it can destroy the tubercle bacillus at will.

The drug is well absorbed by the GI system and therefore is given in tablet form, usually in a dose of between 450mg and 600mg daily prior to eating breakfast. It can gain entry to a wide range of tissues and fluids.

Clinical tip

Rifampicin has the capacity to give an orange tinge to saliva, sputum, tears, sweat and urine. You should forewarn the patient of this to avoid unnecessary concern in relation to this harmless side-effect.

Some patients may suffer skin problems, a raised temperature and GI upsets such as nausea and diarrhoea. Liver damage, with a yellow discoloration of the skin (jaundice), whites of the eyes (sclerae) and mucous membranes, has been reported and can prove fatal.

Clinical tip

Because of the risk of liver damage, patients who are prescribed rifampicin should have their liver enzymes tested prior to commencing therapy.

As with isoniazid, rifampicin affects enzymes in the liver that help to break down certain drugs. Rather than inhibiting the pathways, rifampicin induces them. In other words, drugs such as warfarin, glucocorticoids, opiates, oral hypoglycaemic agents and oestrogen are all broken down more rapidly. This means dosing needs to be adjusted accordingly.

Clinical tip

Rifampicin's ability to break down oestrogen means that if a woman of childbearing years is taking the oral contraceptive, you must inform them that they need extra protection to avoid pregnancy.

Finally, you will find that rifampicin is often given alongside other antibiotics to combat TB. This is in order that we do not give the organism the opportunity to develop resistance.

Pyrazinamide

Pyrazinamide is well absorbed orally and becomes widely distributed in the tissues and fluids of the body. It penetrates well into the meninges, so is particularly useful if the disease spreads there.

Pyrazinamide works in a similar way to rifampicin in that it gains entry to the phagocytes that have ingested the bacteria and destroys it. Side-effects include the raising of plasma uric acid levels, so causing gout. GI symptoms and a raised temperature have also been reported. Liver failure is also a possibility, especially if the drug is given in high doses. However, high doses are uncommon, as a combination of drugs is the preferred technique in treating the organism (see above). Liver function tests should, however, be carried out prior to being commenced on the drug.

Viral infections

Viruses are very different from bacteria. They are a lot smaller and essentially have a core of either DNA or RNA surrounded by a coat of protein (capsid). The coat plus its contents are referred to as the *nucleocapsid*. Some viruses are even more protected in that they develop a further coat of phospholipids from the host cell (the cell in which the virus lives) and some of the virus's own glycoproteins.

At some point in their lifetime, everyone in the world will have been infected by a virus. The common cold, influenza, chickenpox, shingles, warts, measles, mumps and rubella are all caused by viral infections.

Viral mechanisms

Viruses enter a cell and then use the cell's machinery for their own purposes. Viruses do not have the ability to reproduce and replicate themselves, so they have to borrow these mechanisms from their host cell. Infected cells then go on to produce thousands of identical copies of the virus.

The virus gains access to the cell by locking onto a receptor that carries out some normal activity. The virus is then taken into the interior of the cell by a process called *endocytosis*. Once inside the host cell, the nucleic acid centre of the virus starts to use the host cell's machinery to help it replicate. This can take various forms depending on the type of virus.

Some viruses are called DNA viruses. This means that they replicate by latching into and becoming part of the host cell's DNA. Once they have achieved this, they can direct the manufacture of more viruses. Other viruses are called RNA viruses and use the host's RNA, linking with the viral RNA code so that the cell manufactures the proteins that go into building new viruses within the cell. Finally, *retroviruses* work by copying a viral blueprint onto a piece of DNA. This viral DNA is then linked into the host's DNA and so the host starts creating new viruses as part of its normal activity.

Antibiotic drugs are not effective against viruses. A further problem in dealing with viruses is that by the time the body has recognized it has been invaded, a large amount of the virus will have been manufactured and many cells infected.

Human immunodeficiency virus

This is the virus that causes acquired immuno-deficiency syndrome (AIDS). In many cases, the virus is acquired as a sexually transmitted infection (STI) but can be transmitted in infected body fluids such as blood and breast milk and to babies in utero or during delivery.

HIV is the result of the invasion of a particular lymphocyte called a *T-helper cell* (T4 cells). These cells are very important in defending the body and are linked to the immune response.

HIV may remain dormant within the body for many years and most people are quite unaware that they have contracted the disease. However, it is possible by blood testing to confirm within a few weeks of infection whether the person has acquired the virus. The time taken for the virus to progress in terms of loss of immune response in the individual varies from months to years. The virus targets cells with certain receptors on their surface such as CD4 and CCR5. The virus attaches itself to receptors on these cells and is taken in. The host cell then begins to make proteins that will be made into new viruses. These will then eventually leave the cell and gain access to cells of their own by recognizing the receptors on them. As the cells divide, the integrated viral DNA also divides and becomes part of the new cell. This is called *proviral DNA*. It effectively means that any T-helper cell on division passes on the ability to daughter cells to produce more viruses.

Antiretroviral therapy

Antiviral therapy uses a combination of agents that act at different points in the replication of the virus within the human cell. One of the main reasons for using a combination of drugs is to delay the onset of resistance in any one of the therapies. We can now use drugs before HIV infection is confirmed or when it is suspected, using the same drugs we would in treatment with pre-exposure prophylaxis (PrEP) or post-exposure prophylaxis (PEP). Currently, antiviral drugs used in the treatment of AIDS fall into two broad categories: *reverse transcriptase inhibitors* and *protease inhibitors*.

Nucleoside reverse transcriptase inhibitors

Reverse transcription is the second phase in the HIV life cycle. HIV genes are carried on two strands of RNA; however, in order to enter the nucleus of a human cell, the virus must change the genetic code into a strand of DNA. It does this by using a viral enzyme called *reverse transcriptase*. Nucleoside reverse transcriptase inhibitors are designed to block the action of reverse transcriptase.

Examples of this class of drugs are zidovudine, abacavir, didanosine, emtricitabine, stavudine, tenofovir disoproxil and lamividine. All may be given orally but there are some differences in the frequency of administration. Whereas zidovudine and abacavir have short half-lives, lamividine has a long half-life, thus affecting dosing. All these drugs diffuse through a range of tissues. Zidovudine achieves the best concentration in the cerebrospinal fluid, about 65% per cent of that which it achieves in the plasma. Many of these drugs are available now as compound preparations containing two or three drugs for maximum effectiveness.

Adverse reactions to this family of drugs can be serious. Zidovudine can cause bone marrow depression leaving the patient open to all types of infection. Abacavir may cause hypersensitivity reactions including rashes and high temperatures. In comparison, lamividine is associated with mild side-effects only such as headaches and some GI symptoms.

Non-nucleoside reverse transcriptase inhibitors

These drugs have the same effect as the nucleoside reverse transcriptase inhibitors but have a different method of achieving the response. Often, the two types of drugs are given in combination.

The main drugs in this family are nevirapine, etravirine, rilpivirine and efavirenz, all of which are given orally. Nevirapine is highly bioavailable compared with efavirenz, which has between 50 and 60% bioavailability. The half-lives of nevirapine and efavirenz, compared with their relatives, are considerably longer – between 30 and 40 hours.

The main adverse effect of nevirapine is the development of a rash (high incidence and includes Stevens-Johnson syndrome). Other common side-effects include headaches, a high temperature and lethargy. The side-effects of efavirenz also include rash and increased plasma cholesterol, so patients may need to be monitored for this and for potential liver damage. This drug may also lead to disorientation and lack of concentration and, in some patients, drowsiness, so night-time administration is advised.

Protease inhibitors

If the viral RNA manages to make a copy of its genetic blueprint onto DNA, then this is carried into the nucleus of the human cell. Here, another viral enzyme called *integrase* joins the viral DNA onto the human DNA and hides it. Then, when the cell tries to make new proteins, it also makes new viral proteins. Eventually, these proteins are assembled into new HIVs in the endoplasmic reticulum and Golgi apparatus of the cell. This assembly-line relies on an enzyme called *protease* to cut the proteins into either functional units of the virus or viral enzymes.

Protease inhibitors block this stage of viral replication in the cell. Examples of current protease inhibitors include atazanavir, darunavir, fosamprenavir, lopinavir, ritonavir, saquinavir and tipranavir, all of which are given orally and can cause GI disorders, hepatic disorders and endocrine disturbances.

All of the drugs in this family also cause enzyme inhibition, especially to the pathways that break down benzodiazepines. Therefore, the concentration of these drugs will rise if given together with protease inhibitors. It also means there is a high potential for interaction with other drugs using the same enzyme systems for metabolism.

The combination of drugs now given for HIV has dramatically improved the prognosis (see Figure 5.2). This has obviously had a lessening effect on AIDS cases and deaths in industrialized countries. And with advances in the use of drug therapy pre and post exposure reductions in viral contraction are expected.

Other antiviral drugs in HIV treatment and prophylaxis

Enfuvirtide acts by inhibiting the fusion of the HIV to the host cell and is used when other more traditional drugs have proved ineffective. It should be used in combination with another drug.

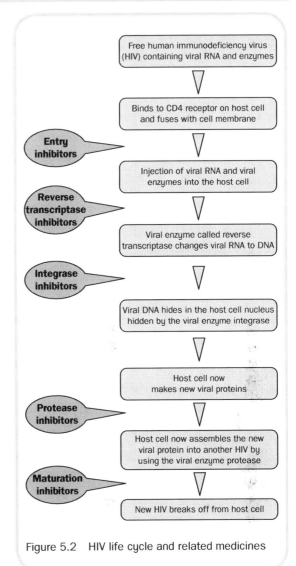

Figure 5.2   HIV life cycle and related medicines

Maraviroc is an antagonist at a chemokine receptor called CCR5 and is restricted to use when the patient is infected with the variant of HIV called CCR5-tropic HIV.

Dolutegravir, elvitegravir and raltegravir are inhibitors of the enzyme HIV integrase which allows the virus to integrate into host cells, therefore inhibition of this enzyme prevents or greatly reduces the ability of the virus to enter and replicate.

Cobicistat has no inherent antiretroviral activity itself but can be given in combination with drugs that do and it enhances their activity.

PrEP and PEP

Post-exposure prophylaxis (PEP) is a short course of HIV medication as outlined above, taken very soon after a possible exposure to HIV to prevent the virus from taking hold in the body. It is intended to be used in an emergency and is not suitable for use in people who are likely to have regular or frequent exposure to the virus. The circumstances in which it should be used include:

- exposure during sexual intercourse where no barrier protection was used or where this failed;
- sharing needles to inject drugs with another person who may be infected;
- needlestick injuries in health care professionals;
- in cases of sexual assault and rape.

Pre-exposure prophylaxis (PrEP) is where people who do not have the HIV virus take HIV medication, as outlined above, on a daily basis to reduce their risk of contracting the virus. It can be used in people who fall into high-risk groups such as:

- people who have an HIV positive sexual partner;
- people who have multiple sexual partners;
- people who regularly inject drugs and share needles.

At the time of writing, PrEP is available on the NHS in Scotland, as part of drug trials in England and Wales and in Northern Ireland as part of a pilot study. It is prescribed in other countries in the world under varying conditions. This picture may well change and you are advised to keep up to date with prescribing restrictions and PrEP availability in the UK at the following website: https://www.iwantprepnow.co.uk/.

Other viral infections and antiviral drug treatments

Aciclovir

You may have come across this drug and used it yourself. The trade name is Zovirax and if you suffer from cold sores you have probably used the product. The drug is used for a number of viral infections including conjunctivitis, genital warts and shingles caused by variants of the herpes and varicella viruses. Occasionally it is used to treat acute chickenpox and encephalitis in immuno-compromised patients.

Aciclovir works by stopping the herpes virus from reproducing and infecting further cells of the body. The drug becomes more active once it has entered the cell that is infected by the virus. The herpes virus works as a DNA virus and aciclovir acts by blocking an enzyme called *DNA polymerase*. The virus needs this enzyme to copy its genetic code from a strand of RNA to a strand of DNA. This process is necessary for the virus to multiply and continue to infect its host. By blocking the action of DNA polymerase, the drug prevents the host cell making copies of the virus. This controls the virus and buys the immune system time to deal with the initial infection.

The drug can be given orally, intravenously or topically (e.g. cream). If a patient is prescribed aciclovir in dispersible form, they should be encouraged to take the tablet dissolved in a full glass of water.

Clinical tip

It is good practice to advise patients to drink plenty of water when taking aciclovir orally to avoid over-concentration of the drug (6 to 8 pints of water per day). It is also important that the patient adheres to the full course of treatment. However, if they miss a dose, they should not double up on the tablets.

The common drug reactions when taking aciclovir include nausea, vomiting, diarrhoea and sometimes headache. In high doses, the drug may cause hallucinations.

Aciclovir should not be given in pregnancy as chromosomal mutations can occur. This is because the foetal cells are dividing rapidly and the tissues are becoming specialized.

Ganciclovir

Ganciclovir also stops the virus passing on its genetic code from a piece of RNA to a piece of DNA. However, it targets a different type of virus, the *cytomegalovirus*. Infection by this virus in people with an intact immune system is usually mild. Therefore, this drug is used only in people whose immune systems are not fully functional (they are immunocompromised). The cytomegalovirus is a problem for people who have AIDS and or who are to undergo an organ transplant.

Ganciclovir is given intravenously and is not rapidly broken down in the cells like aciclovir. It has been shown to remain in infected host cells for as long as 20 hours. However, its side-effects are serious. The medicine causes bone marrow depression leading to depletion in white cells and platelets. This usually recovers once the treatment has stopped. It is also possible that the drug may be carcinogenic, and it is therefore only used to fight life- or sight-threatening disease.

Famciclovir and valaciclovir are further examples of this class of antiviral drugs.

Immunoglobulins

Immunoglobulins contain antibodies against specific viruses. These antibodies set to work on the viral envelope and attempt to destroy it. They also prevent virus attachment to host human cells. If used before the onset of disease, immunoglobulins can be protective to the body. Examples of diseases which immunoglobulins help to prevent are measles, hepatitis, German measles and poliomyelitis.

Interferons

Interferons are a group of proteins that are made by our cells in order to help combat invasion by viruses. These substances have been commercially developed and are given to help us combat infection.

Interferons are not just one substance but a range of proteins with different properties. Some have antiviral properties, particularly interferon-alpha and interferon-beta. These medicines work by influencing the ribosome in the cell to stop making the viral proteins. In this way, they stop the virus from replicating.

These medicines reach optimum capacity in the plasma after 5 hours but do not cross the BBB. Interferon-alpha may be used in the treatment of hepatitis B and AIDS-related Kaposi sarcoma, as well as for hepatitis C.

Side-effects are common and include the development of a high temperature (fever), headaches and pain in the muscles (myalgia). If the therapy must be repeated, more serious side-effects can occur, including bone marrow depression, the development of rashes and dramatic hair loss (alopecia).

Fungal infections

Fungi can be found in our environment and on our skin. Like bacteria, most fungi are not pathogenic unless the immune system becomes depleted. Fungi can invade superficial tissues but more serious damage, sometimes life-threatening, occurs with the invasion of deeper tissues.

It is somewhat ironic that one reason for a significant upturn in fungal infections is the widespread use of broad-spectrum antibiotics, which have decreased the populations of bacteria that normally compete with fungi, therefore allowing the fungi to flourish unchecked. A further reason for the increase in the number of fungal infections is disease processes such as AIDS and the use of more immunosuppressant drugs and cancer therapies. There are three types of fungal organism that can cause disease in the human body and these are discussed below.

Moulds

Moulds grow as long strands called filaments. Once these filaments begin to intertwine, they form a *mycelium*. Moulds that can become infective include the dermatophytes and *Aspergillus*. A typical condition caused by infection with dermatophytes (dermatomycoses) is tinea (better known as ringworm), which can affect the scalp (tinea capitis), the groin (tinea cruris) and the body (tinea corporis). The athlete's foot (tinea pedis) fungus also belongs to this group of fungi.

A more serious condition caused by moulds is aspergillosis, a serious lung infection that is a leading cause of death in patients undergoing bone marrow transplant. Others at risk of developing this condition are immunocompromised patients. *Aspergillus* causes an allergic reaction in the tissues of the lung, which leads to thrombosis and necrosis of the lung tissues as the pulmonary blood vessels are invaded by the fungus.

True yeasts

True yeasts are unicellular and are either round or oval in shape. The yeast *Cryptococcus neoformans* can cause serious meningitis or endocarditis. Again, these mainly occur in individuals whose immune systems have been compromised in some way. This organism is common in soil, especially where there are bird droppings. Infection is usually the result of a person inhaling the fungi.

Yeast-like fungi

These look like yeasts but under certain conditions develop filaments. The most common is *Candida albicans*, which lives quite happily as a commensal organism in our GI system and in the vagina.

> **Clinical tip**
>
> *Candida albicans* becomes problematic (pathogenic) when people become stressed, are immunocompromised or on a course of antibiotics. At such times they may develop oral thrush or vaginitis.

More serious illnesses include inflammation of the lining of the heart (endocarditis) and, in some cases, these fungi can have fatal consequences, as in cases of sepsis.

Antifungal drugs

Most fungal infections are superficial, although they can become systemic (widespread) in immunocompromised patients. Amphotericin has for many years been the first-line antifungal agent, though several other drugs have been developed. This section will focus on two main treatment groups: antifungal antibiotics and synthetic antifungal agents.

Amphotericin

Amphotericin was first used over 50 years ago. It is a macrolide antibiotic, which means that it inhibits protein synthesis in the bacterial cell, and is very complex in its biochemical structure.

It works by targeting fungi and some protozoa. Its specificity is thought to relate to its attraction to a substance called ergosterol. Ergosterol is the main lipid in the membrane of a fungus (in humans, the main lipid is cholesterol). Once the drug has adhered to the membrane of the fungus, it starts to punch holes in it, so causing it to lose potassium. Potassium is the major intracellular positively charged ion (cation) and its loss leads to the death of the organism.

Amphotericin is poorly absorbed from the GI system and so the oral route of administration is only used when the patient has a fungal infection of this system. It can be given topically.

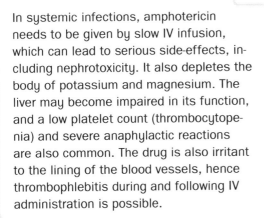

Clinical tip

In systemic infections, amphotericin needs to be given by slow IV infusion, which can lead to serious side-effects, including nephrotoxicity. It also depletes the body of potassium and magnesium. The liver may become impaired in its function, and a low platelet count (thrombocytopenia) and severe anaphylactic reactions are also common. The drug is also irritant to the lining of the blood vessels, hence thrombophlebitis during and following IV administration is possible.

Due to the unwanted effects of amphotericin, researchers have been working on other ways of administering this drug. One reasonably promising development has been to deliver it in little spheres of lipid so that it is in a protected form until it binds with the fungal membrane. Because of its serious side-effects, amphotericin is used mainly for serious and life-threatening fungal infections.

Clotrimazole

This drug is most commonly used topically for fungal skin infections or for vulvar and vaginal infections as a result of *Candida* infection. It is an imidazole antifungal drug which inhibits the synthesis of essential components that contribute to fungal structure and function. It is available as a cream, a liquid, a spray and in pessary form. Treatment can involve a single dose, or multiple applications when using the cream version.

Nystatin

This is an antibiotic that disrupts the membrane of the fungus. It is very poorly absorbed from the GI system and so its use is limited to fungal infections of the GI tract, such as oral thrush. Given in liquid form, it is held in the mouth for a few minutes to help coat the infected areas for best response.

Clinical tip

With oral thrush, nystatin can be given as a liquid preparation or as pastilles that the patient can suck. Oral hygiene and assessment of the mouth is an important aspect of nursing. It is recommended that an oral assessment tool is used. Patients at risk of developing oral candidiasis include those receiving antibiotics and steroids, so it is important that when administering nystatin orally to these individuals you know whether they wear dentures or not. If they do, you should soak them in 1% sodium hypochlorite solution overnight and rinse them well before reinserting.

Griseofulvin

Griseofulvin has a narrow range of activity, which limits its use. The drug is fungistatic and achieves this by stopping the fungus from dividing.

It is used in the treatment of dermatophyte infections of the skin and nails due to its ability to be taken up by the basal cells in the epidermis and concentrate in the protein keratin there. Keratin is the main constituent of our nails and is introduced to our skin cells before we shed them.

Griseofulvin is administered orally and has a peak plasma concentration after 5 hours. It has a long elimination half-life of approximately 24 hours and causes enzyme induction in the liver; therefore, it can affect the metabolism of other drugs the patient may be taking. Side-effects are uncommon but the drug can cause GI upsets as well as headaches and photosensitivity. Treatment needs to continue over a prolonged period to prove effective.

Azoles

This group of drugs is manufactured synthetically. The azoles are fungistatic in nature and have a broad spectrum of activity. Their mode of action is complex and not fully understood. However, what we do know is that they interfere with a fungal enzyme called P450. This prevents lanosterol from converting to ergosterol, thereby affecting the nature of the fungal membrane and its ability to replicate.

One of the disadvantages of using this group of drugs is that humans carry cytochrome P450. As a result, some members of the azole group of drugs can also affect the human cytochrome P450 pathways.

Ketoconazole

This is one of the first of this group of drugs to be given orally in order to treat systemic (generalized) fungal infections. It is well absorbed by the body and disperses widely in human tissues and fluid. However, it does not reach therapeutic levels in the cerebrospinal fluid.

The main unwanted effect of ketoconazole is liver damage, which though rare can be fatal. Other problems that can result from taking this medication include itching of the skin, GI disturbances and inhibition of adrenocorticoids and testosterone.

Fluconazole

This medication is often advertised on television in connection with preventing vaginal thrush. An oral dose of 150mg is often adequate when treating vaginal candidiasis. Side-effects are generally mild, with nausea, abdominal pain and headaches commonplace. However, although rare, diseases of the liver including hepatitis are a possibility.

Miconazole

This drug can be administered in several different ways, including orally for GI infections and as a pessary to treat vaginal candidiasis. It can also be purchased as a gel for the treatment of oropharyngeal candidiasis or as a cream for treating dermatophytosis of the skin.

As with fluconazole, the side-effects when taken orally are mild with GI disturbance, itching, low blood sodium (hyponatraemia) and other blood disorders being reported.

Clinical tip

More problems arise if miconazole is given by IV infusion and you should be alert to irritant reactions at the site of infusion.

Flucytosine

This is a synthetic antifungal agent that can be given orally. It has a narrow scope of activity and is therefore usually given in combination with other antifungal drugs such as amphotericin.

Flucytosine acts on the fungal DNA. Mutations can occur rapidly and as a result the drug is never given alone as the development of resistance would be rapid. The drug can also be given by IV infusion and is widely distributed throughout the body. Most of it is excreted in an unchanged form by the kidneys, thus the dose must be lowered if given to an individual with impaired renal function. It is frequently used as an adjunct to amphotericin in severe systemic infection.

Terbinafine

Terbinafine is given orally for tinea infections of the skin and nails. The drug concentrates itself in the keratin that makes up nail tissue and infuses cells in the epidermis.

It can also be locally (topically) applied and penetrates the skin and mucous membranes effectively. Side-effects are limited and only occur in approximately 10% of all patients. Gastrointestinal disturbances, itching, headaches and muscle pains have been reported (for a summary of administration of antifungal medicines, see Box 5.1).

Protozoa

Protozoa are simple eukaryotic organisms consisting of a single cell ('protozoa' literally means

Box 5.1 Administration of antifungal medicines

Route of administration and type	Name of medicine	Uses and side-effects
TOPICALLY		
Creams	Clotrimazole and miconazole	These are used to treat infections of the skin and vagina. There are usually no side-effects. Some men and women may develop a mild irritation when applying them to the vagina or penis. Sometimes the antifungal cream is combined with a mild steroid preparation (e.g. hydrocortisone)
Shampoos	Ketoconazole	Used to treat infections of the scalp. No side-effects of note
ORALLY		
Liquids and lozenges	Amphotericin and nystatin	Used to treat *Candida* infections of the mouth and throat. No side-effects of note
Tablets	Terbinafine and fluconazole	Terbinafine is used to treat nail infections. Fluconazole is used to treat vaginal candidiasis. Usually no side-effects are reported. Can be bought over the counter
INJECTION	Amphotericin and flucytosine	Used to treat serious fungal infection within the body. Risk of serious side-effects. However, these risks must be balanced against the seriousness of the condition

'first animal'). These cells can reproduce through sexual and asexual means. Some protozoa form protective cysts that are capable of withstanding harsh environmental conditions.

Protozoa are often classified by their structure and ability to move. Sporozoa, for example, are generally capable of limited movement. *Plasmodium* species are an example of this type of parasite and are responsible for malaria in humans.

Some protozoal cells move by wafting an extension called a flagellum. For example, the flagellate protozoan *Trypanasoma* is responsible for diseases such as sleeping sickness and certain forms of vaginitis and urethritis.

Finally, amoebae move by extending parts of their cytoplasm into false limbs called pseudopodia. These organisms are causative agents of dysentery, an acute infection of the intestines, which may spread to other organs, including the liver.

Here, we briefly outline some of the most common protozoal infections. The antiprotozoal medicines used to treat each of these specific infections will be addressed as we proceed. The section is by no means comprehensive and further reading is recommended.

Apicomplexa and malaria

All members of this family of protozoa are parasitic – in other words, they invade and use our cells as hosts. They do not display any visible forms of movement and as a result most of them are intracellular in nature. These organisms have complex life cycles involving sexual and asexual reproduction.

The condition known as malaria is caused by this group of protozoa. Malaria is carried by the female mosquito and remains a major cause of death and disability worldwide.

The symptoms of malaria include a high temperature (fever), shivering, pain in the joints, headaches, vomiting, generalized convulsions and even coma. These symptoms do not become apparent immediately, but usually occur between 7 and 9 days after the host has been bitten by the mosquito. There are four species of protozoa that can cause malaria.

The bite of an infected female mosquito injects the protozoa into the bloodstream. Within a few minutes the organisms find their way to the liver, where they mature for 10–14 days. They then exit the liver cells and re-enter the bloodstream. Here they encounter and invade the red blood cells (erythrocytes) and further their development. Once the red blood cells have burst and given up the fully developed protozoa, these are then free to seek out new red cells to infect. This is how the infection escalates rapidly in the body.

Clinical tip

The periodic fever associated with malaria is due to the intermittent bursting of the erythrocytes. On rupturing, the cells not only release their deadly cargo of parasites but also a chemical which affects the temperature-regulating centre in the hypothalamus.

Quinine

The first effective treatment for malaria, quinine is derived from the natural world, being synthesized from the bark of the cinchona tree. Quinine is effective against the erythrocytic forms of all protozoa that cause malaria. It has no effect against the development of the protozoa in the liver cells.

The drug works by stopping the protozoa using the proteins from the red cells. Haemoglobin, which is contained in the red cells, is toxic to the parasite. The organism has developed ways in which to render the toxic effects of haemoglobin harmless, but quinine interferes with the detoxifying machinery of the protozoa, therefore leading to the death of the organism.

Due to the resistance built up by protozoa to quinine, it is now used only against *Plasmodium falciparum*. The drug is usually given orally as a 7-day course of treatment. It can however be given via the IV route if the patient is very ill. It is not useful in malaria prophylaxis.

Clinical tip

Quinine has a depressant effect on cardiac muscle, so therefore cannot be given as a large one-off dose (bolus). When taken orally, it has a very bitter taste, which is why some patients decide not to take the medicine resulting in poor concordance.

In addition to the depressant effect noted above, the drug also has other side-effects, such as diarrhoea and vomiting. If the dose is increased it can lead to dizziness, ringing in the ears (tinnitus), headaches and blurred vision. If the plasma levels rise still further, the patient may develop low blood pressure (hypotension), disturbances of heart rhythm (dysrhythmias) and severe central nervous system problems such as coma.

Other drugs

Malarone and Riamet can also be used in the treatment and prophylaxis of *P. falciparum* malaria.

Malarone acts by interfering with the pathway required for the parasite to replicate nucleic acids, while Riamet interferes with the conversion of haem. Both drugs can be given orally, with the duration of treatment dependent on whether they are being used for prophylaxis or treatment.

Flagellates

As the names implies, this group of protozoa have flagella which allow them to move. A common sexually transmitted organism, *Trichomonas vaginalis* causes infection in both males and females, although symptoms are more common in women. There are an estimated 7.4 million new cases of trichomoniasis each year across the sexes.

The parasite is sexually transmitted through the penis to the vagina during intercourse or by vulva to vulva contact with an infected partner. Therefore, women can acquire the disease from infected men and women, whereas men usually only contract it from infected women.

Most men do not present many signs and symptoms. Occasionally, they may develop a temporary itch inside the penis, a mild discharge or burning on urinating. Women, on the other hand, develop a frothy green/yellow vaginal discharge which has a strong odour. They may also complain of pain during intercourse and on urinating. Irritation and itching of the vulva are also indications of infection.

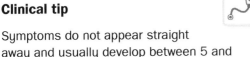

Clinical tip

Symptoms do not appear straight away and usually develop between 5 and 28 days post-exposure.

Metronidazole

This drug interferes with the DNA of the protozoa, so destroying its ability to reproduce. It is usually given orally and is rapidly absorbed, reaching peak plasma levels after 1–3 hours. The drug is also available in rectal and intravenous preparations. For use against trichomoniasis, it is usually given as a single oral dose.

This drug does not have many unwanted effects. The patient should be warned that they may experience a metallic taste when taking the tablet. Minor GI and central nervous symptoms have been reported.

In the treatment of trichomoniasis, the symptoms may suddenly disappear in the male. This does *not* mean that the protozoal infection has disappeared; the male is still capable of infecting a woman. As a result, both partners should be treated at the same time in order to eliminate the organism. Patients being treated should be advised not to have sex until they and their sexual partner both complete the treatment and are symptom-free.

Both parties should also be informed that being treated once does not mean that they cannot become re-infected. Therefore, they should be alert to any signs and symptoms of recurrence.

Clinical tip

The patient should also be informed that metronidazole interferes with the metabolism of alcohol within the body, thus alcohol should be avoided when taking the medication, otherwise they may have a severe reaction.

Amoeboflagellates

These organisms use pseudopodia or flagella to aid their movement. *Entamoeba histolytica* is the cause of amoebic dysentery, an infection of the GI system. This species of protozoa is found in contaminated food and drink. *Entamoeba histolytica* infection is potentially life-threatening, as the protozoa not only take up residence in the bowel but can access the bloodstream and therefore infect other organs such as the liver, lungs and brain.

When the amoeba infects someone, the wall of the large intestine is damaged, so causing ulceration and bleeding. Sometimes the person may complain of abdominal cramps (colic), as well as pain on passing faeces. Bloody, slimy and foul-smelling diarrhoea is also indicative of this infection. The situation becomes much worse if the amoeba breaks through the lining of the gut and invades the peritoneum, causing peritonitis.

The amoeba can now be transported to other organs in the body. This may result in a high temperature and other serious consequences, such as the development of large cysts in the liver and other organs.

Tinidazole

This drug may be used in combination with metronidazole and diloxanide to treat amoebic dysentery. The drug is given orally as a suspension or tablet. It is usually taken with food as a single dose or once a day for between 3 and 5 days. The patient should be encouraged to take the full course even if they feel better. The side-effects are similar to those experienced with metronidazole.

Clinical tip

As the main route of entry for the protozoa into the body is via the mouth, the best way to avoid infection from amoeboflagellates is by ensuring that anything which is eaten is washed or sterilized properly. Fortunately, this disease does not normally occur in the UK and is usually acquired in tropical countries when on holiday and manifests when the person returns home.

Clinical tip

As with metronidazole, patients should not consume alcohol when taking tinidazole. Alcohol may cause the patient to have an upset stomach and suffer from vomiting, stomach cramps (colic) and severe sweating.

Case studies

① Cynthia Day is a 60-year-old woman who has been admitted with a respiratory tract infection. She has been a heavy smoker for 35 years and has been suffering from flu-like symptoms for the past 10 days. On admission, she is pyrexial and dehydrated, although she can eat and drink small quantities. Clarithromycin 550mg BD is commenced orally for 7 days.

- With reference to the anatomy of a bacterium, explain the mechanism of action of clarithromycin.
- Explain the possible reasons why this antibacterial agent is prescribed over other alternatives.
- Explain the clinical observations which you would need to conduct for the duration of Cynthia's treatment.

② Ella Jackson is 18 months old and suffering from an ear infection. The doctor has diagnosed a viral infection and has refused to prescribe antibiotics. Ella's mother does not understand the reason for this and has asked for an explanation. You can reassure her by explaining the difference between viral and bacterial infections. Discuss this with reference to:

- bacterial and viral infections;

←

- mechanism of action of antibiotics;
- alternative medications to relieve Ella's symptoms of pain and fever.

③ Scott Mosier, a 23-year-old man, presented himself to his general practitioner (GP) because he had been coughing, breathless and feeling very tired for the past 4 weeks. In addition, he had weighed himself and was worried as he had lost 5kg. On questioning by his GP, it became apparent that he had recently been on a business trip to Pakistan. The doctor ascertained that he had not been having any night sweats since his return and was not coughing up any blood (haemoptysis).

On general examination, he had a temperature of 37.5°C but had no evidence of anaemia or clubbing of the fingers. The doctor listened to his chest and found crepitations (a crackling or rattling sound) over both lung apices. The doctor then ordered a blood test which showed his haemoglobin and white cell count were normal, but the C-reactive protein was high at 231mg/L. His chest X-ray also showed abnormalities. A sputum specimen that had been sent confirmed that it contained acid-fast bacilli and *Mycobacterium tuberculosis* was subsequently cultured. A diagnosis of *pulmonary tuberculosis* was made.

The patient was treated with isoniazid and rifampicin for 6 months, together with pyrazinamide for the first 2 months. He was allowed home on chemotherapy when his sputum became negative.

With reference to this gentleman's diagnosis of pulmonary TB and the fact that he was taking the antibiotics isoniazid, rifampicin and pyrazinamide, what nursing interventions would you have performed in caring for him?

④ Mr Lorenzo Chopra is a 76-year-old man who has been admitted to the ward with a diagnosis of sepsis probably secondary to a urinary tract infection. He is unwell and the attending health professional prescribes gentamycin 5mg/kg/day intravenously for an initial 5 days in accordance with the local policy.

- What family of antibiotics does gentamycin belong to and what is its mode of action?
- What observations would you be making on the patient's condition?

⑤ Josie is aged 13 and on the autism spectrum. She is prone to pushing things in her ears and often develops ear infections. She has been diagnosed as having otitis media and has been prescribed amoxicillin. She has great difficulty swallowing tablets and capsules and takes any other medication as oral liquids. There is a delay waiting for the stock of amoxicillin suspension, but capsules are available. Her mother suggests that until the suspension arrives, she can open the capsules and mix the contents in Josie's yogurt. Reflect on this and consider the following key points:

- How will opening capsules affect the pharmacokinetics (especially absorption) of the drug?
- How does this affect the legal status of the drug regarding licensing?
- What are the risks and benefits of delaying treatment until the suspension arrives?
- Thinking about capacity and consent, could this be considered covert medicines administration?

Key learning points

Introduction

▶ Infectious diseases are classified as bacterial, viral, fungal or protozoal.
▶ Bacteria are classified as bacilli, cocci or spirochetes.
▶ Bacteria are classified as being gram negative or gram positive.
▶ Antibiotics can be bacteriostatic or bactericidal.

Interference with folate

▶ Bacteria need folate to survive.
▶ Trimethoprim is an antibiotic that stops bacteria using folate.

Beta-lactam antibiotics

▶ Stop the bacteria making a robust cell wall.
▶ Examples include the penicillins and cephalosporins.
▶ Need to check for allergies before giving these medicines.

Interference with protein synthesis

▶ Tetracycline and chloramphenicol work in this way.
▶ Tetracyclines bind to metals (e.g. magnesium), so are not given alongside antacid preparations.
▶ Aminoglycosides (e.g. gentamycin) require regular blood measurement.
▶ Macrolides (e.g. erythromycin) can be used in patients allergic to penicillin.
▶ These drugs cause vomiting and diarrhoea.

Inhibition of bacterial DNA

▶ Ciprofloxacin performs this function.
▶ This drug also binds to metals, so is not given alongside antacids.

Antibiotic resistance

▶ Misuse of antibiotics occurs in medicine, agriculture and household products.
▶ Combinations of bacteria have perpetuated drug-resistant microbes and increased the efficiency with which resistance genes are exchanged.
▶ A lack of economic incentive has led to decreased antibiotic research and development.

Drugs used to treat tuberculosis

▶ Initial infection of the lungs is called primary TB.
▶ Isoniazid, rifampicin and pyrazinamide are the main antibiotics used to treat TB.

←

▶ Isoniazid causes enzyme inhibition in the liver.
▶ Rifampicin can cause orange discoloration of saliva, tears and sweat.
▶ Drugs in this category are often used in combination.

Viral disease

▶ Viruses are essentially DNA or RNA surrounded by a protein capsule.
▶ Viruses invade host cells where they take over the cell's functions.
▶ Treating viral disease is more difficult than treating bacterial disease.
▶ Types of virus include DNA, RNA and retrovirus.

Human immunodeficiency virus

▶ This is a global problem.
▶ The virus attacks T-helper cells (T4 cells).
▶ The T-helper cells display codes which the virus recognizes.
▶ HIV is caused by a retrovirus.
▶ Therapy involves using a combination of drugs.

Nucleoside reverse transcriptase inhibitors

▶ Stop the virus using an enzyme called reverse transcriptase.
▶ Zidovudine and abacavir are examples.

Non-nucleoside reverse transcriptase inhibitors

▶ Have the same mode of action as the nucleoside drugs.
▶ Nevirapine can cause a rash and fever.
▶ Protease inhibitors stop the virus making new viral proteins in the host cell.
▶ Saquinavir is an example.
▶ Drugs in this group can cause enzyme inhibition in the liver.

Other antiviral drugs

▶ Aciclovir is used to treat cold sores and genital herpes.
▶ Works particularly on DNA viruses by blocking an enzyme called DNA polymerase.
▶ Patient should drink plenty of water when taking the medication.
▶ If administered via IV route, you need to monitor the site.
▶ Ganciclovir works on DNA virus by blocking an enzyme called DNA polymerase.
▶ Used in patients who are immunocompromised.
▶ Causes bone marrow depression.
▶ Amantadine is used against influenza A virus.
▶ Immunoglobins are antibodies against specific viruses.
▶ Interferon stops viruses replicating in host cells by interfering with ribosomes.

→

Fungal infections

▶ Caused by moulds, true yeasts and yeast-like fungi.

Antifungal drugs

▶ Amphotericin is a type of macrolide antibiotic.
▶ It cannot be given orally.
▶ When given intravenously, it has serious side-effects.
▶ Nystatin disrupts membranes of the fungus.
▶ Used in *Candida* infections.
▶ Griseofulvin has a narrow range of activity.
▶ Used to treat fungal infections of the nails and skin.
▶ Azoles are synthetically manufactured.
▶ Azoles interfere with fungal P450.
▶ Examples are ketoconazole and fluconazole.
▶ These are both given orally to treat systemic fungal infections.
▶ Flucytosine is another synthetic antifungal drug.
▶ It has a narrow scope of activity.
▶ It acts on fungal DNA.
▶ Terbinafine is given for tinea infections of the skin and nails.

Protozoa

▶ These are simple eukaryotic organisms.
▶ They are classified into apicomplexa, flagellates and amoeboflagellates.
▶ Apicomplexa cause malaria.
▶ The flagellate *Trichomonas vaginalis* causes trichomoniasis.
▶ Metronidazole is used to treat trichomoniasis.
▶ The amoeboflagellate *Entamoeba histolytica* causes amoebic dysentery.
▶ Tinidazole is used alongside metronidazole to treat amoebic dysentery.

Calculations

1. A doctor has prescribed 800mg of erythromycin. You have 500mg in 10mL suspension. How much suspension would you give?

2. What volume is required for an injection if a patient is prescribed 500mg of capreomycin and all you have in stock is 300mg in 1mL?

3. A patient is prescribed 1000mg of chloramphenicol. The stock on hand contains 250mg in 10mL suspension. How much would you administer?

4. You are required to give a dose of an antibiotic in tablet form. The tablets are available in 25mg. The doctor has prescribed 0.05g. How many tablets do you give?

5. A child weighs 12kg and is prescribed an antibiotic at 15mg/kg. If your stock strength is 200mg in 5mL, what volume would you give?

6. A patient has been prescribed erythromycin 250mg tablets. How many tablets are required to complete their 7-day course of 500mg four times a day?

7. Your patient weighs 80kg. How much gentamycin (80mg/2mL) should you give for a dose of 5mg/kg (maximum 400mg)?

8. You have a bottle of amoxicillin syrup containing 250mg in 5mL. How much do you need to give 100mg?

9. You have a vial of gentamycin containing 80mg in 2mL. How much do you need to administer 300mg?

10. You need to give 1g of erythromycin orally. You have erythromycin suspension 250mg in 5mL. How much of the suspension do you give?

Multiple-choice questions

Try answering these multiple-choice questions to test what you have learned from reading this chapter. You can check your answers at the end of the book.

1. What is the mechanism of action of tetracycline antibiotics?

a) They inhibit folate use by the bacteria
b) They destroy the bacterial cell wall
c) They inhibit bacterial protein synthesis
d) They interfere with bacterial DNA

2. What is the drug of choice in treating tuberculosis?

a) Rifampicin
b) Gentamycin
c) Clindamycin
d) Chloramphenicol

3. Why should antacid medicines not be taken with certain antibiotics?

a) The body prefers to absorb antacids
b) Antacids slow down the movement of the bowel
c) They stop the antibiotic being absorbed by the body
d) They increase the side-effects of antibiotics

→

←

4. What is the mechanism of action of the penicillins and cephalosporins?

a) They inhibit folate use by the bacteria
b) They constrict the bacterial cell wall
c) They inhibit bacterial protein synthesis
d) They interfere with bacterial DNA

5. Reverse transcriptase is associated with which virus?

a) Influenza
b) Herpes
c) Human cytomegalovirus
d) HIV

6. Aciclovir is used when treating ...

a) Poliomyelitis
b) German measles
c) Influenza
d) Shingles

7. Viruses are difficult to treat because ...

a) They reproduce in our cells
b) They have very thick walls
c) They are smaller than bacteria
d) The drugs are more expensive

8. Athlete's foot is an example of a ...

a) Mildew
b) True yeast
c) Mould
d) Yeast-like fungi

9. Which of the following drugs is most likely to lead to an infection with thrush?

a) Anticoagulant therapy
b) Morphine
c) Steroid medicines
d) Angiotensin-converting enzyme inhibitors

10. Amphotericin could be described as being ...

a) A newly-developed medicine
b) A synthetic antifungal agent
c) A harmless medicine
d) An antifungal antibiotic

Recommended further reading

Downie, G., Mackenzie, J. and Williams, A. (2007) *Pharmacology and Medicines Management for Nurses*, 4th edition. Edinburgh: Churchill Livingstone.

Jethwa, S. (2015) Penicillin allergy: identification and management, *The Pharmaceutical Journal*, 295 (7878). Available at: https://doi.org/10.1211/PJ.2015.20069170.

Karch, A.M. (2017) *Focus on Nursing Pharmacology*, 7th edition. Philadelphia, PA: Lippincott Williams & Wilkins.

Lapham, R. (2015) *Drug Calculations for Nurses: A Step-by-Step Approach*, 4th edition. London: Arnold.

National Institute for Health and Care Excellence (NICE) (2015) *NICE Guideline NG15: Antimicrobial Stewardship: Systems and Processes for Effective Antimicrobial Medicine Use*. London: NICE.

National Institute for Health and Care Excellence (NICE) (2016) *NICE Guideline NG33: Tuberculosis: Clinical Diagnosis and Management of Tuberculosis, and Measures for its Prevention and Control*. London: NICE. Last updated September 2019.

National Institute for Health and Care Excellence (NICE) (2019) *British National Formulary*. London: NICE. Available at: https://bnf.nice.org.uk.

Simonson, T., Aarbakke, J., Kay, I., Coleman, I., Sinnott, P. and Lyssa, R. (2006) *Illustrated Pharmacology for Nurses*. London: Hodder Arnold.

Anti-inflammatory drugs

6

Chapter contents

Learning objectives

After studying this chapter, you should be able to:

- Describe acute and chronic inflammatory processes.
- Explain the mode of action of non-steroidal anti-inflammatory agents.
- Demonstrate an understanding of what is meant by cyclooxygenase pathway 2 inhibitors.
- Discuss the mode of action and adverse effects of aspirin.
- Define what is meant by the word 'histamine'.
- Describe the mode of action of antihistamine medication.
- Demonstrate an understanding of why steroid drugs are given, their routes of administration and side-effects.
- Explain what information the practitioner should give to a patient taking systemic steroid therapy.
- Define the condition rheumatoid arthritis.
- List three drugs that are categorized as disease-modifying anti-rheumatoid drugs.
- Correctly solve several drug calculations with regard to anti-inflammatory drugs.

Introduction

Inflammation is the body's response mechanism to cellular damage. Without the inflammatory response, our bodies could not survive. Therefore, inflammation is a protective mechanism designed to rid the body of the cause of injury and prepare our tissues to rebuild themselves following injury.

The inflammatory response (see Figure 6.1) is a local reaction that involves release of antibacterial substances that defend the body from attack. The inflammatory process 'protects' the injured area so that toxins cannot affect the whole system. It then provides the infrastructure that enables the body to be restored to its normal functioning. Inflammation could be described as a *homeostatic mechanism*. The main signs and symptoms of inflammation are redness, pain, swelling, heat and loss of function. These are caused by chemicals released by plasma proteins and cells. The plasma proteins and various white cells pass through the walls of capillary vessels to the site of tissue damage, infection or foreign bodies. This response is brought about by a variety of chemicals in the body which dilate blood vessels and act as messengers to attract white blood cells. This is referred to as *chemotaxis*.

Inflammation is classified as being either acute or chronic.

Acute inflammation

Acute inflammation can have many causes, such as an insect bite that can trigger an inflammatory response in susceptible individuals. Acute inflammation is characterized by its rapid onset and short duration. This response is intended to remove debris from the tissue, such as micro-organisms

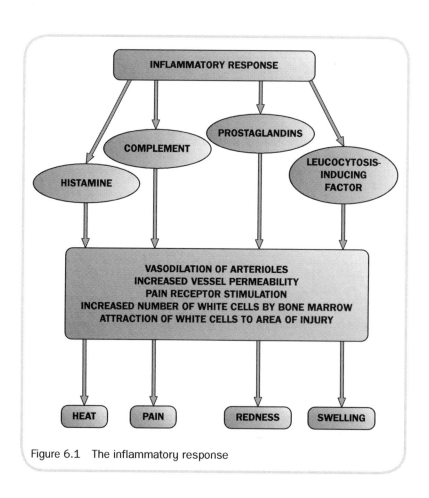

Figure 6.1 The inflammatory response

and other particles of dead tissue. At the same time, the bone marrow is activated, triggering an increased production of phagocytic cells, particularly neutrophils, which can digest invading organisms. Finally, other chemical messengers attract these phagocytic cells from the area of damage through the process of chemotaxis.

One of the first chemicals to be released in the acute inflammatory response is *histamine*, which is released from *mast cells*. The role of histamine in the body is to produce vasodilation and increase the permeability of blood vessels. This in turn allows fluid and phagocytic cells to migrate from the intravascular fluid to the extravascular fluid. The area of damage becomes flooded with fluid, plasma proteins and phagocytic cells. This *acute inflammatory exudate* is part of the signs and symptoms of inflammation discussed earlier.

The flooding of the tissues with fluid and plasma proteins dilutes any toxins that may have been released, especially by bacteria. The excess fluid is drained away by a network of blind capillary-type vessels, which belong to the lymphatic system. Small amounts of bacterial protein are exposed to lymphocytes, which in turn produce antitoxins that we call immunoglobulins. These are attracted to the area of cell injury to neutralize toxins further. A specific group of plasma proteins called the *complement group* assist the inflammatory response by attracting white cells by chemotaxis and promoting the number of phagocytic cells made available to the body.

The primary activators in this response are granular leucocytes known as *neutrophils*. These cells ingest small portions of dead tissue by producing an enzyme, *lysozyme*, that breaks down the bacterial wall. The activity of neutrophils is limited, however, because they do not have the ability to make and store more lysozyme. Therefore, once the neutrophil has used its enzymes and phagocytosis is complete, the cell degenerates and dies.

The secondary activators are two types of agranular white blood cells – *monocytes* and *lymphocytes*. Once monocytes enter the damaged area, they undergo a conformational change, becoming a more specialized type of white cell known as *macrophages*. These cells can mop up any cell debris or bacteria. Unlike neutrophils, they can replenish lysozyme, meaning they are able to sustain their effect, which allows lymphocytes, part of a more specific immune response, to be activated. Specific cells will now have been created to counteract these foreign proteins, or *antigens*. These cells are called lymphocytes: 'T' lymphocytes, which naturally attack any foreign antigens and 'B' lymphocytes, which produce the immunoglobulins to neutralize any toxins produced by the invading bacteria.

Once the area has been cleared, repair can take place. Cells that rebuild tissue, called *fibroblasts*, now start to proliferate and generate collagen, a protein necessary for wound repair. Furthermore, a process known as *angiogenesis* can begin and blood vessels that have been destroyed in the damaged area start to grow again, supplying nutrients and oxygen to the newly forming tissues.

Acute inflammation can be seen as a balance between the damage caused by the invading organisms and the damage caused by the body's response in trying to safeguard surrounding normal tissue. The inflammatory process itself will almost inevitably cause some damage to tissues in its efforts to save other tissues. There are three possible outcomes:

1. **Resolution** – there is complete healing and tissue repair.

2. **Healing by repair** – the tissue is destroyed and now lacks the ability to regenerate. As a result, the previously healthy tissue is replaced by scar tissue, which is fibrous in nature.

3. **Chronic inflammation** – this occurs when the noxious material persists over an extended period, resulting in the continued destruction of tissue.

Chronic inflammation

Chronic inflammation usually arises when a noxious substance is not removed by the acute inflammatory process. There are occasions, however, when chronic inflammation is not preceded by the acute inflammatory process. This is the case in *autoimmune diseases*, for example, where the

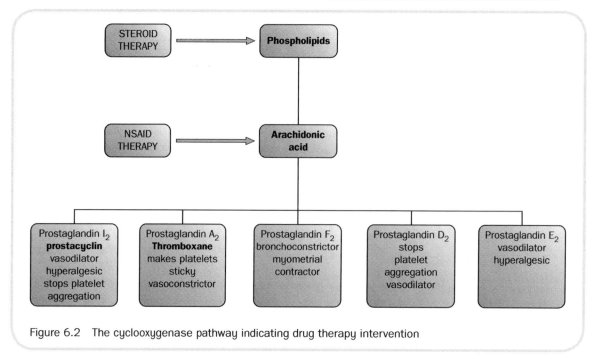

Figure 6.2   The cyclooxygenase pathway indicating drug therapy intervention

body's defence mechanisms appear to be turned on themselves. In this process, autoantibodies are produced by the immune system and directed at normal body tissue, as if that body tissue were foreign.

If the acute inflammatory process cannot remove the foreign material, further tissue destruction will occur. The body will continue to try to repair the damage, but the continued destruction results in those repair efforts being less effective.

In chronic inflammation, the cells that are found at the site of injury differ from those observed in acute inflammation. The more specific defence being mounted is characterized by large amounts of lymphocytes, rather than the neutrophils observed in acute inflammation. In the body's attempts at tissue repair, thick bands of collagen fibres are laid down resulting in fibrosis at the site of injury. For resolution to occur, the patient may require antibiotic therapy, the foreign body to be removed or receive additional pharmacological intervention and support.

To understand the pharmacological action of certain anti-inflammatory drugs, we must revisit a group of substances called *eicosanoids*, which include prostacyclin, thromboxane, prostaglandins

and leukotrienes. These substances are important in the inflammatory response and are formed when a fatty acid, *arachidonic acid*, is released from damaged cells by the action of an enzyme called phospholipase.

Arachidonic acid is a component of two important pathways, the cyclooxygenase pathway and the lipoxygenase pathway. The cyclooxygenase pathway produces prostaglandins (see Figure 6.2), whereas the lipoxygenase pathway results in leukotriene formation. Some anti-inflammatory drugs act on one pathway, while others exert their effects on both.

Non-steroidal anti-inflammatory drugs (NSAIDs)

Non-steroidal anti-inflammatory drugs (NSAIDs) are a group of therapeutic agents whose main use is as an analgesic to treat mild-to-moderate pain (see Chapter 4). Examples include ibuprofen, aspirin and naproxen. They are frequently prescribed for conditions such as osteoarthritis and other musculoskeletal conditions.

This group of drugs works by inhibiting the formation of prostaglandins. Prostaglandins are substances that occur naturally, and the inflammatory variety are released when cell membranes are damaged in some way. They are responsible for dilation of vessels, causing redness and swelling. Some also sensitize the receptors that are responsible for the sensation of pain.

There is more than one cyclooxygenase pathway. Cyclooxygenase pathways in most pharmacological texts are denoted by the prefix COX followed by the number of the pathway (e.g. COX1). The prostaglandins derived from COX1 are involved in the normal management and regulation of body systems. Prostaglandins produced by this pathway are important for maintaining the protective mucous lining of the stomach and intestine, and for the regulation of blood flow to functional cells of the kidney. COX2, in contrast, produces inducible prostaglandins that facilitate the inflammatory response.

Most NSAIDs block both cyclooxygenase pathways. This can be problematic, as they reduce the pain and inflammation associated with the COX2 pathway, while also reducing the homeostatic function of COX1. This can result in GI disturbances, which are common side-effects of the NSAID group of drugs. In some circumstances, these can be severe and peptic ulceration is a risk. The long-term or high-dose use of NDSAIDs should be accompanied by some adjuvant to mitigate this effect, such as the proton pump inhibitor omeprazole. This helps to ensure limited damage to the gastric mucosa.

Another common side-effect of these drugs is the adverse effect they can have on kidney function. Some prostaglandins in the COX1 pathway influence the pressure of blood flow through the kidneys. Patients prescribed these drugs should be monitored for adverse renal effects, and those with reduced renal function should either avoid NSAIDs or be prescribed them for a short time at their lowest therapeutic dose.

NSAIDs may also increase the risk of heart attack, stroke and related conditions. This risk may increase with long-term use and in patients who have underlying risk factors for heart and blood vessel conditions.

> ### Clinical tip
>
> Normal doses of NSAIDs in healthy individuals do not usually pose much of a risk. However, in patients who have other medical conditions such as heart failure, these drugs can cause acute kidney problems. Patients who are likely to react in an adverse way to this group of drugs should have their blood checked at regular intervals for signs of renal impairment.

Naproxen

Naproxen is a commonly used NSAID for the reduction of pain, fever, inflammation and stiffness associated with conditions such as arthritis and ankylosing spondylitis (a chronic arthritis of the spine). It is often the drug of choice when treating an inflammatory condition because it is effective and has relatively few side-effects. However, ibuprofen is still seen as one of the safest drugs in this class (see Chapter 4).

The dose of naproxen will vary depending on the condition it is being used to treat. However, the usual adult dose is 250–500mg twice daily. Because of potential effects on the gastric mucosa, a drug such as omeprazole may also be used.

Naproxen is associated with several suspected or probable interactions that affect the action of other drugs. For example, it may increase circulating levels of lithium by reducing the excretion of lithium by the kidneys. Increased levels of lithium may lead to lithium toxicity. Naproxen may reduce the blood pressure-lowering effects of blood pressure medication because prostaglandins play a role in the regulation of blood pressure.

When naproxen is used in combination with methotrexate or a member of the aminoglycoside group of antimicrobials (e.g. gentamicin), circulating levels of methotrexate or the aminoglycoside may increase, due to their reduced elimination by the kidney. This can lead to toxicity-related side-effects.

Naproxen is not recommended during pregnancy, and caution is advised when breastfeeding.

Cyclooxygenase pathway 2 inhibitors

Celecoxib

Celecoxib belongs to a new generation of NSAIDs that more selectively block the action of COX2. This results in fewer inflammatory prostaglandins being produced, while the prostaglandins that protect the stomach and intestines are not so adversely affected. It therefore reduces pain and inflammation but is less likely than traditional NSAIDs to cause side-effects related to the stomach and renal function.

It is used to treat pain and inflammation in joint and muscular conditions, such as arthritis. The lowest effective dose should be used for each patient. For the management of osteoarthritis, the dose is usually 100mg twice daily or 200mg as a single dose. For rheumatoid arthritis, the dose is usually 100mg or 200mg twice daily.

Allergic reactions can occur with celecoxib. Individuals who have developed allergic reactions (e.g. rash, itching, difficulty breathing) from sulphonamides, aspirin or other NSAIDs may experience an allergic reaction to celecoxib and should not take the drug.

Fluconazole (Diflucan) increases the concentration of celecoxib in the body by preventing the elimination of celecoxib in the liver. Therefore, treatment with celecoxib should be initiated at the lowest recommended dose in patients who are taking fluconazole. As Diflucan can be obtained from a pharmacist, it is important always to ask the patient about other medicines they may be taking prior to dispensing.

Aspirin

Aspirin, due to its anti-inflammatory properties, can be used in the treatment of rheumatoid arthritis and other inflammatory joint conditions. Aspirin is another drug that blocks the COX1 pathway, but also inhibits the COX2 pathway.

Aspirin is a weak acid drug that is readily absorbed in the stomach due to its acid environment. However, much of the absorption takes place in the ileum, the third part of the small intestine, due to its large surface area.

Aspirin is taken orally and can be used in soluble form, where it is mixed with calcium carbonate and citric acid. This aids its rate of absorption into the body.

Adverse effects

Some of the adverse effects of aspirin are similar to those previously described for NSAIDs, such as GI disturbances. There are also a group of symptoms related to central nervous system disruption, including dizziness, tinnitus, loss of hearing, visual disturbances and headache. The drug should not be given to children, as it can cause a life-threatening disorder called Reyes syndrome.

Overdose

Overdose with aspirin has serious consequences. The more serious symptoms of poisoning include high body temperature (hyperthermia), increased respiratory rate (tachypnoea), metabolic acidosis, confusion, cerebral oedema and coma. Aspirin overdose is still classified as a medical emergency.

Histamine

Histamine is a chemical released by cells which contributes to the inflammatory response. The lungs, skin and GI tract have high concentrations of histamine-releasing cells and these systems are where many of the effects of its release are noted. It is also found in mast cells and basophils. Histamine also occurs in cells in the stomach and certain neurones in the brain.

Histamine exerts an effect on several different subtypes of histamine receptors.

Antihistamines

The term 'antihistamine' refers to any drug that blocks the action of histamine on H-receptors. This class of drug is effective in the treatment and management of various inflammatory and allergic responses.

Most drugs in this category are given orally, as they are well absorbed by the body. They reach their peak in the plasma after 1–2 hours. They are well distributed throughout the body and some do not cross the blood–brain barrier and, therefore, cause less sedation than those that do.

Cyclizine, dimenhydrinate and cinnarizine do cross the blood–brain barrier and can be used to treat motion sickness. Non-sedating antihistamines are mainly used for hay fever and mild allergic reactions. Some non-sedating drugs in this category can be purchased as OTC medicines, for example loratadine and cetirizine. Some sedating drugs in this group can be used for this effect, for example, chlorphenamine or promethazine. These may well cause sedation and stop motion sickness, but they will also produce other central nervous system side-effects, such as dizziness, tinnitus and tiredness. The most significant side-effects of antihistamines at a peripheral rather than a central level are dryness of the mouth, blurred vision and, more rarely, constipation and retention of urine.

Steroids

Steroid hormones include a group known as *glucocorticoids*. These are secreted by an area of the adrenal cortex called the *zona fasciculata*. Glucocorticoids are involved in the body's response to stress. They have a pronounced effect on carbohydrate and protein use. The hormones cause a decrease in the uptake of glucose by the body's cells and an increase in glucose production through the breakdown of proteins (gluconeogenesis). This leads to a net increase in blood sugars (hyperglycaemia). At the same time, the body stores more glucose as glycogen in the liver. Protein use is affected because there is a decrease in the production of protein by the cells but an increase in protein breakdown, which is particularly evident in muscle tissue. Use of fats is also affected by glucocorticoids, as they permit fatty tissue to be laid down in a certain way.

Glucocorticoids also affect certain electrolytes within the body. Sodium is retained at the expense of potassium, which is lost via the kidneys. Calcium is another example of a body chemical affected by glucocorticoid activity, as glucocorticoids tend to lower its rate of absorption by the GI tract and increase its loss via the kidneys.

If levels of glucocorticoid remain high in the plasma, this has a negative feedback effect on the hypothalamus and pituitary gland. Basically, the body ceases to stimulate the adrenal cortex

to produce these substances, and over a period of time this will lead to a shrinking of the adrenal cortical area.

The main role of glucocorticoids is their powerful anti-inflammatory and immunosuppressive effects. They reduce redness, pain, heat and swelling but also positively affect the healing and repair process. They can reduce all types of inflammatory response whether caused by physical stimuli or autoimmune responses.

Glucocorticoids have a direct action on the cells involved in the inflammatory response, namely neutrophils, macrophages and fibroblasts. They also have a direct action on the chemicals responsible for inflammation (e.g. COX2 and histamine). It is thought that the production of glucocorticoids is a homeostatic mechanism aimed at regulating the defence systems of the body.

Glucocorticoids can be used to treat conditions where hypersensitivity or unwanted inflammatory processes present. They can be used in a range of conditions from autoimmune disease and organ rejection following transplantation to hay fever and skin conditions. The ability to suppress the normal inflammatory response has consequences for the masking of infections and a reduction in the potential healing properties of all tissues.

Administration

Glucocorticoids can be given several ways. Most types can be administered by mouth and all can be given via the IM or IV routes. They can be applied in a cream to the skin or given as eye drops or nasal sprays. They may be administered directly into joint spaces (intra-articular route) or into the lungs by means of an aerosol. Examples of glucocorticoid drugs are prednisolone, hydrocortisone, dexamethasone and beclomethasone.

Side-effects

The side-effects (see Box 6.1) of glucocorticoids are more likely when they are given systemically rather than locally, and when they are prescribed in high doses over an extended period. Patients on long-term treatment with glucocorticoids are at risk of developing serious side-effects.

Box 6.1 Common side-effects of steroids

Secondary hypertension
Euphoria
Hirsutism
Moon-shaped face
Masked infection
Osteoporosis
Adrenal atrophy
Peptic ulceration
Thinning of the skin
Generalized weakness
Secondary diabetes
Obesity
Striae
Oedema
Poor wound healing

When blood sugar levels are constantly elevated, the body develops a secondary diabetic condition. Elevated blood glucose can lead to muscular weakness and, in children, can affect growth. However, this is unlikely unless the treatment is extended to six months or more. Also, as sodium is retained by the body, so is water, therefore increasing blood volume and leading to a potential hypertensive state.

The action of lowering plasma levels of calcium leads the body to homeostatically replace it from the bones. This in turn can lead to osteoporosis and the potential for an increase in the occurrence of fractures.

As the individual's ability to fight infection is compromised, infection can go undetected. Any infection must be treated early with antibiotics and an increased dose of steroid to compensate for the body's natural response. A particularly problematic side-effect is the inability of wounds to heal. This can lead to extensive long-term therapies being instigated to treat traumatic injuries.

Cortisone injections

Glucocorticoids such as cortisone can be used to treat inflammation. A local injection into the joint space is used to treat a variety of inflammatory musculoskeletal conditions. To treat inflammation that is more widespread in the body, the person may be prescribed systemic injections. Local injections of cortisone may be used to treat a condition known as bursitis. This is inflammation of small sacs containing synovial fluid where muscles and tendons tend to slide over bone, for example, near joints. Thus, local injections are used for bursitis of the hip, knee, elbow or shoulder. You may also see them used to treat tendonitis, such as tennis elbow, or given directly into the joint space in arthritis. Sometimes you may find that injections of cortisone and an anaesthetic such as lidocaine are used to confirm a diagnosis. For example, to assess if a person has arthritis of the hip or lower back, they may well be given a cortisone injection into the hip; if pain in the buttock and the groin improves, the problem is more likely to be arthritis of the hip rather than the lower back.

Giving the corticosteroid by injection allows it to be targeted more directly into tissues that are locally inflamed. Using this more direct route means that the effects of the corticosteroid will be more rapid and powerful than if it were given by the oral route. Thus the likelihood of a single dose will be increased, thus avoiding some of the side-effects mentioned previously.

Short-term complications are uncommon but you may find the skin at the site of the injection begins to become a little lighter in colour – a process known as depigmentation – although this is more common in people with darker skin. Also, the skin at this site begins to shrink (atrophy), due to the effects of the steroid on underlying fat. Pain and inflammation at the injection site, known as post-injection flare, is a relatively uncommon reaction to cortisone injections; it presents with redness, pain and warmth. However, unlike an infective event, these signs occur typically within the first 24 hours following the injection. This phenomenon is due to the crystallizing of the cortisone at the injection site rather than a true allergy to cortisone, which is very unusual. Just as subcutaneous fat can be affected by cortisone, other structures such as tendons may become weakened by corticosteroid injections, especially if repeat injections are given. Tendon ruptures have been reported. Facial flushing may occur in up to 40% of cases but lasts only briefly. Sweating and insomnia are rare side-effects.

In patients who have diabetes, cortisone can increase blood sugar levels. In patients who have underlying infections, cortisone injections can suppress the body's ability to fight the infection, thereby possibly worsening the infection or masking the infection by suppressing the symptoms and signs of inflammation. As a general principle, therefore, cortisone injections ought to be used with caution in cases of diabetes and avoided in people with active infections.

Long-term complications of corticosteroid injections depend on their dose and frequency. At higher doses and with more frequent administration, the potential side-effects begin to include other, more typical side-effects of this class of medicine. For example, the patient may experience thinning of the skin, easy bruising, weight gain, puffiness of the face, acne (steroid acne), elevated blood pressure, cataract formation, thinning of the bones (osteoporosis), and a rare but serious type of damage to the bones of the large joints called avascular necrosis.

Cortisone injections into a joint may have side-effects in addition to those described above. Just as tendons can become weakened by the side-effects of cortisone, other structures within the joint also become affected, particularly with repeated injections. These problems include thinning of the joint cartilage and weakening of the ligaments within the joint, and these overall changes can destabilize the joint itself over time. Therefore, such injections ought to be restricted in number where possible and monitored by medical staff.

Cortisone injections into a joint can rapidly reduce joint pain, therefore aiding restoration of function to a body part immobilized by inflammation. Despite potential side-effects and rarely reported adverse reactions, it is generally the case that low, intermittent doses of corticosteroids pose little significant risk.

Clinical tip

Normal doses of steroids in healthy individuals do not usually pose much of a risk. However, in patients that may have other medical conditions, such as heart failure, these drugs can cause acute kidney problems. Patients who are likely to react in an adverse way to this group of drugs should have their blood checked at regular intervals for signs of renal insufficiency.

The patient must also be educated regarding the risks of suddenly stopping their medication. If the body has stopped stimulating the adrenal cortex, it will lose its ability to make its own corticosteroids. Therefore, any sudden withdrawal will lead to a gross insufficiency and the patient may well enter what is called an 'adrenal crisis'. Patients should be phased off their medication slowly to allow the body to recover its natural abilities. This normally takes about 2 months, although it may take much longer.

All patients receiving long-term therapy are advised to carry a card stating that they are undergoing steroid treatment, which must not be stopped abruptly. They should also inform their dentist about their treatment.

Anti-rheumatoid drugs

Arthritis is inflammation of the joints. Rheumatoid arthritis is a common condition and affects about 400,000 people in the UK according to the National Rheumatoid Arthritis Society. Unlike osteoarthritis, which tends to occur as we get older, rheumatoid arthritis can develop at any age, but usually starts in middle adult life, between the ages of 40 and 60. It affects women more than men.

Rheumatoid arthritis is thought to be an autoimmune disease. In people with this condition, antibodies are formed against the synovial membrane (the capsule which surrounds each joint). This causes inflammation in and around the affected joints. Over time, the inflammation causes damage to the joint, the cartilage and those bones involved in forming the joint.

There are two main classes of drugs that are used in this condition that we have already covered in this chapter: NSAIDs and glucocorticoids. However, another group of drugs frequently used in treating this disease goes under the umbrella term of 'disease-modifying anti-rheumatoid drugs' (DMARDs).

The DMARD group comprises drugs with differing chemical structures and, therefore, modes of action, such as sulfasalazine, gold compounds, penicillamine, chloroquine, methotrexate and leflunomide. The anti-rheumatoid actions of the drugs in this category were discovered mostly by accident – we know that they work but have no conclusive pharmacological evidence to suggest why. DMARDs improve patients' lives by reducing the swelling and tenderness in the joints, and while some years ago this class of drugs was usually used as a last resort, it is now usual to start a DMARD as soon as possible after a diagnosis has been made, to limit disease progression as much as possible.

> ### Clinical tip
>
> Sometimes DMARDs do not have an immediate effect on symptoms and it may take up to 6 months before the patient starts to feel the benefit. Therefore, it is important to inform the patient of the importance of continuing to take the medication as prescribed, even if no effect is felt at first.

The choice of DMARD should take account of the patient's condition, their preference (or not) for certain drugs and any comorbid conditions or other medications. There are a number to choose from and all have similar efficacy but differ in their side-effects and dosing. In acute conditions, a combination of drugs may be of benefit.

Sulfasalazine

Sulfasalazine is an aminosalicylate drug and a pro-drug, which means that it is not active in the

form in which it is given. The drug is broken down into two active components by bacteria that live in the bowel: 5-aminosalicylic acid and sulfapyridine. It is not clear which of these agents is responsible for the beneficial immunosuppressant effect. The effect takes time to become evident and many weeks or months of treatment may be needed before the patient feels the full effect.

Gastrointestinal side-effects are common and include nausea, vomiting and loss of appetite (anorexia). Dizziness can also be experienced by some patients. More serious side-effects include a drop in white cells in the body (leucopenia). Skin rashes and reactions to sunlight (photosensitivity) can also occur. As with any drug, sulfasalazine should be used with caution in patients who have kidney disease, for whom the dose may need to be reduced.

Gold compounds

The earliest use of gold for medicinal purposes can be traced back to 2500 BC in China. As with sulfasalazine, the effect of gold compounds is of slow onset. The patient may not feel any benefit from the medication for 2 months. However, after this time the pain and joint swelling start to lessen. There is also a slowing of bone and cartilage damage within the joint. The mode of action of gold compounds remains unclear.

Gold is given as sodium aurothiomalate and is administered by deep IM injection. After a test dose it should be administered weekly until there is evidence of remission. Then it is given monthly for up to 5 years.

> ### Clinical tip
>
> Several serious adverse reactions to gold compounds can develop, any of which will mean that therapy must be stopped. These include kidney damage, blood disorders, as well as major brain and liver disorders. The patient, nurse and doctor need to be vigilant for adverse signs and symptoms, as early cessation will help to ensure that these serious side-effects do not arise.

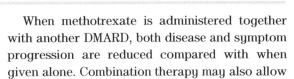

Penicillamine

Penicillamine is used to treat rheumatoid arthritis owing to its immunosuppressive effects. Although the exact nature of its action is unclear, it is thought to reduce the number of circulating T-lymphocytes and macrophages. It also affects chemotactic agents and prevents an important protein called collagen from maturing. Like most of the DMARDs, it takes weeks or months before the patient feels any benefit from the drug. Its onset and activity are similar to that of gold.

Penicillamine is given orally, beginning on a low dose that is increased every 2 months. The maximum dose is about 1500mg per day. The reason for this gradual dosing regime is to avoid unwanted side-effects because at high doses, as many as one in four patients has to stop taking the medication because of unwanted effects.

As with many of the drugs in this section, side-effects include anorexia, nausea and vomiting. Some patients develop a loss of taste because the drug binds to zinc. Rashes and stomatitis are common and serious side-effects include blood disorders such as leucopenia, anaemia and thrombocytopenia.

As penicillamine binds to certain metals (chelation), it should not be given to patients who are taking iron supplements, gold and antacids that contain aluminium or magnesium.

Methotrexate

Methotrexate works on DNA, the genetic material within the nucleus of a cell. As with most drugs in this classification, it is not known how exactly methotrexate works in relation to rheumatoid arthritis, but empirically it has been shown to reduce the amount of inflammation and slow the progression of the disease. It is usually the drug of choice for first-line treatment following diagnosis. The drug has fewer side-effects than the others in this group and because of its favourable results, patients are more likely to be concordant (continue to take the medication). It is given weekly and this unusual dosing regimen must be well explained to patients to prevent them taking the weekly dose on a daily basis. Folic acid is often given concurrently with methotrexate to further reduce any incidence of side-effects.

When methotrexate is administered together with another DMARD, both disease and symptom progression are reduced compared with when given alone. Combination therapy may also allow for lower doses of individual drugs to be given.

Side-effects include nausea, stomatitis, diarrhoea, fatigue and mild inflammation of the liver. As the drug affects the body's ability to fight infection, the patient should be educated to report signs and symptoms, such as sore throat, shortness of breath and frequency of micturition to a health professional. Low blood cell counts are less likely with this drug than others in this group. Rare side-effects such as liver damage and lung damage may be seen.

Chloroquine

This drug is used mainly in the treatment of malaria; however, it has also been shown to reduce progression of disease in rheumatoid arthritis. The drug is generally used in milder cases of the disease or in combination with other DMARDs. It takes around 3–6 months for its effects to become apparent and minor side-effects are like those reported in other DMARDs, such as nausea, diarrhoea and rashes.

Clinical tip

More serious side-effects from chloroquine are ophthalmologic in nature. Prolonged use may lead patients to complain of problems with their peripheral and night-time vision. If patients are prescribed the drug, they should be advised to have a baseline eye test and repeat this on a 6-monthly to yearly basis.

Leflunomide

This drug is thought to work on the cell's DNA and RNA. The immune cells cannot function or reproduce effectively due to the effects of the drug. Hence, leflunomide reduces inflammation in the joints, as well as slowing progressive bone erosion and joint deformity.

The drug can be taken orally and comes in preparations of 10mg, 15mg, 20mg and 100mg tablets. The usual dose is 100mg daily for the first 3 days, then 20mg daily, or 10mg if side-effects arise. These include nausea, diarrhoea and rashes. More severe side-effects are hypertension, chest pain and abnormal heartbeats. Like many of the immunosuppressant DMARDs, leflunomide can mask infections. Liver damage is also a possibility and if liver enzyme tests remain abnormal, the drug should be discontinued. It has a similar efficacy to sulfasalazine and methotrexate and can be prescribed when neither of these drugs is an option for the patient.

Case studies

① Radu Beligan, a 28-year-old professional musician, has been admitted to the ward for medical treatment following an exacerbation of his ulcerative colitis. On admission he was pale with obvious signs of weight loss. During his stay on the ward it is decided to commence oral steroid medication. You have been asked by your mentor to help prepare the patient for discharge. What information would you give to Radu about his new medication with reference to:

■ the action of steroids on the body?

■ the side-effects?

■ any other information?

② Louise Mason is 12 years old. She has juvenile chronic arthritis that is being treated with ibuprofen. The doctor now wishes to give her a 'short burst' of high-dose steroid to bridge her transition onto methotrexate. You have to explain to Louise and her concerned parents how these drugs work and why the steroids need to be given as a bridge from one set of medication to another. Think how you would put the following information into terms that Louise and her parents will understand:

■ the mode of action of these three classes of medicine;

■ the need for Louise to maintain drug therapy between stopping one drug and starting another;

■ the possible side-effects that the high-dose steroid treatment will have.

③ Darinda Novak is a 47-year-old woman who had been diagnosed with rheumatoid arthritis following a fall. After the diagnosis the consultant rheumatologist had tried a medicine called sulfasalazine. This had not helped, however, and her inflammatory condition was worsening. Darinda reluctantly agreed to start a course of oral methotrexate, especially as her pain was increasing.

With reference to this choice of drug, what information will the patient require regarding side-effects?

④ Phyllis Johnson is a 63-year-old woman who has been diagnosed with osteoarthritis of her knees. In the past this lady has had problems with dyspepsia, gastric irritation and ulcer formation. As a result, the GP has decided to prescribe her celecoxib.

With reference to the inflammatory process and the medicine celecoxib, describe the difference between cyclooxygenase 1 and 2 inhibitors.

Key learning points

Introduction

- ▶ Inflammation is a protective mechanism.
- ▶ The inflammatory response is a local reaction.
- ▶ The cardinal signs and symptoms of inflammation are redness, pain, swelling, heat and loss of function.
- ▶ Acute inflammation is characterized by rapid onset and short duration.
- ▶ Histamine is released and is a vasodilator.
- ▶ Area of damage becomes flooded with exudate.
- ▶ Complement proteins are involved in chemotaxis.
- ▶ A variety of leucocytes are attracted to the area.
- ▶ Eventually repair takes place.
- ▶ Chronic inflammation occurs when noxious substances are not removed by the acute phase.
- ▶ Large amounts of lymphocytes are found in the area of chronic inflammation.
- ▶ Attempts to repair tissue often result in fibrosis.
- ▶ Inflammation is caused by the liberation of arachidonic acid.
- ▶ Cyclo-oxygenase and lipo-oxygenase pathways are triggered.

Non-steroidal anti-inflammatory drugs

- ▶ Popular group of drugs.
- ▶ Work by inhibiting prostaglandin formation.
- ▶ Stop the initiation of the cyclooxygenase pathway.
- ▶ Cause renal and gastrointestinal side-effects.

Naproxen

- ▶ Is often the drug of choice when treating an inflammatory condition.
- ▶ May increase circulating levels of lithium.
- ▶ May increase the levels of methotrexate or aminoglycoside.
- ▶ Is associated with the lowest overall cardiovascular risks but may increase the risk of heart attacks, stroke and related conditions.

Cyclooxygenase pathway 2 inhibitors

- ▶ New class of drugs.
- ▶ Sometimes have serious side-effects due to prostaglandin inhibition.

Celecoxib

- ▶ Commonly used for joint and muscular conditions, such as arthritis.
- ▶ Like other NSAIDs may cause serious stomach and intestinal ulcers.

→

Aspirin

▶ Versatile drug.
▶ Blocks COX1.
▶ Is a weak acid that is well absorbed in the stomach.
▶ Should not be given to children.
▶ Causes many side-effects.
▶ Serious in overdose.

Histamine

▶ Found in high concentrations in the lungs, skin and GI tract.
▶ Released by mast cells.
▶ Brings about vasodilation and increased permeability.

Antihistamines

▶ Block action of histamine.
▶ Modify inflammatory response.
▶ Some are used to treat motion sickness, others for allergic responses.
▶ Some have more sedating effects than others.
▶ Side-effects include dryness of mouth, blurred vision, constipation and retention of urine.

Steroids

▶ Produced naturally by the adrenal cortex.
▶ Involved in the body's response to stress.
▶ Effect metabolism of fats, carbohydrates and proteins.
▶ Steroid hormones also affect certain electrolytes (e.g. calcium and sodium).
▶ Giving replacement steroids causes atrophy of the adrenal gland.
▶ Steroids are powerful anti-inflammatory agents.
▶ Have a direct action on all cells involved in the inflammatory response.
▶ Have many side-effects.
▶ May be given by several routes.
▶ Can cause secondary diabetes and hypertension.
▶ Can cause osteoporosis and fractures.
▶ Can cause infection to go undetected and wounds not to heal.
▶ Patients must carry a card and have good discharge advice.

Anti-rheumatoid drugs

▶ Rheumatoid arthritis is an autoimmune condition.
▶ Drugs used in its treatment are called disease-modifying anti-rheumatoid drugs (DMARDs).
▶ These drugs improve patients' lives by reducing swelling and tenderness in the joints.

- ▶ Examples are methotrexate, penicillamine and gold.
- ▶ Often patients have no improvement in symptoms until a few months into treatment.
- ▶ Side-effects are serious and may lead to the patient discontinuing treatment

Calculations

1. A doctor has prescribed 30mg of prednisolone. You have 5mg tablets on the ward. How many should you give?

2. 5mg of prednisolone is equivalent to 20mg of hydrocortisone. How many 5mg prednisolone tablets is equivalent to a dose of 100mg of hydrocortisone?

3. A 3-year-old who weighs 13.5kg has been prescribed ibuprofen 5mg per kg three times daily. Ibuprofen is available as a suspension of 100mg in 5mL. How much should the child receive on each occasion?

4. The doctor prescribes a patient nefopam 60mg. This drug is available as 30mg tablets. How many do you give the patient?

5. A patient requires 85mg of cortisone. The stock ampoule is 100mg in 5mL. How much volume is required?

6. The doctor prescribes a patient 1g of paracetamol. The tablets come in 500mg. How many tablets will you give?

7. A child weighing 30kg is prescribed 60mg per kg per day of paracetamol to be given every 6 hours. What is the size of each dose?

8. Methylprednisolone 60mg is to be given by IM injection. The solution available is 80mg in 1mL. How much do you draw up?

9. The qualified nurse on the ward has to prepare hydrocortisone 400mg for IV injection. She has ampoules consisting of a solution 250mg in 2mL. How many mL will she draw up for you to check?

10. Phenergan 25mg IM is prescribed for a patient. The stock on the ward is 50mg in 1mL. How much fluid do you draw into the syringe?

Multiple-choice questions

Try answering these multiple-choice questions to test what you have learned from reading this chapter. You can check your answers at the end of this book.

1. **The role of histamine in the inflammatory response is ...**

a) To attract white blood cells to the area of inflammation
b) To increase the amount of neutrophils being produced
c) To produce immunoglobulins
d) To produce vasodilation and increase permeability of blood vessels

2. **In chronic inflammation, what type of cells are found at the site of injury?**

a) Lymphocytes
b) Neutrophils
c) Macrophages
d) Erythrocytes

3. **Why do NSAIDs affect kidney function?**

a) Because they are excreted by the kidneys
b) Because they cause widespread vasodilation
c) Because they interfere with normal homeostatic functions of prostaglandins
d) Because they are toxic to the kidney tubules

4. **Why would you not give aspirin to children?**

a) Because it could cause problems with the liver and brain
b) Because it is not effective in children
c) Because it damages children's kidneys
d) Because the drug has been superseded by modern drugs

5. **Steroid hormones are produced by ...**

a) The hypothalamus
b) The adrenal glands
c) The thymus gland
d) The spleen

6. **Steroids may cause secondary hypertension because ...**

a) They lower calcium levels
b) They cause glycogen to break down to glucose
c) They retain sodium
d) They retain potassium

$\longrightarrow$

←

7. **Why should steroid drugs not suddenly be discontinued?**

a) Because only a consultant physician can do this
b) Because this should only be carried out in hospital
c) The body becomes tolerant to the drug
d) The body needs time to recover its natural steroid-making capacity

8. **Which of the following is a DMARD?**

a) Prostacyclin
b) Penicillin
c) Penicillamine
d) Paracetamol

9. **What is usually the drug of choice in treating rheumatoid arthritis?**

a) Gold compounds
b) Methotrexate
c) Sulfasalazine
d) Chloroquine

10. **What is the mode of action of DMARDs?**

a) Mostly it is unknown
b) They promote secretion of steroid hormones
c) They inhibit stem cell production
d) They inhibit action of white cells

Recommended further reading

Barber, P. (ed.) (2013) *Medicine Management for Nurses Case Book.* Maidenhead: Open University Press.

Downie, G., Mackenzie, J. and Williams, A. (2007) *Pharmacology and Medicines Management for Nurses,* 4th edition. Edinburgh: Churchill Livingstone.

Greenstein, B. and Gould, D. (2008) *Trounce's Clinical Pharmacology for Nurses,* 18th edition. New York: Churchill Livingstone.

Karch, A.M. (2017) *Focus on Nursing Pharmacology,* 7th edition. Philadelphia, PA: Lippincott Williams & Wilkins.

Lapham, R. (2015) *Drug Calculations for Nurses: A Step-by-Step Approach,* 4th edition. London: Arnold.

Simonson, T., Aarbakke, J., Kay, I., Coleman, I., Sinnott, P. and Lyssa, R. (2006) *Illustrated Pharmacology for Nurses.* London: Hodder Arnold.

Anticoagulant therapy

7

Chapter contents

Learning objectives

After studying this chapter, you should be able to:

- Describe the four processes involved in normal blood clotting.
- List the factors that increase the likelihood of thrombosis occurring.
- Describe what is meant by the term acute coronary syndromes.
- Identify at least six drugs that act on the clotting cascade.
- Compare the modes of action of aspirin, heparin and warfarin.
- List the drugs that would be used to reverse the effects of heparin and warfarin.
- Define what is meant by the term 'international normalized ratio'.
- Describe the information given to a patient who is taking anticoagulant therapy, in particular warfarin.
- Demonstrate an understanding of fibrinolytic drugs and suggest in which circumstances they may be given.
- Identify a circumstance when a fibrinolytic drug would be contraindicated.
- Correctly solve several drug calculations about anticoagulant therapy.

Introduction

Blood clotting is a normal homeostatic mechanism, the purpose of which is to prevent the loss of blood from the cardiovascular system and to ensure that blood vessels remain intact. This mechanism works very well in preventing haemorrhage from smaller blood vessels (e.g. capillaries, arterioles and venules). However, the mechanism is overwhelmed if bleeding occurs from the large vessels such as major veins or arteries. If such bleeding occurs, interventions from a first aid, medical or surgical perspective must be employed to control the bleeding.

The word used for stopping bleeding or haemorrhage from the body is *haemostasis* and, as stated above, is a normal homeostatic function of the body. The blood and damaged blood vessels release factors that work together to form a plug of solid matter which blocks the tear in the blood vessel. Haemostasis is divided into four processes:

Constriction of the blood vessel

Following the tearing of a blood vessel, the body reflexively constricts the size of the vessel, which also leads to the contraction of the severed ends. The constriction of vessels spreads to affect other local small vessels. The blood flow through these small vessels is now reduced and this allows the platelets and the plasma to contact the damaged area of the blood vessel. When this occurs, the body is setting in motion a state of events, the first being a reduction in the likelihood of the plug of platelets being washed away.

Formation of a platelet plug

Damage to the wall of a blood vessel exposes proteins within the vessel wall. These are collagen and elastin fibres and lie underneath the thin inside layer of the vessel. The exposure of these important proteins causes platelets to adhere to the site of injury. Adhesion of the platelets to themselves and the site of injury is further helped by one of the *plasma clotting factors* called factor VIII.

The process of platelet adhesion is reversible up to a point. Once the platelets have released the granules which they contain, white blood cells begin to stick to the platelets. During this build-up of the foundation of the clot, the platelets also release a substance known as thromboxane (TXA). This has two effects: first, it increases the ability of the cells to stick together; second, it makes the blood vessel smaller through vasoconstriction. At this point, the cells that have been exposed under the intima lining of the blood vessels start to produce a substance known as prostacyclin. This works in the opposite way to thromboxane in that it stimulates vasodilation and stops the cells sticking together. This is an important point, as certain drugs are given to affect the balance between thromboxane and prostacyclin (e.g. dipyridamole and aspirin).

As the platelet cells continue to stick together, they release a platelet factor that acts as a platform on which various blood clotting factors can bind. The foundation is now secured for the next process to begin.

Formation of the fibrin/blood clot

This process involves an insoluble protein called *fibrin*, which plugs the tear in the vessel wall. Insoluble fibrin lays down a mesh of white fibres which stick to each other and to tissue cells. This mesh traps other blood cells and more platelets. The clot gradually constricts, squeezing out any serum and leaving a solid but elastic plug.

To achieve this outcome, the blood and platelets must go through a complex chain reaction. Each phase of this reaction is brought about by what are called 'plasma clotting factors' (always referred to using Roman numerals – see Table 7.1).

This cascade of events can be triggered in two distinct ways. First, damaged cells release a substance called *thromboplastin* or factor III. As thromboplastin is not part of the blood, this blood clotting pathway is known as the *extrinsic pathway*. The extrinsic pathway is therefore triggered by events such as physical injury to the blood vessels. The second trigger involves contact of the blood with exposed collagen fibres, which are not usually exposed since they lie under the inner surface of the blood vessel. However, if damage occurs to this delicate lining, collagen fibres meet blood products and the clotting cascade mechanism

Factor	Name
I	Fibrinogen
II	Prothrombin
III	Tissue factor
IV	Calcium
V	Proaccelerin
VII	Stabilizing factor
VIII	Antihemophilic factor A
IX	Christmas factor
X (a)	Stuart-Prower factor
XI	Plasma thromboplastin antecedent
XII	Hageman factor
XIII	Fibrin stabilizing factor

Table 7.1   Plasma clotting factors (adapted from Barmore and Burns 2019)

commences. This set of events is known as the *intrinsic pathway*. The triggering of the extrinsic pathway occurs with pathological states such as atherosclerosis (fatty deposits being laid down in the walls of arteries).

The key step in both systems is activation of a plasma factor called factor X. These systems work together to ensure that the body produces large enough amounts of thrombin to be effective in stemming blood loss.

A point to remember here is that the blood is thought to contain natural inhibitors of the clotting factors. These inhibitors are believed to stop widespread clotting from taking place, thus localizing events. The best known of these natural anticoagulants is *antithrombin III*.

Dissolving of the fibrin clot

Dissolving of a clot takes place much more slowly than does the building of one and the slow removal of the clot is part of life's normal process. Fibrin is dissolved by a substance called *plasmin*. This product is not normally present in the plasma but is derived from an inactive protein called *plasmin*ogen. Plasminogen can be activated by a number of triggers, including plasma clotting factor VII, red, white and certain renal cells. The

body has natural plasmin inhibitors, such as *antiplasmin*. These ensure that widespread destruction of fibrin does not take place.

Blood clotting and the development of thrombosis

Thrombosis is the formation of a clot in a vessel within the cardiovascular system, which relates to or arises from a disease process. There are three factors that increase the likelihood of thrombosis:

1. injury to the vessel wall;
2. altered blood flow;
3. increased likelihood of the blood to clot.

For example, people who have developed fatty plaques, who are physically immobile or who are being treated with certain contraceptives are more at risk of developing thrombosis. Thrombosis can occur in both arteries and veins. In arteries, the clot is usually associated with a build-up of fatty plaques (atherosclerosis) and has a large platelet component. Veins, in contrast, are usually associated with slow flow of blood through the vessels and there is a large fibrin component. Due to the make-up of the venous thrombosis, the clot has a large jelly-like tail that floats in the vessel. If this breaks off, it becomes an 'embolus', which may lodge in smaller vessels, resulting in the death of tissue.

There are three categories of drugs that affect blood clotting and the formation of thrombosis:

1. drugs that affect fibrin formation;
2. drugs that affect platelet function;
3. drugs that affect dissolving of the clot.

Acute coronary syndromes

Acute coronary syndromes (ACS) arise from narrowing of the blood vessels that supply the heart. This narrowing is caused by atheroma, which builds up within the lining of the artery so that the space inside (lumen) becomes diminished. Atheroma is a fatty (lipid) substance that occurs in patches within the vessel; these patches are usually referred to as plaques. These plaques of atheroma form gradually over several years in one or more places in the coronary arteries. Each plaque has a similar presentation: a soft inner fatty centre with a firm outer shell.

The narrowing in the coronary vessel as a result of these fatty deposits causes a sudden reduction in the blood flow to the heart. The signs and symptoms of ACS include chest pain, which some patients describe as a feeling of pressure in their chest rather than a pain, while others describe it as a central crushing pain. Some patients will experience this type of chest pain even when they are at rest or doing light physical activity, and this is known as unstable angina. Indeed, the first sign of acute coronary syndrome can be a sudden stopping of the heart (myocardial infarction).

ACS refers to a group of signs and symptoms caused by this decreased blood flow in the coronary arteries and subsequent effects on the cardiac muscle. This spectrum of clinical presentations includes changes on a patient's electrocardiogram ranging from ST-segment elevation myocardial infarction (STEMI) to presentations found in non–ST-segment elevation myocardial infarction (NSTEMI) or in unstable angina. As we have indicated, ST elevations refer to a finding on an electrocardiogram, wherein the trace in the ST segment is abnormally far above what is known as the isoelectric line. The elevation of the ST-segment signals that a rupture of an atherosclerotic plaque and partial or complete thrombosis of the infarct-related artery has occurred. However, as with any medical condition, one must proceed with caution, as you may come across patients who do not report any chest pain, particularly elderly and diabetic patients.

Because of the risk of thrombosis in patients who have atheroma, antiplatelet and anticoagulant therapy are key in treating ACS; the National Institute for Health and Care Excellence (NICE) has incorporated this therapy into treatment pathways and quality standards (NICE 2014b).

Drugs that act on the clotting cascade

Drugs in this category can be used to manipulate the cascade system when there is a defect in the process of clotting, or when unwanted coagulation has taken place. Fortunately, deficiencies in clotting factors rarely occur. However, two examples need to be mentioned here: haemophilia A, caused by lack of factor VIII and 'Christmas' disease or haemophilia B, caused by lack of factor IX or the 'Christmas' factor (named after Stephen Christmas, the first patient to be diagnosed). These missing factors can be replaced by either giving fresh plasma or giving concentrated preparations of factors VIII and IX. Other problems that lead to an inability of the cascade mechanism to produce clotting are acquired. These tend to be more common in origin and include liver diseases, vitamin K deficiency (especially in neonates) and excessive prescription of oral anticoagulants. These three situations require the person to be administered vitamin K.

Vitamin K

This vitamin takes its 'K' from the German word 'Koagulation'. It occurs naturally in plants and is essential for the plasma clotting factors we discussed earlier. It is particularly important for the formation of factors II, VII, IX and X.

Naturally occurring vitamin K or *phytomenadiole* can be given by mouth or by IV infusion. If given orally, its absorption will rely on the person's digestive system being normal, as it is necessary for *bile salts* to be produced and excreted into the duodenum. However, if this is not the case, such as in obstructive jaundice, a synthetic preparation is available that does not require these bile salts in order to be absorbed into the body. This drug is known as *menadiol sodium phosphate*. Vitamin K is used clinically in a range of situations, including:

- overdose with warfarin;
- in babies to prevent haemorrhagic disease;
- in diseases that cause vitamin K deficiency.

Heparin (unfractionated)

Heparin is a complex protein found in the liver and mast cells. It is comprised of many chains of varying molecular weights. It is a powerful anticoagulant but is broken down by digestive enzymes, and thus it is given by IV infusion. Heparin results in anticoagulation of blood both inside and outside the blood vessels. It works by activating antithrombin III. Antithrombin III is a naturally occurring anticoagulant in the body and heparin accelerates its rate of action significantly. This in turn stops the cascade at the thrombin stage, so inhibiting the fibrinogen-to-fibrin stage of blood clotting from taking place.

Heparin acts immediately following IV administration and its elimination half-life is approximately 40–90 minutes. In emergency cases, therefore, it is usually given by a bolus dose, followed by a constant rate infusion via a pump mechanism. It is important that the patient is not given too much heparin, or they will haemorrhage.

Clinical tip

The main concern when administering heparin is haemorrhage. This often appears as blood in the urine (haematuria) but bleeding from other sites should also be treated seriously. Early signs of a problem include ease of bruising. If bleeding does occur, the therapy should be stopped immediately and, if necessary, the patient should be given protamine sulphate, which reverses the action of heparin.

A rare complication of heparin is a decrease in the number of circulating platelets (thrombocytopenia). The patient's platelet count should be ascertained if they remain on heparin therapy for more than 5 days. This can be done by measuring the activated partial plasma thrombin time (aPPT test). Osteoporosis has been reported in people who have been receiving long-term administration of heparin, although why this occurs remains unclear.

Low molecular weight heparins

These are a form of heparin but instead of comprising many chains of varying molecular weight, 60% of their chains are of a lower molecular weight. This group of drugs can be given subcutaneously and can be administered by the patient, a carer or health care professional in the home setting. They also need to be given less frequently than heparin.

Low molecular weight heparins can be given to lessen the risk of thrombosis developing post-surgery (prophylaxis). They are given via the SC route until the patient can mobilize well. They are effective in treating deep vein thrombosis and pulmonary embolism and as they do not cross the placental barrier, they can be used in pregnancy. Drugs in this group include tinzaparin, enoxaparin and dalteparin. Although bleeding can occur, these drugs are less likely than heparin to cause thrombocytopenia.

These drugs bind to and accelerate the activity of antithrombin III. By activating antithrombin III, they speed up the inhibition of coagulation factors Xa (Stuart-Prower) and IIa (prothrombin), where 'a' stands for 'activated'. The anticoagulant effect can be directly related to their ability to inhibit factor Xa. Factor Xa initiates the conversion of prothrombin to thrombin, so the drugs' inhibition of this process results in decreased thrombin and ultimately the prevention of fibrin clot formation.

Clinical tip

Before using a low molecular weight heparin, check it visually for particles or discoloration. If either is present, do not use the drug. To minimize irritation, change the injection site with each dose. To minimize bruising, do not rub the site after injection.

Mild irritation, pain, bruising, redness or swelling at the injection site may occur and the patient should be reassured that this is not unusual. Inform them that fatigue or fever may also occur and that if these effects persist or worsen, they should notify their doctor or pharmacist promptly. Although most people on this medication do not suffer serious side-effects, it can cause bleeding if its effect on blood clotting proteins is too great. The patient should tell their doctor immediately if any of the following unlikely but serious signs occur: unusual pain, swelling, discomfort, unusual or prolonged bleeding, unusual or 'easy' bruising, dark urine, black stools, severe headache, confusion, vision changes, dizziness, fainting, seizures, weakness or numbness. Dose reductions may be required in patients with hepatic impairment and this group of anticoagulants may be less suitable than unfractionated heparins in patients with renal impairment.

Hirudin

This anticoagulant is a naturally occurring protein found in the salivary glands of medicinal leeches. Rather than potentiating the effects of antithrombin III, hirudin is a specific inhibitor of thrombin. Analogues can now be produced synthetically by recombinant techniques. The drug bivalirudin is an analogue used in unstable angina and in the management of ST segment elevation myocardial infarction.

Coumarins

The coumarins (warfarin, acenocoumarol and phenindione) antagonize the action of vitamin K and so reduce the production of prothrombin and clotting factors VII, IX and X. The onset of action of warfarin takes several days, as the plasma factors that have been manufactured prior to commencement of warfarin take time before they are eliminated from the body.

Warfarin is the most common oral anticoagulant and is given in tablet form, as it is easily absorbed by the GI tract. One of the problems with warfarin is that it is strongly attracted to plasma proteins. These proteins normally help maintain the osmotic intravascular pressure. However, as warfarin is bound to these, potential problems occur with stabilizing the dose, treating elderly people and giving other drugs, such as aspirin, that compete for binding sites on the plasma proteins. The peak pharmacological concentration takes approximately 48 hours. The effectiveness of the drug is measured by a blood test known as the *prothrombin time*, now expressed as an international normalized ratio or INR. This laboratory test measures the time it takes for blood to clot

and compares it to an average. The higher the INR value, the longer it takes for blood to clot.

Clinical tip

While taking warfarin, patients will have regular blood tests to establish their INR. For patients diagnosed with atrial fibrillation, the target INR typically should be between 2.0 and 3.0. Patients who have been fitted with mechanical heart valves should have an INR around 3.0 or 4.0.

Warfarin crosses the placenta and therefore should not be given in the first 3 months of pregnancy, as fetal abnormalities may ensue. Intracranial bleeding in the baby may occur during delivery and mothers should be immediately offered prophylaxis with vitamin K.

As with heparin, the most obvious side-effect is bleeding. This may be due to deliberate or accidental overdose or to the interaction of warfarin with other drugs leading to an increase in its anticoagulant effect. If bleeding does occur, the drug should be withdrawn. The anticoagulant effects may be reversed by giving fresh frozen plasma or vitamin K (phytomenadione) intravenously.

A complication of warfarin is a condition referred to as calciphylaxis, which occurs when calcium collects in the small vessels in the skin and produces painful rashes, blood clots and sores. This may seem paradoxical, as warfarin is given for its anticoagulant effect. The MHRA/CHM issued a warning about this in 2016 after an increase in reports of its occurrence and the likelihood of it developing in patients with renal disease.

A variety of disease processes and drugs can modify the action of warfarin. Some potentiate the anticoagulant actions, while others lessen the effect of the drug. Liver disease, thyrotoxicosis and fever may all interfere with the natural manufacture of clotting factors by the body. If warfarin is given in these circumstances, there will be an increase in anticoagulation. Some drugs can also lead to exaggerated anticoagulant effects if given in conjunction with warfarin. Drugs such as cimetidine can reduce the breakdown of warfarin by liver enzymes. NSAIDs compete successfully with warfarin for a place on plasma proteins, therefore leaving more active drugs in the plasma. Antibiotics are another group of drugs that need careful thought before prescribing because broad spectrum antibiotics and some sulfonamides depress the body's natural ability to manufacture vitamin K by intestinal flora.

Anticoagulant effects can also be lessened in some circumstances. Hypothyroidism is associated with a slower breakdown of coagulation factors. Foods and commercially produced preparations containing high vitamin K content will reduce the warfarin effect. Also, drugs that cause the enzymes in the liver that break down warfarin to increase, such as carbamazepine, will have the same effect. Warfarin is a complex drug that needs to be monitored carefully, and good discharge advice is crucial.

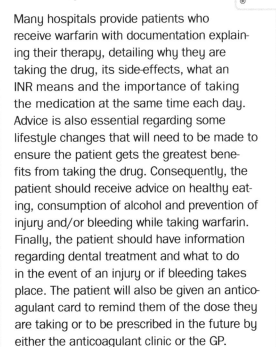

Clinical tip

Many hospitals provide patients who receive warfarin with documentation explaining their therapy, detailing why they are taking the drug, its side-effects, what an INR means and the importance of taking the medication at the same time each day. Advice is also essential regarding some lifestyle changes that will need to be made to ensure the patient gets the greatest benefits from taking the drug. Consequently, the patient should receive advice on healthy eating, consumption of alcohol and prevention of injury and/or bleeding while taking warfarin. Finally, the patient should have information regarding dental treatment and what to do in the event of an injury or if bleeding takes place. The patient will also be given an anticoagulant card to remind them of the dose they are taking or to be prescribed in the future by either the anticoagulant clinic or the GP.

Antiplatelet drugs

Earlier in this chapter we discussed the importance of the formation of a platelet plug in haemostasis. Drugs that affect this important process have strong therapeutic value. Probably the most common and popular in this category is aspirin.

Aspirin

In discussing the platelet plug, we highlighted two important substances that work in opposing ways on the stickiness of blood. These are thromboxane, which increases the stickiness and prostacyclin, which decreases the stickiness. Aspirin alters the fine balance between these two prostaglandins. It reduces both substances in the body but because prostacyclin can be made by endothelial cells and thromboxane levels require 7–10 days for new platelets to be formed, prostacyclin levels are improved at the expense of thromboxane. Therefore, an anticoagulant effect is achieved. Aspirin does have a few serious side-effects, but these are limited as it is given at a low dose for its anticoagulant effect. A dose of 75mg daily is sufficient to achieve anticoagulation, as opposed to a dose of 300mg daily which would be prescribed in its role as an analgesic. Aspirin may be given for a number of conditions, including coronary thrombosis, angina and following transient ischaemic attacks or stroke.

Clopidogrel

This is a powerful antiplatelet medicine used for a variety of conditions, including coronary artery disease, peripheral vascular disease and cerebrovascular disease.

The drug works by blocking receptor sites on the platelets. This means that when fibrin is formed it cannot stick to the platelet, and so the plug to block bleeding does not occur as the platelets cannot clump together. It is sometimes used alongside aspirin.

Clopidogrel can be given orally and is normally prescribed at 75mg once per day. It is a pro-drug activated by the liver when it first passes through. Once the drug has been activated, its elimination half-life is 8 hours. The drug reaches a peak level in the blood after one hour. It should be used with caution in patients with renal or hepatic impairment.

Clinical tip

Haemorrhage is by far the most common side-effect of this class of drug. You should ask the patient to report any unusual bleeding or bruising. Another side-effect is neutropenia (low level of a type of white blood cell called a neutrophil in the bloodstream). Therefore, you should encourage the patient to contact their doctor if they experience fever, signs of infection or extreme tiredness.

Fibrinolytic drugs

These drugs mimic the body's own ability to dissolve blood clots. A number of drugs are used in practice that dissolve clots in order to allow free passage of blood back to an area that has been starved of blood (i.e. ischaemic). Their main use is in patients who have had acute myocardial infarction following blockages of the coronary artery, but these can also be given to patients who have had an ischaemic stroke caused by thrombus formation.

Clinical tip

In practice, you will often hear fibrinolytic drugs referred to as 'clot busters'.

Streptokinase

This drug is used to dissolve the fibrin of blood clots, especially those that occur in the heart and lungs. Acute myocardial infarction results from blockage of a coronary artery, which results in an area of heart muscle being deprived of blood. Streptokinase is used to break down such clots in the coronary vessels.

The drug triggers the plasma protein plasminogen to liberate plasmin, which breaks down fibrin, so dissolving the clot. The drug is extracted from bacteria called *haemolytic streptococci*. It has a short half-life of less than 20 minutes and is therefore given by continuous IV infusion. Most people will have developed antibodies to streptococcal proteins, so often a large bolus dose is used to start therapy, followed by a maintenance infusion. As antibodies form against the streptococcal proteins, it is usually best not to provide a further treatment with the drug until a year has elapsed. Also, due to the body's immune response, other drugs, such as chlorphenamine or hydrocortisone, may be given to reduce any allergic response.

Clinical tip

The main risk of streptokinase is haemorrhage. This normally occurs near the injection site or a site of recent trauma. You must constantly monitor the site of administration and document any untoward signs and symptoms. It is contraindicated in patients in whom it may cause bleeding, such as those with peptic ulcer. Therefore, it is important to ask the patient about their past medical history before administration of this drug.

Alteplase

This drug is derived from human tissue plasminogen activator, and thus directly converts plasminogen to plasmin. It binds strongly with fibrin and digests clots in coronary arteries at least as well if not better than streptokinase. It has the advantages of not causing immune responses and, having a greater attraction to fibrin-bound plasminogen rather than circulating plasma fibrinogen, is said to be 'clot selective'. As with streptokinase, the drug has a short half-life and is therefore given by IV infusion. Although alteplase is less likely to cause bleeding, it is contraindicated in pregnancy, uncontrolled hypertension, haemorrhagic cerebrovascular disease and active internal bleeding. If bleeding occurs, it can be treated with tranexamic acid. This stops plasminogen activation and therefore prevents clots dissolving. The patient may also be given fresh plasma or coagulation factors.

Direct acting anticoagulant drugs (DOACs)

Rivaroxaban and apixaban are members of the class of drugs known as oral factor Xa inhibitors. By inhibiting factor Xa, thrombin production and the formation of clots are ultimately inhibited. Currently, these drugs are licensed for the prevention of venous thromboembolism (VTE) in adults undergoing elective hip or knee replacement surgery, at a fixed dose of 10mg daily. They can also be used for treatment of deep vein thrombosis (DVT), and pulmonary embolism as well as in ACS.

These drugs have predictable pharmacokinetics, with little variation of plasma concentration with age, weight or renal function following a fixed dose. With a fixed dose, a wide therapeutic window, few drug interactions and predictable pharmacodynamics, no routine monitoring of coagulation parameters is required. They are well absorbed from the gut and maximum inhibition of factor Xa occurs 4 hours after a dose. The effects last 8–12 hours, but factor Xa activity does not return to normal within 24 hours, so once-daily dosing is possible.

The anticoagulant dabigatran is a member of the class of drugs known as direct thrombin inhibitors. It offers an alternative to warfarin as an orally administered anticoagulant, since it does not require frequent blood tests for INR monitoring while offering similar results in terms of efficacy.

Dabigatran is a pro-drug with no anticoagulant activity; once absorbed, it is rapidly converted by enzymes in the GI tract, blood and liver into dabigatran, a thrombin inhibitor. Although costly, dabigatran has several potential advantages over warfarin. The pharmacokinetics are quite predictable, simplifying dosing and eliminating the need for frequent blood tests and monitoring. In addition, the drug necessitates no dietary restrictions, although potential drug interactions include those with quinidine, ketoconazole, amiodarone, rifampicin and verapamil. Peak anticoagulation effects occur between 30 minutes and 2 hours after ingestion and dabigatran is primarily eliminated by the kidneys.

Case studies

① Olek Krupa is a 65-year-old widower and owns a roofing company. His aim is to retire in a couple of years' time, so he is increasingly leaving his sons to manage the business while he enjoys more golfing holidays. He lives on his own but has a wide circle of friends. He enjoys watching football and having a few pints at his local pub. He does this on a few nights or afternoons in the week. He recently visited his GP for a check-up but prior to this had not seen his doctor for a number of years. He was found to have high blood pressure, be overweight and to have a heart condition for which the GP prescribed aspirin. Further to this, he was referred to his local cardiologist, who recommended that he stop the aspirin in favour of commencing warfarin.

What advice would you give to Mr Krupa with regard to his warfarin therapy?

② Mr Patel is a 70-year-old man who has been on warfarin for some years for his atrial fibrillation. His condition had been well controlled by the warfarin and his regular blood tests had shown that his INR readings reflected a time in the therapeutic range (TTR) of 74%. He has now been referred to the surgeon by his GP since he has been displaying certain gastrointestinal signs and symptoms. Following his consultation with the consultant surgeon, he has been given a date for an endoscopic removal of colonic polyps.

- ■ What is the difference in the modes of action of warfarin and enoxaparin?
- ■ Mr Patel is anxious regarding this surgery and he asks you to tell him what will happen to his warfarin therapy before, during and after the procedure. What do you tell him?

③ Bo Wong is a 72-year-old female who has a history of osteoarthritis. She has had a right total hip replacement and is now ready for discharge. She has agreed to administer her own enoxaparin at home for 4 weeks post-operatively to prevent deep vein thrombosis formation.

Your mentor has asked you to teach the lady how to do this, so she is confident. What instructions would you give her?

Key learning points

Introduction

- ▶ Blood clotting is a normal homeostatic mechanism.
- ▶ Haemostasis is divided into four processes: constriction of blood vessel, formation of platelet plug, formation of fibrin clot and dissolving of the clot.
- ▶ Constriction of the vessel reduces blood flow.
- ▶ Constriction allows clotting factors to contact the damaged vessels.
- ▶ Formation of a platelet plug begins with exposure to collagen and elastin fibres.
- ▶ Platelets release thromboxane.
- ▶ The formation of a fibrin clot is a complex chain reaction triggered in one of two ways: extrinsically or intrinsically.
- ▶ The clot dissolves more slowly than it was formed.
- ▶ Fibrin is dissolved by plasmin.

Blood clotting and the development of thrombosis

- ▶ Thrombosis is the formation of a clot in a vessel within the cardiovascular system, which relates to or arises from a disease process.
- ▶ In arteries, the clot is usually associated with a build-up of fatty plaques (atherosclerosis).
- ▶ Acute coronary syndromes arise due to narrowing of the blood vessels supplying the heart by these fatty plaques leading to thrombus formation.

Drugs that act on the clotting cascade

Heparin

- ▶ Heparin is a complex protein that cannot be given orally.
- ▶ It works by activating antithrombin III.

→

▶ It stops the clotting cascade at the thrombin stage.
▶ The activated partial plasma thrombin time (aPPT) test is used to measure efficacy.
▶ Low molecular weight heparins are more predictable.
▶ They are given subcutaneously twice daily.
▶ Examples are tinzaparin and enoxaparin.

Enoxaparin

▶ Enoxaparin binds to and accelerates the activity of antithrombin III.
▶ The dose to prevent thromboembolism is 40mg subcutaneously once a day.
▶ The usual duration of administration is 6–11 days, but up to 14 days.
▶ To minimize irritation, use a different injection site for each dose.
▶ To minimize bruising, do not rub the injection site following administration.
▶ The patient should tell their doctor immediately if signs of bleeding occur.

Warfarin

▶ Warfarin is a vitamin K antagonist.
▶ It reduces the manufacture of a range of clotting factors.
▶ It takes several days to achieve its effects.
▶ It is highly protein bound.
▶ It is measured by the INR.
▶ Can cross placental barrier.
▶ Haemorrhage is a major side-effect.
▶ A number of disease processes and other drugs can potentiate or inhibit its action.
▶ Patients should be given detailed discharge advice.

Aspirin

▶ Aspirin alters the fine balance between thromboxane and prostacyclin.
▶ It is given in low dosages to limit side-effects.
▶ It is suitable for a number of conditions (e.g. coronary thrombosis).

Clopidogrel

▶ Stops fibrin attaching to platelets.
▶ Often given alongside low-dose aspirin.
▶ Haemorrhage is a common side-effect.

Streptokinase

▶ Dissolves fibrin.
▶ Liberates plasmin from plasminogen.
▶ One treatment is given per year.
▶ Risk of haemorrhage.

→

←

Alteplase

▶ Converts plasminogen to plasmin.
▶ Does not cause immune response like streptokinase.
▶ Has to be given intravenously.
▶ Contraindicated in pregnancy, haemorrhagic cerebrovascular disease and internal bleeding.

Direct acting anticoagulant drugs

▶ Rivaroxaban and apixaban are oral factor Xa (Stuart-Prower) inhibitors.
▶ Dabigatran is an option for primary prevention of venous thromboembolic event.

Calculations

1. A doctor orders a patient to have 25,000 international units (iu) of heparin which is to be given intravenously. On the ward you only have 5000iu of heparin in 1mL. How many mL of heparin would you give?

2. A patient has been prescribed 300mg of aspirin. You have 75mg tablets. How many would you need to administer?

3. The dose of tinzaparin for the treatment of deep vein thrombosis is 175 units per kg. The injection is 20,000 units per mL. What dose would be required to treat a 60kg patient?

4. A doctor orders heparin 9000iu to be given subcutaneously twice daily. The ward stock only consists of 10,000iu per mL. How many mL of heparin would you give?

5. Warfarin is available as 0.5mg, 1mg, 3mg and 5mg tablets. You need to administer a 7mg dose. What is the least number of tablets you can give?

6. 20,000iu of heparin is added to 500mL of 0.9% saline. The dose prescribed is 200iu per hour. Calculate the rate of the infusion in mL per hour.

7. You need to give 1mg of vitamin K orally. How many mL of a 10mg per mL vitamin K injection would you give?

8. You have been asked to prepare a heparin syringe for intravenous infusion; 40mL of solution is required, containing 500 units of heparin per mL. The heparin ampoules stocked on the ward contain 5000 units per mL. What volume of heparin and saline would be required to prepare the syringe?

9. You have a syringe of enoxaparin containing 150 mg per mL. How much is required to give a 90kg man a dose of 1.5mg per kg?

10. An anaesthetist prescribes a patient 2500iu of dalteparin sodium 2 hours prior to surgery, 2500iu 4–8 hours post-surgery and 5000iu daily for 5–10 days post-operatively. How many mL from a vial containing 10,000iu per mL should be administered: (a) prior to surgery, (b) after surgery and (c) the following day after surgery?

Multiple-choice questions

Try answering these multiple-choice questions to test what you have learned from reading this chapter. You can check your answers at the end of this book.

1. **Haemophilia A is caused by a lack of which clotting factor?**

a) Factor X
b) Factor VII
c) Factor VIII
d) Factor III

2. **Where in the body is heparin normally manufactured?**

a) Liver
b) Kidney
c) Spleen
d) Pancreas

3. **What substance does heparin activate in order to produce its anticoagulant effect?**

a) Antithrombin
b) Thromboxane
c) Prostacyclin
d) Fibrinogen

4. **What drug reverses the effects of heparin?**

a) Warfarin
b) Aspirin
c) Vitamin K
d) Protamine sulphate

5. **How does warfarin work?**

a) Decreases the amount of circulating platelets
b) Increases the amount of antithrombin
c) Antagonizes vitamin K
d) Increases the amount of prostacyclin

6. **Which of the following drugs is a low molecular weight heparin?**

a) Clopidogrel
b) Tinzaparin
c) Dipyridamole
d) Hirudin

→

7. What blood test is used to measure the effectiveness of warfarin?

a) International normalized ratio
b) International notifiable ratio
c) Internal negative report
d) Integrated notice of randomization

8. Aspirin has an effect on the balance of which two substances?

a) Thromboxane and fibrinogen
b) Prostacyclin and calcium
c) Thromboxane and prostacyclin
d) Antithrombin and thrombin

9. Which of the following is a fibrinolytic medicine?

a) Beconase
b) Lipase
c) Alteplase
d) Mono amine oxidase

10. The main mode of action of fibrinolytic drugs is to ...

a) Increase the amount of vitamin K
b) Decrease the amount of platelets
c) Decrease the amount of plasmin
d) Increase the amount of plasmin

Recommended further reading

Barmore, W. and Burns, B (2019) *Biochemistry, Clotting Factors*, StatPearls. Available at: https://www.ncbi.nlm.nih.gov/books/NBK507850/.

Downie, G., Mackenzie, J. and Williams, A. (2007) *Pharmacology and Medicines Management for Nurses*, 4th edition. Edinburgh: Churchill Livingstone.

Greenstein, B. and Gould, D. (2008) *Trounce's Clinical Pharmacology for Nurses*, 18th edition. New York: Churchill Livingstone.

Karch, A.M. (2017) *Focus on Nursing Pharmacology*, 7th edition. Philadelphia, PA: Lippincott Williams & Wilkins.

Lapham, R. (2015) *Drug Calculations for Nurses: A Step-by-Step Approach*, 4th edition. London: Arnold.

National Institute for Health and Care Excellence (NICE) (2008) *Technology Appraisal TA157: Dabigatran Etexilate for the Prevention of Venous Thromboembolism after Hip or Knee Replacement Surgery in Adults*. London: NICE.

National Institute for Health and Care Excellence (NICE) (2009) *Technology Appraisal TA170: Rivaroxaban for the Prevention of Venous Thromboembolism after Total Hip or Knee Replacement in Adults*. London: NICE.

National Institute for Health and Care Excellence (NICE) (2013) *Clinical Guideline CG172: Myocardial Infarction: Cardiac Rehabilitation and Prevention of Further Cardiovascular Disease*. London: NICE.

National Institute for Health and Care Excellence (NICE) (2014a) *Clinical Guideline CG180: Atrial Fibrillation: Management*. London: NICE.

National Institute for Health and Care Excellence (NICE) (2014b) *Quality Standard QS68: Acute Coronary Syndrome in Adults*. London NICE.

Simonson, T., Aarbakke, J., Kay, I., Coleman, I., Sinnott, P. and Lyssa, R. (2006) *Illustrated Pharmacology for Nurses*. London: Hodder Arnold.

Drugs for respiratory conditions

8

Chapter contents

Learning objectives

After studying this chapter, you should be able to:

- Describe the basic pathology involved in asthma and COPD.
- Explain the mode of action of medicines used in treating these conditions.
- Demonstrate an understanding of the unwanted effects of medicines used in treating these conditions.
- Discuss the correct technique involved when teaching a person to use an inhaler.
- Demonstrate an understanding of the links between the pharmacology of therapies used in treating respiratory conditions and the care given by the health practitioner.

Introduction

Many chronic diseases are brought about by demographic, environmental and lifestyle changes and the chronic conditions of the respiratory system are a good example of this. This chapter will look at asthma and chronic obstructive pulmonary disease (COPD), as these constitute most diagnoses of respiratory conditions.

Asthma

Asthma is the leading chronic disease in developed countries and its incidence is increasing. Asthma UK reports that there are 5.4 million people currently living in the UK with asthma. Asthma has also been responsible for around 1200 deaths per year in England and Wales since 2001. This is based on information retrieved from the Office of National Statistics) death registrations summary of 2016 (ONS 2017). The condition is characterized by a reversible obstruction of the airways, which, in turn, causes the individual to become breathless and start to cough or wheeze. Asthma can be acute or chronic. Severe acute asthma (known as *status asthmaticus*) is not reversed very easily and, as a result, continues to be fatal and requires prompt treatment. Chronic asthma usually has an intermittent pattern of breathlessness (dyspnoea), coughing and wheezing.

In acute asthma, the main reason for obstruction of the airways is *bronchoconstriction*. Further significant obstruction of the airways is brought about by inflammatory changes in the mucosa, which cause an increase in mucous production, more epithelial cells being shed and swelling of the tissues within the respiratory passages.

Symptoms

Asthma symptoms are thought to be caused by hyper-reactivity or hyper-responsiveness of the cells lining the air passages. It seems that bronchiolar tissue in some individuals is more sensitive to certain trigger factors than in others. Trigger factors differ from person to person and include irritant chemicals, exposure to foreign proteins called allergens, dust and/or dust mites, and cold air. The British Lung Foundation (2019a) provides useful and medically reviewed information on the causes and triggers of asthma.

Symptoms typically include:

- cough;
- wheezing;
- shortness of breath;
- tightness of the chest.

Numerous cells and chemicals play a part in the changes that take place in the tissues of a person with asthma. This pathophysiology is complex and can involve many structures and mediators.

Pathological changes in asthma

The changes in the respiratory system that bring about asthma are the result of an antigen triggering the immune response. This results in the stimulation of *T-lymphocytes*, a type of white cell. These T cells (known as T-helper cells) stimulate the release of cytokines and interleukin production and release, which is responsible for the inflammation (Kudo et al. 2013).

Another specific group of white cells thought to be involved in asthma are the *eosinophils*. These cells are implicated in the inflammatory response triggered by T-cell activation and cause the release of a range of chemicals that contribute to the contraction of bronchial smooth muscle, permeability of small blood vessels and excessive secretion of mucous. It is also suggested that the eosinophils produce chemicals that have a toxic effect on the epithelial lining of the airways and are responsible for the excessive epithelial shedding associated with this condition (Possa et al. 2013).

Macrophages are a type of bacteria-engulfing cell or phagocyte which have a protective function. However, in asthma these cells are responsible for releasing pro-inflammatory cytokines, leukotrienes and interleukins, which sustain the bronchial hyperactivity (Fricker and Gibson 2017). This is thought to occur by increasing mucosal oedema, facilitating the number of eosinophils in the airway tissues.

The swelling of the local tissues from oedema is compounded by extra mucous production. Mucous is part of our general defence strategy in that it provides us with a mechanism to trap particles

Normal airway   Asthmatic airway   Airway during attack

Figure 8.1   Airway lumen sizes

and bacteria and clear them from the upper respiratory tract. However, in asthma the size of the bronchial glands and goblet cells is increased, and they subsequently produce large amounts of mucous that is thickened by cell debris from the epithelial shedding. The cilia that normally move debris towards the pharynx also have their capability curtailed, contributing to the overall narrowing of the air passages (see Figure 8.1).

Asthma in children

Asthma is the leading cause of chronic illness in children. It affects as many as 1 in 11 children in the UK and the UK has one of the highest prevalence rates in the world (Asthma UK 2019). It can begin at any age, but most children have their first symptoms by age 5. Children still die from asthma – there were 13 recorded deaths in 2016 in England and Wales (ONS 2017) – and there is still significant disability associated with the disease, particularly severe childhood asthma, despite pharmacological advances.

There are many risk factors for developing childhood asthma, including:

- presence of allergies;
- family history of asthma and/or allergies;
- frequent respiratory infections;
- low birth weight or prematurity;
- exposure to tobacco smoke before and/or after birth;
- link to atopic conditions such as eczema (NHS 2019).

The diagnosis of asthma in children is difficult because of the complex nature of the disorder in the young. In an adult, a wheeze is a very important sign in the diagnosis of asthma; in children, however, there are many different causes of wheezing. In addition, children younger than 5 are generally unable to perform pulmonary function tests with the result that those involved in diagnosis rely heavily on history, symptoms and medical examination.

Most asthma medications that are given to adults and older children can also safely be prescribed to toddlers and younger children. Drugs that are approved for younger children are given in doses adjusted for their age and weight. In the case of inhaled drugs, a different delivery device based on the child's age and ability may be required because many children are not able to coordinate their breathing well enough to use a standard inhaler.

Clinical tip

While on placement, you may be asked to give a child their inhaled asthma medication using a nebulizer. A nebulizer delivers asthma drugs, usually bronchodilators, by changing them from a liquid to a mist. The child gets the drug by breathing it in through a facemask. These breathing treatments usually take 10–15 minutes and are given several times a day. Children may be able to use a metered dose inhaler (MDI) with a spacer. A spacer is a chamber that attaches to the MDI and holds the burst of medication (see Figure 8.2).

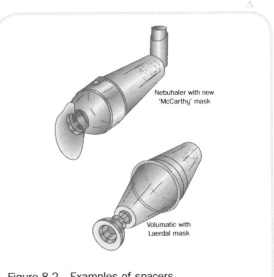

Nebuhaler with new 'McCarthy' mask

Volumatic with Laerdal mask

Figure 8.2   Examples of spacers

Drugs used in treating asthma

There are two basic drug groups given to patients who have asthma: *bronchodilators* and *anti-inflammatory agents*. They are not mutually exclusive, i.e. some bronchodilators may have an effect on inflammatory cells. Drugs and their use are outlined in the BTS/SIGN Guidance of 2016. For adults, the stepwise progression can be seen in Box 8.1 and for children in Box 8.2.

Beta 2 adrenoreceptor agonists

These drugs are referred to as *bronchodilators*. They open the air passages by directly activating beta receptors, relaxing the smooth muscle in the walls of the bronchioles. This allows a more normal movement of air between the atmosphere and the alveoli. This group of drugs is available in both short- and long-acting forms. An example of a short-acting form in this class is salbutamol and it is the one you will encounter most often.

Box 8.1 Summary of management of asthma in adults

Steps	Actions
Regular preventer	Low-dose inhaled corticosteroid
Initial add-on preventer	Low-dose inhaled corticosteroid
	PLUS
	Long-acting beta 2 agonist often in a combination preparation
Additional add-on therapies	IF no response to long-acting beta 2 agonist, STOP and consider increased dose of inhaled corticosteroid
	IF benefit seen from long-acting beta 2 agonist but control still inadequate, continue long-acting beta 2 agonist and increase inhaled corticosteroid to medium dose
	IF benefit seen from long-acting beta 2 agonist but control still inadequate, continue long-acting beta 2 agonist and inhaled corticosteroid and consider trial of leukotriene receptor antagonist OR slow-release theophylline OR long-acting muscarinic antagonists
High-dose therapies	Consider trials of increasing inhaled corticosteroid up to high dose
	Add a fourth drug leukotriene receptor antagonist OR slow-release theophylline OR long-acting muscarinic antagonist OR beta agonist tablet
	Refer for specialist care
Continuous or frequent use of oral steroids	Use daily steroid tablet in lowest dose providing adequate control
	Maintain high-dose inhaled corticosteroid
	Consider other treatments to minimize the use of steroid tablets
	Refer for specialist care
Short-acting beta 2 agonists as required at all steps	

Source: Based on BTS/SIGN (2016)

Box 8.2 Summary of management of asthma in children

Steps	Actions
Regular preventer	Very low-dose inhaled corticosteroid OR leukotriene receptor antagonist if < 5 years
Initial add-on preventer	Very low-dose inhaled corticosteroid PLUS Long-acting beta 2 agonist if child > 5 years Leukotriene receptor antagonist if child < 5 years
Additional add-on therapies	IF no response to long-acting beta 2 agonist, STOP and consider increased dose of inhaled corticosteroid IF benefit seen from long-acting beta 2 agonist but control still inadequate, continue long-acting beta 2 agonist and increase dose of inhaled corticosteroid IF benefit seen from long-acting beta 2 agonist but control still inadequate, continue long-acting beta 2 agonist and inhaled corticosteroid and consider trial of leukotriene receptor antagonist
High-dose therapies	Consider trials of increasing inhaled corticosteroid up to medium dose Add a fourth drug (e.g. slow-release theophylline) Refer for specialist care
Continuous or frequent use of oral steroids	Use daily steroid tablet in lowest dose providing adequate control Maintain medium-dose inhaled corticosteroid Consider other treatments to minimize the use of steroid tablets Refer for specialist care
Short-acting beta 2 agonists as required at all steps	

Source: Based on BTS/SIGN (2016)

Clinical tip

Beta 2 adrenoreceptor agonists are often referred to as 'relievers' because they relieve the difficult breathing (dyspnoea), shortness of breath and wheezing associated with an asthma attack. Generally, these drugs have a short period of action.

Most short-acting beta 2 agonists are available as aerosols to inhale by mouth several times a day. Most are also available as solutions that can be used with a special apparatus called a *nebulizer*. The maximum effect occurs within 30 minutes and the duration of action is between 4 and 6 hours. The patient is usually prescribed the drug on a 'prn' (*pro re nata* – as required) basis. Long-acting beta 2 agonists such as salmeterol and formoterol are now very common in the management of asthma, as they are recommended by the BTS/SIGN Guidance (2016). They are sometimes prescribed in a combination inhaler with a prevented corticosteroid. This allows for a more manageable regime for patients rather than having multiple inhalers. Their action is the same as that of the short-acting beta 2 receptor agonists, but the duration is longer, providing relief for a more sustained period of time. This often reduces the need for the person to use their relieving short-acting inhaler.

Clinical tip

The longer-acting drugs in this class are often called 'controllers' because they help people with moderate-to-severe asthma control their symptoms. The effects of these drugs are longer-lasting at around 12 hours.

These medications are also available as dry powders, administered by inhalation. However, they are not prescribed on a prn basis but are taken regularly, such as twice daily.

Although very well tolerated, the beta 2 adrenoceptor agonists are not without side-effects, the most common of which are tremor and tachycardia.

Methylxanthines

The drug from this family most commonly employed in the clinical setting is theophylline, which works as a bronchodilator by relaxing the bronchial smooth muscle. Several mechanisms of action have been proposed but it is still unclear how this drug produces its effects. Recently, theophylline has also been shown to have some anti-inflammatory properties, especially with regard to mast cell activity. Theophylline is a useful drug in that it produces bronchial dilation, so reducing the symptoms of chronic asthma, reducing the dosage of oral corticosteroids and reducing the requirement for symptomatic use of beta 2 adrenoreceptor agonists.

Theophylline has a relatively short half-life and therefore you will come across a variety of sustained-release preparations. It is metabolized in the liver by a group of enzymes called *cytochrome P450*. Therefore, if the patient is taking other drugs using the same enzyme system, theophylline will accumulate. Two examples of drugs that might cause this interaction are erythromycin and ciprofloxacin.

Theophylline is used both in chronic asthma and chronic obstructive pulmonary disease (COPD) and as an emergency treatment in acute severe asthma. Despite its effectiveness, it is not used as a first-line treatment but rather a third- or fourth-line option in adults. One of the factors that limits its use is the high incidence of side-effects within its therapeutic range and narrow therapeutic index. As the plasma levels of the drug increase, so do the side-effects, and concordance with this drug can be poor because of these side-effects. Theophylline has a stimulant effect on the central nervous system, causing increased alertness and can interfere with sleep. It also stimulates the cardiovascular system by increasing heart rate as well as the force of contraction and thereby the patient's blood pressure. Indigestion is also a common side-effect, probably due to the drug increasing gastric secretion and relaxation of the cardiac sphincter, thus leading to reflux.

Muscarinic receptor antagonists

The parasympathetic nervous system has a role in bronchoconstriction; therefore, if these effects on the bronchioles of the lungs were blocked, dilatation would take place. This is the basic premise of this group of drugs. The compounds are used mainly in asthma, chronic bronchitis and COPD.

Ipratropium

Ipratropium comes as a solution to inhale by mouth, either as an aerosol or in a nebulizer. The aerosol is usually prescribed four times a day. The bronchodilator effect begins after approximately 45 minutes and lasts for 3–5 hours. This drug can cause side-effects ranging from leaving an unpleasant taste in the mouth and/or a dry mouth to rashes, hoarseness and chest pain. Other anti-muscarinic drugs such as tiotropium and gly-copyrronium are available but ipratropium bromide is the most widely used in asthma.

Inhaled corticosteroids

Inhaled *corticosteroids* are now a regular therapy in asthma management. Two drugs commonly used are beclometasone dipropionate and fluticasone. Both have anti-inflammatory and immuno-suppressive activity. When inhaled they prevent the production of a chemical called *arachidonic acid*, which, in turn, leads to reduced formation of prostaglandins and leukotrienes, reducing the inflammatory response. Both drugs when taken regularly reduce the frequency of 'reliever' bronchodilator intake.

Inhaled corticosteroids are now preferred to oral steroids because of the lower risk of side-effects. However, side-effects do still occur but are usually only local in nature, for example sore and dry throat, and occasionally patients may develop oral thrush (candidiasis).

Clinical tip

It is recommended that an asthmatic patient who needs to use a bronchodilator more than once or twice daily on a regular basis should be prescribed inhaled corticosteroids. Patients should be advised that inhaled corticosteroids will have no effect when taken for acute symptoms. Patients should also understand that it will take a number of weeks before they start to feel the benefit of these medicines.

Clinical tip

The fungal infection candidiasis can be prevented to some extent by rinsing the mouth after inhaling the drug or using a special device called a spacer, which reduces the deposits of the drug in the tissues of the mouth and throat. The patient may have to be treated with antifungal lozenges.

More serious local side-effects are hoarseness and changes of the voice (dysphonia). General or systemic side-effects are seen in high dosages. Beclometasone may cause weakening of bone (osteoporosis), while other side-effects may include skin reactions and blurred vision. Blurred vision should be reported to the prescriber, as it may be an indicator of central serious chorioretinopathy. Furthermore, the Medicines and Healthcare Products Regulatory Agency (MHRA) have issued important safety information on this since 2017 (NICE 2019).

Leukotriene receptor antagonists

As outlined above, leukotrienes are involved in the inflammatory pathways involved in the pathophysiology of asthma. Therefore, using drugs to block their effects can have a very positive effect in asthma management. The drugs currently available are two oral medications called montelukast and zafirlukast. Montelukast is favoured, as it has a range of licensed medicinal forms making its use appropriate in both children and adults.

Clinical tip

Inhaler technique
As inhaled medicines are so important in the management of asthma, it is equally important that nurses educate their patients in a systematic manner.

→

←

1. Get the patient to hold the inhaler with the clear end pointing upwards. Place the metal canister inside the clear end, ensuring that it is fully and firmly in place and that the canister is at room temperature.

2. Remove the protective dust cap from the end of the mouthpiece. If the cap was not placed on the mouthpiece, check the mouthpiece for dirt or other particles.

3. If the patient is using the inhaler for the first time or has not used it in the last 3 days, get them to prime it by pressing down on the canister to release two sprays into the air, away from their face. Ensure they do not spray the medication into their eyes.

4. Ask the patient to breathe out as completely as possible through their mouth, then to hold the inhaler between the thumb and the next two fingers with the mouthpiece at the bottom and facing them. The patient should then place the open end of the mouthpiece into their mouth and avoid covering the drug outlet piece with their tongue. The patient should close their lips tightly around the mouthpiece and close their eyes.

5. The patient should now breathe in slowly and deeply through the mouthpiece at the same time pressing down firmly on the top of the canister.

6. The patient should hold their breath for a count of 10, then remove the inhaler and breathe out slowly.

7. If the patient is to take another dose, ask them to wait for approximately 15 seconds and then repeat as above.

8. Finally, ask the patient to replace the protective cap on the inhaler.

Chronic obstructive pulmonary disease

Chronic obstructive pulmonary disease (COPD) is a general term that includes the conditions chronic bronchitis and emphysema. Chronic bronchitis and emphysema commonly occur alongside each other, leading to a narrowing of the airways and interruption of the flow of air to and from the lungs, resulting in shortness of breath. In clinical practice, COPD is defined by its characteristically low airflow in lung function tests, or spirometry. In contrast to asthma, this limitation is poorly reversible and usually becomes progressively worse over time. The British Lung Foundation, using figures produced by a project on the respiratory health of the nation, reports that upward of 1.2 million people are living with COPD in the UK. These figures and more are available from the British Lung Foundation (BLF 2019b).

The cause of COPD is long-term exposure to lung irritants. The most common irritant implicated in COPD is tobacco smoke. This is primarily a disease of smokers but inhaling passive cigarette smoke, air pollution and workplace or environmental causes also contribute to its incidence.

The symptoms of COPD include:

- ongoing and persistent cough with mucous production;
- shortness of breath, especially on exertion;
- wheeze;
- chest tightness;
- increased incidence of respiratory infections.

Although these symptoms are similar to those seen in asthma, the productive cough is usually the first symptom to develop, meaning that the patient produces sputum (phlegm). This cough tends to come and go at first, and then gradually becomes more persistent (chronic). The patient may actually refer to this cough as being a 'smoker's cough' in the early stages of the disease. When breathlessness begins, people often become more concerned and this is the point at which they may seek medical advice, allowing a diagnosis to be made.

Breathlessness and a wheeze may at first occur only when the person is exerting themselves, such as when they climb stairs. The symptoms become gradually worse over the years especially if the person continues to smoke. Difficulty with breathing may eventually become quite distressing.

Chest infections are more common in a person who has COPD. A sudden worsening of symptoms (such as when the patient has an infection) is called an *exacerbation*. Wheezing with a cough and breathlessness worsens and the patient may cough up more sputum than normal. Such infections can be bacterial *or* viral in nature, which will determine the management required.

Stopping smoking is the most important intervention in early COPD to reduce and arrest symptom progression. Patients may need support with smoking cessation. If symptoms become troublesome, pharmacological treatment may be prescribed (treatments are not curative, but may relieve symptoms.

Drugs used in treating COPD

Pharmacological interventions are aimed at reducing the incidence of symptoms and allowing the patient to maximize remaining lung function to lead as full a life as possible. Many of the drugs used were covered under the section on asthma such as beta 2 adrenoreceptor agonists, methylxanthines, muscarinic receptor antagonists and inhaled corticosteroids.

For patients with moderate-to-severe COPD, long-acting bronchodilators are the mainstay of therapy; as symptoms progress, guidelines recommend combining bronchodilators from different classes to improve efficacy.

Inhaled long-acting beta 2 agonists (LABAs)
Examples of medicines in this category that you are likely to come across are formoterol and salmeterol. They improve the function of the lungs and the patient will state that they find breathing easier and they generally feel less breathless.

They may also report that they do not get as out of breath as they used to when carrying out daily activities. The medicines have also been associated with the patient having fewer occurrences of acute signs and symptoms (exacerbations) from their COPD. Because COPD is not curable, not all patients will see an improvement in their signs and symptoms.

Formoterol and salmeterol have a duration of action of 12 hours, compared to 4–6 hours for salbutamol, allowing a more sustained opening of the bronchioles (bronchodilation).

Clinical tip

The more long-acting beta 2 agonist the patient takes, the more likely are side-effects such as fine tremor, tachycardia, headache and muscle cramp; therefore the nurse should ask the patient to report and document these, as palpitations and tremor may limit the dose that can be tolerated.

Indacaterol is a newer LABA that can be given once daily due to its 24-hour duration of action. With a rapid onset of action as well, it is currently the most advanced drug in this class. It is also available as a combined preparation with the anti-muscarinic drug glycopyrronium.

Long-acting muscarinic antagonists (LAMAs)
The advent of long-acting anti-muscarinic drugs such as tiotropium, aclidinium and glycopyrronium has also increased the quality of life for patients with COPD.

Tiotropium was the first of this class of drugs to be formulated. Providing consistent 24-hour bronchodilation, tiotropium improves the symptoms of COPD and, like the LABAs, it improves quality of life. As with the LABAs, it has also been found to lower the rate of exacerbation. Aclidinium bromide is another LAMA that is administered twice daily to relieve symptoms in COPD.

Phosphodiesterase 4 inhibitors

With inflammatory changes occurring in the lung tissues of a patient with COPD, cells associated with inflammatory changes will be present. The main inflammatory cells found in the tissues in COPD patients are macrophages and lymphocytes. As the COPD progresses, so does the severity of inflammation in the small airways and lung tissue. These physiological alterations contribute to tissue in the airways becoming thicker, narrowing the air passages. Due to lung tissue destruction, the elastic recoil of the lungs becomes diminished. Another physiological response in inflammation is hypersecretion of mucus, which diminishes airway size even further and makes gaseous exchange more difficult.

If we could pharmacologically inhibit the inflammatory response in COPD, then we would alleviate the symptoms and improve the quality of life of the individual. This is what the phosphodiesterase 4 inhibitors attempt to compensate for. They are an adjunct to bronchodilators in the treatment of COPD and their mode of action is anti-inflammatory in nature. Drugs in this class include roflumilast, a potent and selective phosphodiesterase (PDE) 4 inhibitor, and the previously mentioned drug theophylline, a weak non-selective PDE4 inhibitor. The selective PDE4 inhibitors are generally much better tolerated than non-selective PDE4 inhibitors, have been shown to improve lung function, decrease the rate of exacerbations and improve quality of life, and to have proven anti-inflammatory effects in patients with COPD. Also, the selective PDE4 inhibitors are more convenient to use for both patients and nurses, as they require less monitoring and management than, say, theophylline.

Case studies

① Joseph Olita, a 30-year-old man, has been on salbutamol inhaler and inhaled steroids for many years. His asthma has never really been under control and his steroid and beta-agonist usage has increased steadily. It is suspected that Joseph has not been using his inhalers properly. You are asked to reinforce this patient's technique. What steps would you take the patient through and what advice would you give? Discuss with reference to:

- the mode of action of the two medicines;
- the correct inhaler technique;
- the language you would use in teaching Joseph this technique.

② Elizabeth Jones is 11 years old and is asthmatic. Her asthma is well controlled on the following medications: a salbutamol 'easibreath' device, two puffs as required for breathlessness; an inhaled corticosteroid prophylaxis. Elizabeth is moving up to high school and is embarrassed about using her inhalers in front of her classmates. Explain to her the benefits of preventative use of her steroid inhaler and the need to use her salbutamol to prevent a severe asthma attack. Discuss with reference to:

- corticosteroid action on the airways and bronchodilation produced by salbutamol;
- assuaging Elizabeth's concerns.

③ Faustina Olamba is 23 years old and lives in supported accommodation. She has Down's syndrome and asthma and has been on long-term inhalers which she is helped to take by her carers.

Recently, she has been suffering from recurrent bouts of oral candidiasis. Her GP attributes this to her inhaled medication and has been treating her with nystatin.

Outline what drug is likely to be responsible and the measures that she and her carers can take to minimize the occurrence of the infections.

Key learning points

Introduction

▶ Chronic diseases are brought about by demographic, environmental and lifestyle changes.

Asthma

▶ Can either be acute or chronic.
▶ Triggered by chemicals, antigens or cold air.
▶ Respiratory changes triggered by an allergic response.
▶ Cytokines and inflammatory mediators are released causing bronchoconstriction.
▶ Swelling and excess mucous production is present.

Asthma in children

▶ Affects as many as 1 in 11 children in the UK.
▶ There are many risk factors for developing childhood asthma.
▶ A diagnosis of asthma in children is difficult because of its complex nature.
▶ Most asthma medications can safely be prescribed for younger children.

Drugs used in treating asthma

▶ Two groups are used: bronchodilators and inhaled anti-inflammatories.
▶ Examples of bronchodilators are salbutamol, salmeterol and theophylline.
▶ Examples of inhaled corticosteroids are beclomethasone and fluticasone.
▶ Candidiasis can be a problem with inhaled corticosteroids.
▶ Inhaler technique is an important part of patient education.

Chronic obstructive pulmonary disease

▶ A general term that includes the conditions chronic bronchitis and emphysema.
▶ The most common cause is smoking.
▶ Difficulty with breathing may eventually become distressing.
▶ Drugs that may be considered are beta-agonists, antimuscarinics and theophylline.

Calculations

1. A patient requires oral theophylline at a dose of 10mg/kg twice daily. They weigh 25kg. Your stock tablets are 250mg. How many would need for a 28-day supply?

2. Seratide inhaler contains 3000mcg of salmeterol. It contains 60 doses. How much salmeterol is in each dose?

3. A child requires fluticasone 100mcg twice daily and is prescribed an inhaler with 50mcg per dose. How many doses of this are required for the day?

4. Your mentor asks you to check a dose of medication for IV injection. The patient requires aminophylline 50mg and the ampoule comes as 250mg in 10mL. How much should have been drawn into the syringe?

5. Your patient is prescribed salbutamol tablets at a dose of 4mg three times per day. You only have access to 2mg tablets for preparing a 7-day supply. How many will you need?

6. Your patient is prescribed indacaterol for COPD. They should take 150mcg daily for 4 days, then increase the dose to 300mcg. Each dose in the inhaler contains 150mcg and there are 30 actuations. How long will this inhaler last?

7. A patient requires 125mcg of ipratropium by nebulizer. You have 500mcg in 2mL solution. How much do you put into the nebulizer chamber?

8. Your patient has been prescribed a salbutamol 'easyhaler' which has 100mcg per dose and 200 doses per device. They can take the 100mcg up to eight times per day. How many inhalers should be prescribed to guarantee a 30-day supply?

9. Roflumilast 500mcg tablets come in a pack of 30 costing £37.71. The patient requires 13 of these per year to cover all days of treatment. What is the annual cost of this drug??

10. Montelukast 4mg sachets cost £4.85 for 28 but the 4mg chewable tablets cost £0.89. How much more expensive would it be for 13 prescriptions per year to give the granules?

Multiple-choice questions

Try answering these multiple-choice questions to test what you have learned from reading this chapter. You can check your answers at the end of this book.

1. **Which of the following drugs is a beta 2 agonist used in the treatment of asthma?**

a) Ipratropium
b) Salbutamol
c) Beclometasone
d) Theophylline

2. **What measures might be employed to help reduce the possibility of developing oral candidiasis when using inhaled corticosteroids?**

a) Using a spacer and altering the inhaler technique
b) Altering the inhaler technique and taking antifungal lozenges
c) Rinsing the mouth and altering the inhaler technique
d) Using a spacer and rinsing the mouth after taking the medication

3. **Which of these drugs is a weak inhibitor of phosphodiesterase?**

a) Theophylline
b) Salbutamol
c) Roflumilast
d) Fluticasone

4. **Tiotropium is an example of which class of drug?**

a) LABA
b) Corticosteroid
c) Anti-muscarinic
d) PDE4 inhibitor

5. **Which of the following drugs acts at leukotriene receptors?**

a) Salmeterol
b) Salbutamol
c) Montelukast
d) Fluticasone

6. **Which drug group would be the first-line management of asthma after a short-acting beta 2 receptor agonist is prescribed?**

a) Long-acting beta-adrenoreceptor agonists
b) Inhaled corticosteroids
c) Leukotriene receptor antagonists
d) Oral corticosteroids

7. **Fluticasone with salmeterol is an example of a combination of which two classes of drug?**

a) Corticosteroid + leukotriene receptor antagonist
b) Corticosteroid + short-acting beta 2 agonist
c) Corticosteroid + LAMA
d) Corticosteroid + LABA

←

8. **The most common cause of COPD is …**

a) Previous diagnosis of asthma
b) Smoking
c) Air pollution
d) Genetic predisposition

9. **Asthma diagnosis in children is difficult because …**

a) It is a complex condition in the young
b) Children's lungs are not mature
c) Children cannot perform spirometry
d) They often grow out of it

10. **Which of the following are risk factors for childhood asthma?**

a) Prematurity
b) Presence of atopic condition
c) Parents who smoke
d) All of the above

Recommended further reading

Asthma UK (2019) *The Reality of Asthma Care in the UK: Annual Asthma Survey 2018 Report*. London: Asthma UK. Available at: https://www.asthma.org.uk/support-us/campaigns/publications/survey/.

Bourke, S.J. and Burns, G.P. (2011) *Respiratory Medicine*, 11th edition. Malden, MA: Blackwell.

British Lung Foundation (BLF) (2019a) *Asthma*. London: BLF. Available at: https://www.blf.org.uk/support-for-you/asthma.

British Lung Foundation (BLF) (2019b) *Chronic Obstructive Pulmonary Disease (COPD) Statistics*. London: BLF. Available at: https://statistics.blf.org.uk/copd.

British Thoracic Society (BTS) and Scottish Intercollegiate Guidelines Network (SIGN) (2016) *British Guideline on the Management of Asthma: A National Clinical Guideline*. London/Edinburgh: BTS/SIGN.

Downie, G., Mackenzie, J. and Williams, A. (2007) *Pharmacology and Medicines Management for Nurses*, 4th edition. Edinburgh: Churchill Livingstone.

Fricker, M. and Gibson, P.G. (2017) Macrophage dysfunction in the pathogenesis and treatment of asthma, *European Respiratory Journal*, 50: 1700196. Available at: https://doi.org/10.1183/13993003.00196-2017.

Greenstein, B. and Gould, D. (2008) *Trounce's Clinical Pharmacology for Nurses*, 18th edition. New York: Churchill Livingstone.

Karch, A.M. (2017) *Focus on Nursing Pharmacology*, 7th edition. Philadelphia, PA: Lippincott Williams & Wilkins.

Kudo, M., Ishigatsubo, Y. and Aoki, I. (2013) Pathology of asthma, *Frontiers in Microbiology*, 4: 263. Available at: https://doi.org/10.3389/fmicb.2013.00263.

Lapham, R. (2015) *Drug Calculations for Nurses: A Step-by-Step Approach*, 4th edition. London: Arnold.

National Institute for Health and Care Excellence (NICE) (2019) *British National Formulary*. London: NICE. Available at: https://bnf.nice.org.uk.

NHS (2019) Available at https://www.gosh.nhs.uk/conditions-and-treatments/conditions-we-treat/asthma.

Office for National Statistics (ONS) (2017) *Death Registrations in England and Wales: Summary Tables: 2016*. London: ONS.

Possa, S.S., Leick, E.A., Prado, C.M., Martins, M.A. and Tibério, I.F.L.C. (2013) Eosinophilic inflammation in allergic asthma, *Frontiers in Pharmacology*, 4: 46. Available at: https://doi.org/10.3389/fphar.2013.00046.

Simonson, T., Aarbakke, J., Kay, I., Coleman, I., Sinnott, P. and Lyssa, R. (2006) *Illustrated Pharmacology for Nurses*. London: Hodder Arnold.

Drugs for diabetes mellitus

9

Chapter contents

Learning objectives

After studying this chapter, you should be able to:

- Describe the basic pathology involved in diabetes mellitus.
- Discuss the differences in onset and progression of type I and type II diabetes.
- Explain the mode of action of medicines used in treating these conditions.
- Demonstrate an understanding of the unwanted effects of medicines used in treating these conditions.
- Discuss the differences in medication use between type I and type II diabetes.
- Demonstrate an understanding of the links between the pharmacology of therapies used in treating diabetes and the care given by the health practitioner.

Introduction

In this chapter, you will learn about the two types of diabetes and their similarities and differences. Diabetes is a common condition across the UK and the developed world. The Diabetes Prevalence Survey of 2018 (Diabetes UK 2019) showed that 3.8 million people were diagnosed with diabetes in the UK. These figures are extrapolated from the Quality and Outcomes Framework (QOF) registers compiled by general practices throughout the UK.

Part of the nurse's role is the need to ensure that medicines are administered appropriately. The Nursing and Midwifery Council's Standards for Pre-Registration Nursing Programmes published in May 2018 state that education must

> *ensure that field-specific content in relation to the law, safeguarding, consent, pharmacology and medicines administration and optimisation is included for entry to the register in one or more fields of nursing practice*

This is backed up by the Standards of Proficiency for Registered Nurses in the area of skills:

Annexe A: Communication and relationship management skills

2. Evidence-based, best practice approaches to communication for supporting people of all ages, their families and carers in preventing ill health and in managing their care

2.1 share information and check understanding about the causes, implications and treatment of a range of common health conditions including anxiety, depression, memory loss, diabetes, dementia, respiratory disease, cardiac disease, neurological disease, cancer, skin problems, immune deficiencies, psychosis, stroke and arthritis

Diabetes

Diabetes mellitus is a chronic disease of metabolism caused by either an insufficient production of insulin in the body or an insufficient effect of insulin in the peripheral tissues. The main problems stem from a wide fluctuation in the range of blood glucose levels, which leads to several short- and long-term difficulties for the individual. There are two main forms of diabetes: type I and type II (see Box 9.1).

Box 9.1   The two types of diabetes

	Type I	Type II
Description	Little or no insulin is produced by the pancreas; insulin is required to sustain life, thus the need for daily insulin in order to survive	Pancreas doesn't make enough insulin, or body doesn't use insulin correctly, thus the need to control the intake of carbohydrates. Some people can maintain normoglycaemia with diet alone, some need oral hypoglycaemic drugs, while some will eventually require insulin
Usual age of onset	Less than 20 years	Typically, 40–60 years
Control by oral antidiabetic drugs	No	Possible

←

Control by insulin	Yes	May be required as the disease progresses or if the patient remains unresponsive to oral therapy
Symptoms	Symptoms appear rapidly: frequent micturition; extreme hunger; extreme thirst; extreme weight loss; weakness and tiredness; feeling edgy and mood changes; nausea; vomiting; blurred vision	Symptoms appear slowly (the person may not feel any symptoms at all): increased thirst; increased micturition; feeling tired; feeling edgy; nausea; loss of weight; slow wound healing; recurrent infections of the skin, gums, vagina/penis and bladder; blurred vision; tingling or loss of sensation in hands or feet
Complications	Diabetic coma or keto-acidosis from hyperglycaemia; hypoglycaemia; nephropathy; blindness; myocardial infarction; cerebrovascular accident; peripheral vascular disease; neuropathy	Diabetic coma from hyperglycaemia; hypoglycaemia; nephropathy; blindness; myocardial infarction; cerebrovascular accident; peripheral vascular disease; neuropathy
Treatment	Carbohydrate-controlled healthy diet; exercise; daily insulin; regular monitoring of blood glucose levels; monitoring of urine	Carbohydrate-controlled healthy diet; exercise; regular monitoring of blood glucose levels; monitoring of urine

In type I diabetes, the body produces little or no insulin in cells contained in the pancreas known as the 'Islets of Langerhans' or the beta cells. The pancreas is a specialized gland that lies just behind the stomach. Its functions range from regulating the amount of sugar (glucose) in the blood to producing enzymes that help break down and digest proteins, carbohydrates and fats. It is thought that the beta cells in the pancreas are destroyed by the body's own immune response – hence diabetes is an autoimmune disease. Someone with type I diabetes will be required to take insulin for the rest of their lives.

In type II diabetes, the beta cells may produce small amounts of insulin but not enough to control the levels of glucose in the plasma. In addition, the cells of the body, and particularly in the periphery, cannot utilize insulin properly. This means that glucose is stopped from entering peripheral cells, so increasing the glucose levels in the plasma. This type of diabetes is linked to the problem of obesity.

As stated in the Introduction, an estimated 3.8 million people in the UK are currently living with diabetes (Diabetes UK 2019). However, it is suggested that there are as many people again who go undiagnosed. The figures suggest that around 90% those diagnosed have type II diabetes, 8% have type I and around 2% have rarer types of diabetes.

The risk of type II diabetes is higher if it runs in the family or if the patient is overweight. From this perspective, prevention of obesity will also lead to prevention of type II diabetes.

Without treatment, the main symptoms of diabetes can be divided into two main types: acute symptoms and chronic complications. There are a number of symptoms that could be referred to as 'classic'. These are excessive thirst (polydipsia), producing lots of urine requiring many trips to the bathroom (polyuria), blurring of vision, tiredness and weight loss due to muscle wasting (loss of muscle mass).

The chronic complications of diabetes are caused by long-term raised glucose levels in the body. This leads to damage, particularly to blood vessels and peripheral nerves.

Clinical tip

Macrovascular disease refers to damage to the larger blood vessels resulting in coronary heart disease or peripheral vascular disease. *Microvascular disease*, in contrast, refers to damage to smaller vessels resulting in eye problems (retinopathy) and kidney damage (nephropathy). Damage to the outside of the nerves (the nerve sheaths) is also a problematic complication; this process is referred to as 'neuropathy', a major cause of diabetic foot problems including amputation.

Diabetic ketoacidosis

Diabetic ketoacidosis (DKA) is a complication of diabetes. A patient with DKA will have high blood glucose levels (hyperglycaemia), high levels of ketone bodies in their plasma (ketosis), and because these ketone bodies are acidic, the patient's blood becomes more acidic (metabolic acidosis). DKA occurs mostly in people with type I diabetes mellitus (DM).

The patient often reports feeling nauseous and may actually start to vomit. Another common symptom is abdominal pain. If these signs and symptoms are left unchecked, the condition can progress to cerebral oedema, coma, even death. DKA, therefore, will be diagnosed with the detection of ketosis and metabolic acidosis in the presence of hyperglycaemia. Treatment of DKA involves replacing fluids, administrating insulin and preventing the patient's potassium levels from dropping (hypokalaemia).

As we have indicated, DKA is most common among patients with type I DM and develops when their ability to produce insulin is insufficient to meet the body's basic metabolic requirements. In a small minority of patients, DKA is the first indication of type I DM. Insulin deficiency can be described as absolute, such as when a patient does not administer their insulin. Insulin deficiency can also be described as relative, such as when the usual level of insulin is not enough to meet the body's metabolic demands from physiological stress. Stressors that can cause this relative imbalance and cause DKA include acute infection such as pneumonia or the development of a urinary tract infection. Myocardial infarction is another complication that can trigger DKA. Certain drugs are also implicated in causing DKA, including corticosteroids, thiazide diuretics and sympathomimetics.

In type II diabetes, DKA is less common, but it can occur in individuals under abnormal physiological stress.

Treatment

The management of DKA involves the replacement of fluid and electrolytes and the administration of insulin. Such management should follow the Guidelines for the Management of Diabetic Ketoacidosis in Adults (2013), published by the Joint British Diabetes Societies Inpatient Care Group. Such treatment should ideally be given in high-dependency settings because clinical and laboratory assessments are at first required every 1–2 hours, with appropriate adjustments in treatment.

Intravenous fluids are needed immediately, as intravascular volume should be restored in order to raise blood pressure and therefore ensure kidney perfusion. Once this immediate intravenous fluid has been given, the team needs to ensure that the remaining total body water deficits are corrected more slowly. This may take place over the next 24 hours. When blood pressure is over 90mmHg, sodium chloride 0.9% should be given by intravenous infusion at a rate that addresses the deficit and provides maintenance; see Joint British Diabetes Societies Inpatient Care Group (2013) for suggested regimen.

The usual way to correct hyperglycaemia is to give the patient regular insulin, such as insulin detemir or insulin glargine. Initially, the patient may require 0.1 unit/kg as an IV bolus of soluble insulin. This is then followed by a continuous IV infusion of 0.1 unit/kg/hour in 0.9% saline solution. During this time the patient's blood sugar will be regularly monitored. If the plasma concentration of glucose does not fall by 50 to 75mg/dL (2.8 to 4.2mmol/L) in the first hour, insulin doses should be doubled. Children should be given a continuous IV insulin infusion of 0.1 unit/kg/hour or higher with or without a bolus.

If the doses of insulin are sufficient, you should begin to see an improvement in the levels of circulating ketones. Sometimes an improvement in ketosis is linked to an improvement in the pH of the blood. This means that ketone decline may take some time until the blood pH improves.

As the patient's condition improves, attention will turn to the type of insulin to be given next. The patient will be switched to regular insulin 5–10 units every 4–6 hours, with the route of administration being by subcutaneous injection. When the patient's condition has been stabilized and they are able to eat and drink normally, a typical split-mixed or basal-bolus insulin regimen is begun. During this transitional period, the patient should continue intravenous insulin for 1–4 hours after the initial dose of subcutaneous insulin is given. In contrast, children should continue to receive 0.05 unit/kg/hour insulin infusion until subcutaneous insulin is initiated and pH exceeds 7.3.

Hypokalaemia, or low potassium levels, needs to be prevented. This occurs in DKA because of urinary loss. Prevention requires close monitoring and replacement of potassium, which will be given alongside the patient's intravenous fluids. Levels should be checked every 1–2 hours in the initial stages of treatment.

Medicine management of diabetes

The overall aim of the treatment of diabetes is to maintain blood glucose levels within the normal range (normoglycaemia) and achieve the required HBA1c target for the patient based on their condition and in line with guidelines. The HBA1c measurement gives an understanding of the diabetic control over the past 8–12 weeks and is a better indicator for the prescriber than a spot blood glucose check. This will relieve the acute symptoms and should minimize the impact of chronic complications on the individual. Achieving normoglycaemia is very difficult and drug treatment is on an individual basis. An increase in exercise and cessation of smoking are advisable in order to reduce high blood pressure (hypertension) and high fat content in the blood (hyperlipidaemia). These measures have been shown to reduce the risk of long-term complications of this disease. However, the most important key to treatment of diabetes is diet. This can be done alone or in combination with insulin or other oral hypoglycaemic agents.

Insulin

The hormone insulin is released in the body as a direct response to raised levels of blood glucose. Insulin is released directly into the bloodstream and stimulates the uptake of glucose; it is the key that allows glucose to enter cells, and without it the door remains locked and glucose builds up in the blood. Insulin also promotes conversion of glucose to a substance called *glycogen*, which allows the body to store glucose for periods when the person is not eating but still requires glucose for bodily functions.

Insulin also limits the amount of fat breakdown in the body, a process called *lipolysis*. Triglycerides (large fat molecules), which are normally stored in fatty (adipose) tissue, are broken down into their constituent fatty acids and glycerol. These are then transported to the liver where they are used to fuel certain metabolic pathways. As insulin is either absent or low in quantity in diabetes, these metabolic pathways soon become saturated, resulting in the production by the body of acidic compounds such as ketone bodies and acetate.

Treatment with insulin

At one time, insulin was extracted from the pancreas of cattle (bovine insulin) or pigs (porcine insulin). However, today it is almost entirely human in nature. This is possible through use of a process called *recombinant DNA technology*, which involves inserting the DNA code for human insulin production into bacteria so that they then produce commercial amounts of insulin (see Box 9.2).

Insulin is destroyed in the GI system, which is why you never see it given by mouth as a tablet, for example.

Once absorbed, insulin has a short half-life of approximately 10 minutes. Therefore, for longer-term control, long-acting insulin is required. Insulin doses need to be drawn up precisely and injected subcutaneously at times determined by the prescriber in line with the patient's lifestyle and needs. Insulin doses can be varied in line with blood glucose readings.

Clinical tip

Insulin is usually given by injection. The most common method of administration is subcutaneously. It can be auto-injected by means of a device called a 'pen', although some patients prefer to use a small insulin pump. The most recent device available is the insulin jet system, which can be used on the abdomen, thighs or buttocks. It forces a very small stream of insulin through a nozzle placed on the skin. The jet of insulin is propelled with such force that it penetrates the skin without the need for a needle.

Box 9.2   Types of insulin

Rapid-acting analogue (clear)
Onset: 10–15 minutes
Peak: 60–90 minutes
Duration: 4–5 hours
Fast-acting (clear)
Onset: 30 minutes–1 hour
Peak: 2–4 hours
Duration: 5–8 hours
Intermediate-acting (cloudy)
Onset: 1–3 hours
Peak: 5–8 hours
Duration: up to 18 hours
Long-acting (cloudy)
Onset: 3–4 hours
Peak: 8–15 hours
Duration: 22–26 hours
Extended long-acting analogue
Onset: 90 minutes
Duration: 24 hours
Premixed (cloudy)
Presented as a single vial containing a fixed ratio (a percentage of rapid-/fast-acting to a percentage of intermediate-/long-acting)

Rapid-acting insulins

Soluble insulin produces a quick and short-lived effect. It works in the same way as natural insulin by binding to the receptors on the cells and allowing glucose to enter. It also causes the cells in the liver, muscles and fat to increase their uptake of glucose from the blood. *Insulin lispro* is a special form of human insulin that works more rapidly but for a shorter period of time. This enables people to inject themselves just prior to eating a meal if they so wish. These types of insulins are the only ones suitable for IV injection.

Clinical tip

Examples of rapid-acting soluble insulins include insulin aspart, insulin glulisine and insulin lispro. When given subcutaneously, they work within 30–60 minutes with a peak action between 1 and 4 hours, and their effects last for around 9 hours. They are usually injected 15–30 minutes before a meal so that the increasing blood glucose levels after eating can be controlled. You will see these sorts of insulins being used in clinical practice as treatment for ketoacidosis where the regime is also called a 'sliding scale'. This means the insulin dose is determined by the person's blood glucose value, which is obtained at predetermined times (e.g. every 2 hours).

Intermediate-acting insulins

Longer-acting preparations of insulin are made possible by mixing the insulin with a substance that slows its use in the body. An example of this is *isophane insulin*, which starts working about 90 minutes after administration. Its maximum effect occurs 4–8 hours after administration and keeps working for as long as 24 hours.

Clinical tip

Isophane insulin is naturally white and cloudy in appearance and should not be used if it is not uniformly this colour after mixing. To mix the vial, gently roll it in your hands at least 10 times before administration.

The *biphasic insulins* are a combination of soluble insulin and isophane insulin. Examples of these include *biphasic isophane insulin, biphasic*

insulin aspart and *biphasic insulin lispro*. Premixed combinations provide a rapid initial lowering of blood glucose, followed by a more prolonged effect that lasts throughout the day. This is thought to mimic the body's own insulin production more closely.

Long-acting insulins

Like intermediate-acting insulins, long-acting insulins (examples of which include protamine zinc insulin, insulin zinc suspension, insulin detemir, insulin glargine and insulin degludec) function like the body's normal insulin production, but their duration of action may last up to 36 hours. Insulin glargine and insulin degludec are given once daily and insulin detemir is given once or twice daily according to individual requirements. The older long-acting insulins (insulin zinc suspension and protamine zinc insulin) are rarely prescribed these days.

Side-effects

The main problem when giving insulin is that the blood sugar may be lowered too much, a state we call hypoglycaemia, which can cause brain damage. A person using insulin is three times more likely to be at risk from the effects of hypoglycaemia than a non-user.

Clinical tip

Patients with hypoglycaemia become dizzy, feel faint, begin to sweat and often appear to be drunk. The obvious way to treat this is to give sugar in the form of sweet drinks, glucose tablets or sugary snacks. If the person is unconscious, and this can occur relatively quickly, they will need IV glucose or intramuscular glucagon. Glucagon is a hormone that works in the opposite way to insulin and raises the blood glucose level by promoting the breakdown of stored glucose in the liver and muscles.

Insulin pumps

An insulin pump is portable and attached to the patient (Figure 9.1). It consists of a main pump unit which holds an insulin reservoir (usually 3mL capacity like the cartridges used in an insulin pen). The reservoir is attached to a long, thin piece of tubing with a needle or cannula at one end which is known as the 'infusion set'.

To use the pump, the cartridge is filled with fast-acting insulin and fitted inside. There is no need to take long-acting insulin because the insulin pump delivers constant amounts to the body. The needle or cannula is inserted under the skin and held in place with an adhesive patch, which fixes to the surrounding skin. The other end of the tube is connected to the pump, which then delivers insulin through the infusion set according to its programming.

Using a pump, patients can instantly change the insulin dose, and fast-acting insulin is more easily absorbed by the body. Because the body receives a constant, regular flow of insulin, the effect is more stable also.

There are two types of dose with an insulin pump, basal and bolus. Modern insulin pumps allow users to regulate the doses simultaneously and adjust the basal rate at any point. The *basal dose* is the same as a long-acting insulin regime

for those diabetics without an insulin pump. This programme is consistent and regular and controls the level of insulin into the bloodstream. The *bolus dose* is designed to counteract food being consumed. Therefore, when a diabetic snacks or eats a meal, the insulin pump can be programmed to provide an extra boost of insulin. Pumps can also be programmed to release a bolus dose over a longer period, which is ideal for meals in restaurants and on other similar occasions.

Many patients can now monitor their blood glucose levels more quickly and easily using a scanner system linked to an app on their phones called FreeStyle Libre, which allows them to adjust their pumps and be more responsive to changing glucose levels. Other devices such as Omnipod and Dexcom G5 are available.

Oral antidiabetic drugs

These drugs are usually given to people with type II diabetes. Dietary control and lifestyle change can mitigate some of the changes in blood sugar but they are often not sufficient to control levels. There are several classes of non-insulin antidiabetic drugs and their prescription is made in line with NICE Guideline NG28 based on effectiveness, safety, tolerability and the patient's individual circumstances (NICE 2019a). The aim of treatment is to reduce the long-term risk of complications and control blood glucose effectively. This can be determined by measuring HbA1c levels.

NICE guidelines start with first line treatments and then step up, referred to as treatment intensification steps. They outline such steps as in Table 9.1.

Metformin hydrochloride

Metformin is an antidiabetic medicine from a drug group called biguanides. It works in people with type II diabetes in three ways. First, it reduces the amount of glucose produced by cells in the liver. Second, it increases the sensitivity of muscle cells to insulin. Third, it delays movement of glucose from the GI tract to the blood following a meal. The cumulative effect of these processes is to lower the person's blood glucose level.

Metformin is a first-line medicine in the treatment of type II diabetes due to its ability to help

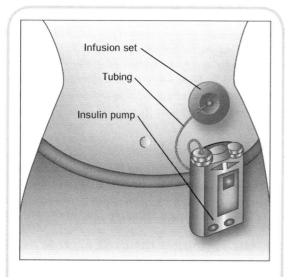

Figure 9.1   An insulin pump

Initial drug treatment	Treatment with a single non-insulin blood-glucose-lowering therapy (monotherapy)
First intensification of drug treatment	Treatment with 2 non-insulin blood-glucose-lowering therapies in combination (dual therapy)
Second intensification of drug treatment	Treatment with either 3 non-insulin blood-glucose-lowering therapies in combination (triple therapy) or any treatment combination including insulin

Table 9.1   Stages of oral antidiabetic drug treatment

with weight loss, as well as its low risk of inducing hypoglycaemic events. It can be used in combination with other antidiabetic medicines to provide better normoglycaemia.

The drug, which has a half-life of approximately 3 hours, is initially given at a dose of 500mg three times a day either with or after food; it is then titrated up over a few weeks to maximum effect while trying to maintain the lowest effective dose so as not produce side-effects. The most common side-effects are anorexia (lack of appetite), diarrhoea and nausea. An increase in lactic acid in the blood is a rare but potentially fatal consequence of taking the medication. This is more common in patients who already have kidney, liver or heart failure who should not be prescribed the drug.

Sulfonylureas
This class of drugs is also used in the treatment of type II diabetes, particularly in people whose diabetes cannot be controlled by diet alone. They work by stimulating the beta cells in the pancreas to secrete insulin. Examples of drugs in this class are glibenclamide, gliclazide, glipizide and tolbutamide.

These drugs come in tablet form and are usually taken two or three times a day. They may lead

to hypoglycaemia, and patients should monitor their blood glucose. They are also associated with modest weight gain.

> **Clinical tip**
>
> Patients should be alerted to report symptoms such as shakiness, dizziness, sweating, sudden changes in behaviour and mood, and weakness, as these may indicate a low blood glucose.

There are some significant drug interactions with sulfonylureas, and certain drugs potentiate the hypoglycaemic effects. NSAIDs will lead to hypoglycaemia when given with sulfonylureas. However, drugs such as thiazide diuretics and corticosteroids lessen the hypoglycaemic effects. This means that patients should have their blood glucose monitored more closely to ensure adequate control is maintained.

Meglitinides
Some drugs such as the meglitinides that are not based on the sulfonylureas have also been developed to expand the range of therapy. Examples include repaglinide and nateglinide, which work in a similar way to the sulfonylureas in that they enhance secretion of insulin from the beta cells in the pancreas. They are not as potent as most of the sulfonylureas, are rapidly absorbed and have a short elimination half-life of 3 hours. This means that they have a short duration of action and there is therefore a lower risk of hypoglycaemia as a side-effect.

> **Clinical tip**
>
> Nateglinide comes in tablet form and is usually taken three times daily. It can be taken up to 30 minutes before or just before a meal. If a meal is missed, the patient should not take the tablet; equally, an extra meal will require an extra tablet.

Thiazolidinediones (glitazones)

The action of this class of drugs is complex. They reduce the breakdown of stored glucose in the liver and increase the amount of glucose entering muscle tissue. Insulin that is circulating is enhanced by these drugs. The accumulation of these actions leads to a lowering of the blood glucose level. They do not cause hypoglycaemia as a side-effect when used on their own but may do so if combined with insulin or a sulfonylurea.

The only tablet in this group is pioglitazone. It is used on its own or together with metformin and/or another antidiabetic medicine to treat type II diabetes. It can also be used with insulin. Pioglitazone comes as a tablet to take by mouth. It is usually taken once daily with or without meals. It should be taken at around the same time every day.

> ### Clinical tip
>
> You should inform the patient that it may take 2 weeks for their blood sugar to decrease and several weeks more for them to feel the full effect of pioglitazone.

Common side-effects include nausea, difficulty in focusing, ankle swelling, an increase in appetite and weight gain. Pioglitazone and other similar medications for diabetes may cause or worsen congestive heart failure (a condition in which the heart is unable to pump enough blood to the other parts of the body).

Alpha-glucosidase inhibitors

A drug called acarbose is used from this family of medicines to treat type II diabetes. It works by slowing down the action of chemicals in the body that break down foods which release glucose. Slowing food digestion helps to keep the blood glucose from rising to a very high level after a meal. It is given as a tablet, usually three times a day. It is important that the patient takes each dose with the first bite of their meal. Side-effects include flatulence, diarrhoea, abdominal pain and bloating due to the amount of unabsorbed carbohydrates left in the GI system. Acarbose is not a treatment for diabetes that you will encounter often in a hospital setting, although it is an option for patients.

Diapeptidylpeptidase-4 inhibitors (gliptins)

These drugs are relatively new in the management of type II diabetes and include alogliptin, linagliptin, sitagliptin, saxagliptin and vildagliptin. They work by acting on diapeptidylpeptidase-4, an enzyme that affects glucagon and insulin levels. Their action leads to increased glucagon release, which subsequently causes a rise in insulin secretion and a decrease in blood glucose. They can be used as monotherapy or in combination with other drugs or insulin. In the case of renal or hepatic impairment, some of these drugs have a better safety profile than others.

Sodium glucose co-transporter 2 inhibitors

These drugs, which include canagliflozin, dapagliflozin and empagliflozin, are again relatively new drugs for the treatment of diabetes. They can be used as an initial treatment in patients where metformin is not appropriate, but they are associated with a higher risk of DKA than other oral antidiabetic agents. These drugs directly but reversibly inhibit the transporter found in the proximal convoluted tubule of the nephron in the kidney, which in turn causes reduced reabsorption of glucose in the tubule and increases glucose excretion in the urine. These drugs should be used with caution in the elderly and in patients with renal impairment, and the BNF clearly lays out dose reductions that should be used in this instance.

Glucagon-like peptide-1 receptor agonist

This class of drugs should be used only as part of dual or triple therapy when other combinations of drugs have not produced the required reduction and stabilization of blood glucose. These drugs, which include albiglutide, dulaglutide, exenatide, liraglutide and lixisenatide, act by augmenting glucose-dependent insulin secretion and by slowing gastric emptying time. They can be given as monotherapy or in combination. They should be avoided in patients with an estimated glomerular filtration rate of less than 30mL/min. They must be discontinued, and drug therapy changed, in women of childbearing potential who wish to try to conceive. They need to be given by injection.

Case studies

① Hannah is 23 years old and a type I diabetic maintained on insulin via a pump and she is independent in managing her blood glucose levels. She also suffers from anxiety. She has to go into hospital for a planned surgical procedure and is worried about what will happen when she has to fast before the operation and who will manage her blood glucose. Using the guidance in the BNF, discuss the important aspects to outline to Hannah and the likely changes she will encounter before, during and after her minor procedure.

② Olly Phillips is 12 years old and has mild learning difficulties and cerebral palsy. He is a type I diabetic and his mother manages his insulin injections and his diet. Olly wants to start injecting himself and is learning how to do this with your support and his mother in attendance. Outline what you would need to assess and consider when teaching Olly how to do his injections.

Key learning points

Introduction

▶ Diabetes is a common long-term condition in the UK.

Diabetes

▶ A chronic metabolic disease.
▶ Two types: type I and type II (insulin dependent and non-insulin dependent).
▶ Complications of the disease produce macrovascular and microvascular problems.

Medicine management of diabetes

▶ Treatment aims to achieve normoglycaemia.
▶ Insulin preparations have different lengths of action.
▶ Insulin is given by SC injection.
▶ Doses must be drawn up precisely and injected when needed.
▶ Giving insulin can cause hypoglycaemia.
▶ Oral hypoglycaemics can be used in type II diabetes mellitus.

Calculations

1. A patient requires metformin 500mg daily for 1 week followed by 500mg twice daily for 1 week, then 500mg twice daily as a maintenance. How many tablets will they need for a 28-day supply for the first month of treatment?

2. Your patient requires dulaglutide 0.75mg by injection. You have 3mg per mL solution. How much should be given?

3. Exenatide comes in pre-filled syringes at a strength of 0.25mg/mL. The dose required with each injection is 10mcg. How many mL will the pen deliver per dose?

4. The exenatide pen in question (3) contains 2.4mL. How many doses does this equate to?

5. Repaglinide can be given at a maximum of 4mg in any single dose and up to 16mg maximum per day. If the patient requires 16mg, what is the minimum number of doses per day to ensure 4mg per dose is not exceeded?

6. Your patient requires 15mg per day of glibenclamide. You have only got 2.5mg tablets in stock. How many are required to give the dose?

7. An adult patient has been commenced on 1.5g of tolbutamide daily in 3 divided doses. You have 500mg tablets. How many tablets per dose?

8. The doctor has prescribed pioglitazone 45mg daily. The drug trolley has 15mg tablets and 30mg tablets. What combination do you need to give the fewest number of tablets?

9. You have a vial of rapid-acting insulin containing 100 units/mL. How much do you need to give 28 units?

10. Accu-check testing strips come in packs of 50. Your patient tests their blood glucose 3 times per day. How many FULL days will they get from one pack?

Multiple-choice questions

Try answering these multiple-choice questions to test what you have learned from reading this chapter. You can check your answers at the end of the book.

1. Glipizide belongs to which family of hypoglycaemics?

a) Sulfonylureas
b) Biguanides
c) Meglitinides
d) Glitazones

2. Insulin is given by injection because ...

a) It is cheaper to give it that way
b) It takes a long time to absorb it from the GI tract

→

c) It is destroyed in the GI tract

d) A tablet has yet to be developed

3. **Metformin acts by ...**

a) Reducing the glucose produced by the liver

b) Increasing the sensitivity of muscles to insulin

c) Delaying glucose movement from the GI tract

d) All of the above

4. **In DKA, the patient will have which of the following symptoms?**

a) Increased blood glucose

b) Decreased blood glucose

c) Increased blood glucose and high ketones

d) Decreased blood glucose and low ketones

5. **An example of a microvascular complication of diabetes is ...**

a) Coronary heart disease

b) Peripheral vascular disease

c) Neuropathy

d) Nephropathy

6. **Insulin is produced by ...**

a) The liver

b) The pancreas

c) The kidney

d) The bowel

7. **The age of onset of type I diabetes is typically ...**

a) At birth

b) Under 20 years

c) Over 40 years

d) Over 65 years

8. **Oral antidiabetic drugs are given when ...**

a) Type I is diagnosed

b) Type II is diagnosed

c) Type I and insulin not wanted

d) Type II and dietary control inadequate

9. **Which of the following should be avoided in pregnancy?**

a) Exenatide

b) Metformin

c) Insulin

d) All of the above

10. Of which of the following is dapagliflozin?

a) A competitive antagonist

b) A reversible inhibitor

c) An irreversible inhibitor

d) A non-competitive antagonist

Recommended further reading

Diabetes UK (2019) *Diabetes Prevalence 2018*. Available at: https://www.diabetes.org.uk/professionals/position-statements-reports/statistics/diabetes-prevalence-2018.

Downie, G., Mackenzie, J. and Williams, A. (2007) *Pharmacology and Medicines Management for Nurses*, 4th edition. Edinburgh: Churchill Livingstone.

Greenstein, B. and Gould, D. (2008) *Trounce's Clinical Pharmacology for Nurses*, 18th edition. New York: Churchill Livingstone.

Joint British Diabetes Societies Inpatient Care Group (2013) *The Management of Diabetic Ketoacidosis in Adults*, 2nd edn. Available at: https://www.diabetes.org.uk/Professionals/Position-statements-reports/Specialist-care-for-children-and-adults-and-complications/The-Management-of-Diabetic-Ketoacidosis-in-Adults.

Karch, A.M. (2017) *Focus on Nursing Pharmacology*, 7th edition. Philadelphia, PA: Lippincott Williams & Wilkins.

Lapham, R. (2015) *Drug Calculations for Nurses: A Step-by-Step Approach*, 4th edition. London: Arnold.

National Institute for Health and Care Excellence (NICE) (2015) *NICE Guideline NG17: Type 1 Diabetes in Adults: Diagnosis and Management*. London: NICE. Last updated July 2016.

National Institute for Health and Care Excellence (NICE) (2019a) *NICE Guideline NG28: Type 2 Diabetes in Adults: Management*. London: NICE.

National Institute for Health and Care Excellence (NICE) (2019b) *British National Formulary*. London: NICE. Available at: https://bnf.nice.org.uk.

Simonson, T., Aarbakke, J., Kay, I., Coleman, I., Sinnott, P. and Lyssa, R. (2006) *Illustrated Pharmacology for Nurses*. London: Hodder Arnold.

Cardiovascular drugs

10

Chapter contents

Learning objectives

After studying this chapter, you should be able to:

- Describe the basic conditions classified as cardiovascular diseases.
- Explain the mode of action of medicines used in treating cardiovascular disease and relate these to physiology.
- Demonstrate an understanding of the unwanted effects of medicines used in treating these conditions.
- Demonstrate an understanding of the links between the pharmacology of therapies used in treating disorders and the care given by the health practitioner

Introduction

Cardiovascular disease is a major cause of morbidity and mortality in the UK and is linked with other comorbidities and mortality. According to the British Heart Foundation (BHF 2019), it kills more than 1 in 4 people in the UK:

- Heart and circulatory diseases cause more than a quarter of all deaths in the UK, that's nearly 170,000 deaths each year – an average of 460 deaths each day or one every three minutes in the UK.
- There are around 7.4 million people living with heart and circulatory disease in the UK: 3.9 million men and 3.5 million women.
- Coronary heart disease (CHD) is the most common type of heart and circulatory disease. It is also the most common cause of heart attack and the single biggest killer worldwide.
- In the UK there are more than 100,000 hospital admissions yearly due to heart attacks: that's one every five minutes.
- Around 1.4 million people alive in the UK today have survived a heart attack.
- Over 900,000 people in the UK are living with heart failure.
- Strokes cause over 36,000 deaths in the UK each year and are the biggest cause of severe disability.
- People with a history of heart diseases are at least twice as likely to develop vascular dementia.
- There are more than 30,000 out-of-hospital cardiac arrests in the UK each year. The survival rate is less than 1 in 10.
- More than 3.9 million adults in the UK have been diagnosed with diabetes.

Many of the drugs prescribed in cardiovascular disease can be used for more than one of the different conditions we discuss here.

Hypertension

Hypertension (high blood pressure) is associated with a risk of coronary artery disease, which we will discuss later in this chapter. Increased pressure in

the blood vessels has a direct effect on the heart and vasculature. One of the major problems with hypertension is that it often has few or no symptoms and many individuals only discover they have the condition on routine screening. The effects of raised blood pressure have a pronounced effect on the heart, particularly the left ventricle. This increases in size (ventricular hypertrophy) as it attempts to pump against an increased peripheral resistance.

The arteries also respond to the increased pressure within them by enlargement of their muscular walls. This hypertrophy both in the heart and vessels leads to cardiac failure, as a muscle cannot restore its normal contractility.

The risk of cerebral vascular accident (stroke) also increases significantly with elevation in systolic and diastolic pressures. Hypertensive disease is also associated with the formation of fatty plaques in the walls of blood vessels, a condition we call atherosclerosis, which can lead to further increases in hypertension. The combination of high pressure and atherosclerosis leads to weakness in the walls of arteries and increases the risk of their rupture. The blood vessels most commonly affected are the cerebral, coronary and renal vessels. Therefore, as well as the increased risk of cerebral vascular accident and myocardial infarction, the individual is also at risk of renal disease.

There are two classes of hypertension: primary and secondary. In secondary hypertension, the elevated blood pressure is caused by renal or endocrine disease. However, most cases of hypertension are primary or 'essential' hypertension, and this condition is still not fully understood. Hypertension is most likely due to several interrelated factors, which might be genetic or environmental.

Regardless of cause, hypertension can be fatal if left untreated. In most instances, the disease process is protracted and this is known as *benign hypertension*. However, in a small minority of cases, the disease progresses very rapidly and is very difficult to control. This is referred to as *malignant hypertension* and is usually triggered by kidney disease arising from essential hypertension or other causes.

Arterial pressure is regulated by the performance of the heart (measured as cardiac output) and the diameter of the arterioles (total peripheral resistance). Hypertension involves an increase in either cardiac output or the peripheral resistance. Mechanisms that seem to be involved affect the extracellular fluid volume and expand the circulating blood volume. This involves excessive renin secretion from the kidneys. Renin is a hormone that raises blood pressure in the body. Increased sympathetic activity that activates stress hormones and an excessive dietary salt intake, possibly associated with a low potassium intake, are also implicated in the pathogenesis of this disease.

Non-pharmacological remedies for hypertension are usually the first to be prescribed before commencing medicines. Weight reduction, salt restriction, moderation in alcohol consumption and cessation of smoking are all recommended before prescribing treatment. A GP may also prescribe a regime of moderate exercise, which has been shown to be beneficial in helping to lower systolic pressure. Relaxation and biofeedback could also be considered before commencing drug therapy. It is

important that the disease is diagnosed and treated early, as intervention – whether pharmacological or non-pharmacological – can reduce the risk of much cardiovascular disease associated with hypertension.

In the past, the treatment of hypertension involved giving patients medicines that had many side-effects, but as medicine has progressed, so has the pharmacology. Generally, patients are commenced on a thiazide diuretic. If this does not provide adequate control, then the patient may be prescribed drugs from the beta-adrenoreceptor antagonist (beta blocker) group. If the blood pressure remains elevated, then the individual will progress onto more potent groups of drugs such as angiotensin-converting enzyme inhibitors or calcium antagonists (calcium channel blockers). Finally, a blockade of alpha adrenoreceptors would be commenced. Typically, drug regimens for people with hypertension consist of a number of these drugs used in combination according to NICE clinical guideline NG136 (2019a) and are given in a stepwise manner (see Box 10.1 for Step 1 key recommendations).

Box 10.1 Drugs used in hypertension: Step 1

Angiotensin-converting enzyme (ACE) inhibitor or an angiotensin II receptor blocker (ARB) to adults starting step 1 antihypertensive treatment who:

- have type II diabetes and are of any age or family origin (see also recommendation 1.4.29 for adults of black African or African-Caribbean family origin) **or**
- are aged under 55 but not of black African or African-Caribbean family origin.

If an ACE inhibitor is not tolerated, use an ARB to treat hypertension.

Offer a calcium-channel blocker (CCB) to adults starting step 1 antihypertensive treatment who:

- are aged 55 or over and do not have type II diabetes **or**
- are of black African or African-Caribbean family origin and do not have type II diabetes (of any age).

(adapted from NICE 2019a)

Thiazide diuretics

Thiazide diuretics are usually the first-line treatment for mild-to-moderate hypertension, providing there are no contraindications. One such drug is bendroflumethiazide, which works by stopping

the body from selectively reabsorbing sodium. This affects the circulating blood volume, causing it to decrease. It has also been noted that this group of diuretics has an effect on blood vessels, causing them to vasodilate and lower blood pressure.

Bendroflumethiazide is well absorbed from the GI tract, so is usually given as a tablet. A dose of 2.5mg daily is usually prescribed. Higher doses will not necessarily lead to a greater fall in blood pressure but will increase the side-effects. Its maximum effect takes is seen at 4–6 hours and its duration of action is between 8 and 12 hours.

Problems can arise with this drug. First, it increases the amount of uric acid present in the plasma because it prevents that acid from being secreted from the body. Therefore, anybody suffering from gout should not take bendroflumethiazide. Another common side-effect is potassium depletion.

Clinical tip

If a patient is a diabetic, controlling their blood sugar will become more difficult when taking drugs for high blood pressure. Male impotence is known to be caused by thiazide diuretics in some individuals. However, this is reversible by stopping the medication. Caution should also be taken if the patient is receiving lithium for bipolar disorder, as the diuretic can cause blood levels of lithium to become elevated.

Even on a small dose of 2.5mg bendroflumethiazide, routine urea and electrolyte blood investigations should be carried out on a yearly basis. More significant side-effects can occur, and the drug can cause hyperglycaemia.

Beta-adrenoreceptor antagonists

In practice, these drugs are usually referred to as *beta blockers*. If a patient develops hypertension, taking a beta blocker will result in a gradual fall in arterial pressure. However, this will take several days or weeks to occur. How these drugs work is not fully understood but they appear to have actions that reduce the cardiac output, reduce renin production from the kidney and reduce the release of stress-related hormones such as adrenaline.

There are at least two types of beta-adreno-receptors in the body, some in the heart (beta 1 receptors) and some in the lungs (beta 2 receptors). Beta blockers are either selective, whereby they block the effect of adrenaline at beta 1 receptors, or non-selective, whereby adrenaline is blocked at both beta 1 and beta 2 receptors. This is an important consideration because beta 2 receptors bring about bronchodilation. Therefore, blocking this effect in patients with airway disease is not desirable. Such patients should be given a selective drug such as atenolol.

This group of medicines can be given in tablet form. Some are taken once daily (e.g. atenolol) while others need to be taken more often (e.g. propranolol). Serious side-effects are not common but are important when imparting information to patients.

Patients with diabetes need to be informed that they might not be aware of becoming hypoglycaemic. The signs and symptoms of hypoglycaemia are mediated through the sympathetic nervous system. This group of drugs inhibits sympathetic responses and the patient may therefore have little warning of an impending lowering of blood glucose levels.

Due to the fall in circulating blood volume, peripheral perfusion of tissues is a consideration. Often a person will complain of having cold hands and feet. Therefore, patients with peripheral vascular disease pose a particular problem and this type of medicine should be avoided. Other side-effects may include fatigue, a low pulse rate (bradycardia) and very vivid dreams and nightmares.

Clinical tip

One way of identifying a drug from this group is that its name ends in 'olol' (e.g. atenolol).

Angiotensin-converting enzyme inhibitors

Angiotensin-converting enzyme (ACE) inhibitors work by stopping the powerful vasoconstricting effects of angiotensin II on the blood vessels. In order to become active, angiotensin II has to convert from angiotensin I. This group of drugs, which includes captopril, stops this conversion from taking place, thus lowering blood pressure.

It is important that the patient drinks plenty of fluids while on these drugs. Dehydration lowers the blood pressure further, so causing an unwanted severe hypotensive state. Captopril can be used on its own or in combination with other antihypertensive agents. It is a powerful hypotensive drug and therefore patients usually commenced on a low dose.

It is sometimes advisable to take the initial dose of the drug before going to bed, so removing any chance of fainting or falling due to hypotension.

Clinical tip

Most drugs ending in 'pril' are a member of the ACE inhibitor group (e.g. captopril).

A dry cough from irritation of the bronchial mucosa is a common side-effect with some patients going on to experience bronchospasm. Captopril has certain individual side-effects due to the nature of its biochemistry. It can cause rashes, changes in taste, a lowering of a group of white cells called neutrophils (neutropenia), and the appearance of protein in the urine (proteinuria).

Other drugs in this group such as lisinopril and ramipril will not cause the same degree of side-effects as captopril because their chemical structure is slightly different. Patients who have a narrowing of their renal artery (renal artery stenosis) will develop renal failure if treated with this group of drugs, as their bodies depend on a fully functioning renin angiotensin cycle.

Calcium channel blockers

These drugs act by limiting the amount of calcium that enters smooth and cardiac muscle. This causes the blood vessels to dilate, resulting in a fall in blood pressure. Some of these drugs are more effective in their action on the heart muscle (e.g.

verapamil) while others work better on smooth muscle of the blood vessels (e.g. nifedipine and amlodipine).

Calcium antagonists are well absorbed by the GI system and are given in tablet form. However, drugs differ in how short- or long-acting they are, and this has an effect on dosage and unwanted side-effects. For example, nifedipine has a short half-life and needs to be taken more frequently than amlodipine, which is taken once a day. However, slow-release preparations of nifedipine are available.

Unwanted side-effects are an extension of the drug's therapeutic activities. Shorter-acting medicines may cause flushing and headaches and if used over a long period of time can cause ankle swelling. Apart from these predictable side-effects, these drugs are relatively trouble-free.

Alpha-adrenoreceptor antagonists

A drug called prazosin was the first selective alpha antagonist to be developed and was used for many years. However, other drugs have now been developed, such as doxazosin and terazosin, which can be taken once a day.

Like beta blockers, these drugs work by inhibiting the action of adrenaline and noradrenaline on body systems. The drugs mentioned above are highly selective, which means they can affect vessels, so causing dilatation, but do not speed up the heart rate (tachycardia). Nor do they lead to any appreciable severe lowering of blood pressure when standing (postural hypotension). Perhaps it is for these reasons that they have become more popular, especially in combination with other antihypertensive therapies.

Angiotensin II receptor blockers (ARBs)

Although angiotensin II receptor blockers (ARBs) work on the renin-angiotensin system, their mechanism of action is very different from that of ACE inhibitors, which inhibit the formation of angiotensin II. ARBs are receptor antagonists that block type 1 angiotensin II (AT1) receptors on bloods vessels and other tissues such as the heart. These receptors stimulate vascular smooth muscle contraction. Because ARBs do not inhibit ACE, they do not cause an increase in bradykinin, which contributes to the vasodilation produced by ACE inhibitors and also some of the side-effects of ACE inhibitors (cough and angioedema). Therapeutic uses include hypertension and heart failure. Examples of this class of drugs are candesartan and irbesartan.

Heart failure

Heart failure can affect the left or right side of the heart and can have many causes, some of which are listed below:

- ischaemic heart disease
- disease of the valves of the heart
- idiopathic cardiomyopathy
- viral or bacterial cardiomyopathy
- myocarditis or pericarditis
- arrhythmias
- hypertension
- thyroid disease
- pregnancy – can induce heart failure
- septic shock – leads to multi-organ failure, which can include the heart.

There are changes that we can see which indicate that the heart is failing. These can be seen in the heart itself and are classed as cardiac, or can be seen in the vascular system itself:

- *Cardiac*
  - Decreased stroke volume and cardiac output
  - Increased end-diastolic pressure
- *Vascular*
  - Increased systemic vascular resistance
  - Decreased arterial pressure
  - Decreased venous compliance
  - Increased venous pressure
  - Increased blood volume

The primary goal of drug therapy in heart failure is to improve cardiac function and reduce the clinical symptoms associated with the condition (e.g. oedema, shortness of breath, exercise intolerance). Improving cardiac function together with reducing circulating volume can dramatically improve the clinical symptoms.

Systolic dysfunction is the most common type of heart failure, accounting for 60–70% of cases. It is characterized by a decreased ejection fraction (> 45%). The strength of ventricular contraction is not able to produce an adequate stroke volume, which, in turn, leads to a reduction in cardiac output. This is usually caused by destruction or dysfunction of the cardiac muscle cells. This can occur as a result of an inflammatory process such as myocarditis, infiltration of the muscle structure as seen in amyloidosis, or, most commonly, ischaemic changes associated with myocardial infarction. Because the left ventricle does not empty properly, there is an increase in the ventricular end diastolic pressure, which, in turn, causes an increase in the pressure within the vasculature of the lungs, resulting in the seeping of fluid into the tissues of the lungs (pulmonary oedema). The increased pressure on the right ventricle causes an increase in the pressure in the systemic circulation, which, in turn, causes fluid to seep out of the capillary beds producing peripheral oedema.

Stroke volume can be improved by several means:

- increasing preload, or the amount of blood in the ventricle just prior to contraction;
- decreasing afterload, therefore reducing the pressure opposing ventricular emptying;
- increasing inotropy, that is increasing the force of the ventricular contraction.

In heart failure (particularly systolic dysfunction), preload is already elevated due to ventricular dilation and/or increased blood volume. Increasing preload will exacerbate pulmonary or systemic congestion and oedema, thus increasing preload is not a viable option for increasing cardiac output in heart failure patients.

Decreasing afterload with vasodilator drugs can significantly enhance ventricular stroke volume. The afterload is often elevated in heart failure, so reducing afterload has been found to be very effective in the treatment of systolic dysfunction. It increases stroke volume and thus decreases preload, thereby improving ejection fraction.

Diastolic dysfunction occurs when the ventricle cannot fill properly because it cannot relax or because the ventricular wall has become thick or rigid. Diastolic failure is characterized by an elevated diastolic pressure in the left ventricle, despite an essentially normal/physiological end-diastolic volume. Diastolic dysfunction results in a large increase in ventricular end-diastolic pressure, which can lead to pulmonary oedema. Despite a large end-diastolic pressure, the end-diastolic volume may be reduced because of the decreased ventricular compliance.

It is important to note that diastolic dysfunction may be a normal part of ageing and does not always constitute part of a disease process. Diastolic dysfunction is more difficult to treat than systolic dysfunction. It is important to note that while pharmacologic intervention can improve the clinical status of heart failure patients, cardiac function and organ perfusion are generally not restored to normal values. In the later stages of heart failure or in severe acute failure, a patient may be very refractory to drug therapy. When this occurs, the only option may be surgical correction of the underlying problem (if identified), mechanical cardiac assist devices or heart transplant.

Drugs used in heart failure fall into the following categories:

- *Diuretics*:
    - thiazide diuretics
    - loop diuretics
    - potassium sparing diuretics
- *Vasodilators* (dilate arteries and veins):
    - angiotensin-converting enzyme (ACE) inhibitors
    - angiotensin II receptor blockers (ARBs)
    - direct acting arterial dilators
    - vasodilators
    - natriuretic peptides
    - phosphodiesterase inhibitors
- *Cardio-stimulatory or inotropic drugs* (stimulate contractility):
    - digoxin
    - beta agonists (sympathomimetic drugs)
    - phosphodiesterase inhibitors

- *Cardio-inhibitory drugs*:
    - beta blockers
    - calcium channel blockers (for diastolic dysfunction)

Coronary artery disease

As stated in the Introduction, cardiovascular disease is a major cause of morbidity and mortality in the UK, and coronary artery disease is one of the primary causes. It is often also called ischaemic heart disease and you may come across these two terms being used interchangeably.

Coronary heart disease describes what happens when the blood supply to the heart is blocked or interrupted. This can be caused by a build-up of fatty substances and deposits in the coronary arteries, a process called atherosclerosis. Over time, the walls of the arteries can become narrowed or clogged by these fatty deposits This causes symptoms such as chest pain, palpitations and breathlessness. The progress and severity of the narrowing or blockage often dictates the outcome for the patient. Some experience angina, while some can go on to have a myocardial infarction (commonly known as a heart attack).

Angina

The main symptom of angina is the onset of central chest pain, which has the following characteristics:

- it feels tight, dull or heavy – it starts centrally but may spread to the left arm, neck, jaw or back;
- it is often triggered by physical exertion or stress;
- it usually stops within a few minutes of resting or of taking relieving medication.

Some patients may experience other symptoms, such as nausea or breathlessness.

There are two main types of angina:

- *Stable angina* (the more common of the two), where the angina attacks have a trigger (such as stress or exercise) and stop within a few minutes of resting or taking relieving medication.

- *Unstable angina* (less common but more serious), in which the attacks are more unpredictable (they may not have a trigger) and can continue despite resting or initial relieving medication.

Some patients may go on to develop unstable angina after having had stable angina for some time, whereas others do not progress from the stable variety.

The use of medication in the treatment and management of angina is aimed at the following:

- treating attacks when they happen (medication only taken when needed);
- preventing further attacks;
- reducing the risk of heart attack and stroke.

If the medications used do not successfully manage the condition, then surgery to improve blood flow to the heart muscles may be recommended. This is usually in the form of a stent to widen the narrowed vessels, or a coronary artery bypass operation.

The drugs used in angina increase blood flow to the heart muscle by dilating the blood vessels. The main drug given to treat an attack is glyceryl trinitrate (GTN), which is taken in the form of a spray or dispersible tablet under the tongue (sublingual route) upon the onset of pain not relieved by rest. It is a nitrate derivative that acts by relaxing vascular smooth muscle in arteries and veins, resulting in dilation of the vessels to improve the narrowing that is causing the pain. Patients should be counselled about when and how to take the medication, to repeat if necessary and at what point they should seek medical attention if the pain is not relieved by rest and medication use.

Many patients will also need to take regular medication to prevent angina attacks. This may not stop angina attacks but usually reduces their frequency and severity. These drugs are also nitrate derivatives. Isosorbide dinitrate and isosorbide-5-mononitrate are organic nitrate esters that can be taken orally to prevent angina attacks.

For long-term prevention of chest pain in patients with stable angina, a beta blocker (such as atenolol, bisoprolol fumarate, metoprolol tartrate or propranolol hydrochloride) should be given as first-line therapy. A rate-limiting calcium channel blocker (such as verapamil hydrochloride or diltiazem hydrochloride) should be considered as an alternative if beta blockers are contraindicated. Dihydropyridine derivative calcium channel blockers (such as amlodipine) may be effective in some patients.

If a beta blocker alone fails to control symptoms adequately, one in combination with a calcium channel blocker should be considered. If this combination is not appropriate due to intolerance of, or contraindication to, either beta blockers or calcium channel blockers, NICE (2011) recommends adding a long-acting nitrate, ivabradine, nicorandil or ranolazine.

A long-acting nitrate, ivabradine, nicorandil or ranolazine should also be considered as monotherapy in patients who cannot tolerate beta blockers or calcium channel blockers, if both are contraindicated, or when they both fail to adequately control angina symptoms.

All patients with angina are at high risk for other significant cardiovascular events such as heart attack and stroke. The risk of these events occurring can be prevented by active management of risk factors through lifestyle changes (such as stopping smoking, losing weight, increasing physical activity and reducing blood pressure), psychological support and drug treatment.

All patients with stable angina due to atherosclerosis should be on long-term treatment with low-dose aspirin (75mg once a day orally) and a statin (such as simvastatin or atorvastatin) to reduce cholesterol. Treatment with an ACE inhibitor can also be considered, especially if the patient has diabetes.

Myocardial infarction

Myocardial Infarction (MI) or heart attack is a serious cardiovascular event and without prompt treatment may result in cardiac arrest and death. A heart attack is caused when a clot or atheroma completely occludes the arteries supplying the heart muscle and no blood reaches the area of myocardium served by the artery affected.

Patients suffering a heart attack should be given opioid analgesia such as morphine for their chest pain while other management is being decided upon. The treatment can be pharmacological or surgical.

Thrombolytic drugs, also called 'clot busters', are drugs used immediately when a heart attack is confirmed (must be given within 12 hours of onset of chest pain). They act to dissolve the clot that is occluding the artery. If atheroma is the cause, then surgical intervention in the form of stent or bypass is required. Intravenous administration of clot-dissolving drugs such as tissue plasminogen activator (TPA) can open up to 80% of acutely blocked coronary arteries.

After treatment and management for a myocardial infarction, patients should be assessed for their cardiovascular risk factors. It may be that they require ongoing management to prevent further coronary artery events. Any existing condition such as angina, heart failure or hypertension should be treated as above, and the patient educated on lifestyle adjustments that may be necessary to mitigate any risk.

Arrhythmias

There are a range of conduction disorders which affect the heart and can lead to arrythmias, the most common being atrial fibrillation (AF).

Atrial fibrillation

This is where the atria (the two upper chambers of the heart) beat out of synchrony with the ventricles (the two lower chambers of the heart) and in an irregular fashion. This irregular conduction can often be rapid in nature. This irregularity results in palpitations, dizziness, shortness of breath and fatigue. If the condition is not managed or left untreated, the person is at a greater risk of stroke or embolism. Atrial fibrillation can be classified as follows (NHS 2018):

- *Paroxysmal atrial fibrillation* – episodes come and go, and usually cease within 48 hours without any treatment.
- *Persistent atrial fibrillation* – each episode lasts for more than 7 days (or less when it's treated).

- *Long-standing persistent atrial fibrillation* – where there has been continuous atrial fibrillation for a year or more.
- *Permanent atrial fibrillation* – where atrial fibrillation is present all the time.

The aims of drug treatment, as part of a personalized package of care, are to return the heart rate to a regular (sinus) rhythm and reduce the risk of stroke or other complications. The type of treatment used can be tailored to individual needs. Reduction of stroke risk is by use of anticoagulants (outlined in Chapter 7), so we will concentrate here on drugs used for rate management.

Digoxin

Digoxin belongs to the group of drugs known as cardiac glycosides and was originally derived from the foxglove plant in the form of digitalis. It has been used to treat heart conditions for many years and remains a valuable drug in treating conduction disorders. Digoxin increases the levels of calcium inside myocardial cells and causes a change to cardiac muscle contractility, increasing the force of contraction. It has a secondary action on movement of sodium and potassium which slows electrical conduction. This can slow and steady the heart rate, but the drug can be toxic in large amounts, so monitoring of heart rate during treatment in necessary and dose adjustments should be made as required to maintain the heart rate between 60 and 100 beats per minute.

According to the 2014 NICE guidance on managing atrial fibrillation, digoxin should be offered as a single therapy to patients with non-paroxysmal atrial fibrillation who are largely sedentary.

Clinical tip

It is important to check the pulse of a patient before giving them their dose of digoxin. If they are found to be bradycardic (a pulse < 60), then the dose should be omitted until the prescriber has been informed. The patient can self-monitor this at home.

Other drugs

Calcium channel blockers, beta blockers and angiotensin II receptor blockers can all be used in patients with atrial fibrillation to stabilize ventricular rate. The choice of the drug used should be based on the patient's symptoms, heart rate, comorbidities and patient preference.

Flecainide acetate acts by decreasing the sensitivity of the heart muscles to electrical impulses, thereby slowing and regulating electrical conduction producing a steady rate and rhythm. The drug can be given by slow intravenous injection in new-onset life-threatening fibrillation where urgent rate control is required and is a pharmacological alternative to electrical cardioversion. This must only be done under close specialist supervision in hospital with a cardiac monitor and resuscitation equipment available. The drug can also be used orally for longer-term benefit in recurrent fibrillation.

Case studies

① Tom McBrayer is a 55-year-old man who presented to his GP with elevated blood pressure, which had been monitored by the practice nurse in the preceding 3 months. A mean score of 185/95 mmHg had been recorded at varying times of the day. His GP starts him on perindopril 10mg, an ACE inhibitor. Explain how angiotensin-converting enzyme inhibitors work.

② Kevin Todd is a 68-year-old gentleman who has been having recurrent episodes of atrial fibrillation. He has had flecainide for cardioversion on numerous occasions and the decision has been made to start him on digoxin therapy. Mr Todd has heard of this drug and is concerned that it may slow his heart too much and he is reluctant to take it. Reflect on how you might reassure him by giving him information on how the drug works and what monitoring he can do at home to ensure he is taking the correct dose to treat his condition.

③ Chuck Andrews is a 49-year-old man who has attention deficit hyperactivity disorder (ADHD) and moderate learning difficulties. He has suffered a myocardial infarction and as a result of investigations has been diagnosed with coronary artery disease and has had bypass surgery. He has now to take an ARB to reduce his blood pressure and is confused as he doesn't understand why he still needs medicine after his operation. What are the key points to discuss with Chuck with regard to:

■ the need for the medication?

■ explaining the action of the medicine?

■ ensuring Chuck understands the information given him?

■ helping him attain adherence to the medication regime?

Key learning points

Hypertension

▶ High blood pressure has pronounced effects on the heart.
▶ It is associated with atherosclerosis.
▶ Lifestyle changes are the first course of action in treatment.
▶ The main classes of drugs are thiazide, diuretics, beta-adrenoreceptor antagonists, angiotensin-converting enzyme inhibitors, calcium antagonists or blockers and alpha-adrenoreceptor antagonists.
▶ Drugs are often given in combination therapy.
▶ Patients usually start with thiazides and progress to more powerful agents.

Heart failure

▶ Heart failure can be caused by systolic or diastolic dysfunction.
▶ Changes can be seen in the heart itself or in the vascular system in general.
▶ Drugs used aim to improve cardiac function and manage symptoms.

Coronary artery disease

Angina

▶ Angina can be stable or unstable.
▶ Main treatment drugs are nitrate derivatives which relax smooth muscle and dilate blood vessels.
▶ Patients with angina should be on drug treatment to prevent secondary events such as MI and stroke.

Myocardial infarction

▶ MI is caused by occlusion of one or more coronary arteries by clots or atheroma.
▶ Thrombolytic drugs can be used in the case of clot occlusion.
▶ Ongoing treatment may be needed for any underlying cardiovascular disease

Arrhythmias

▶ Atrial fibrillation is the most common conduction disorder.
▶ Arrhythmias increase the risk of embolic disease such as stroke.
▶ The aim of treatment is to correct heart rate and prevent secondary complications.
▶ Flecainide acts to chemically cardiovert the heart.

Calculations

1. A patient requires intramuscular furosemide 20mg. Your stock ampoule contains 40mg in 4mL. How many mL would you draw up?

2. Your patient requires flecainide at a dose of 2mg/kg with a maximum per dose of 150mg. Your patient weighs 65kg. You have a solution of 150mg/15mL. How much is required to give the dose?

3. The dose of flecainide calculated in question (2) needs to be given over 30 minutes. What rate in mL/hour should it be given at?

4. Bendroflumethiazide 7.5mg is prescribed orally. Your stock tablets are 2.5mg. How many tablets would you give?

5. Your mentor asks you to check a dose of medication for a patient who is prescribed a loading dose of digoxin by IV infusion. The dose is 1mg and you have 250mcg/mL to add to a bag to make up 100mL of infusion solution. How many mL of digoxin solution needs to be added to how many mL of fluid to get 100mL? What should the rate per hour be to deliver the 1mg dose in 2 hours?

6. You must explain to a patient their medication titration of ramipril and they are wondering how many tablets they will need to take with them as they are off to stay with their family for 28 days. They have to take 2.5mg daily for the first 14 days and then 5mg daily for the next 14 days. They have 2.5mg tablets.

7. Your patient is prescribed candesartan 8mg once daily to be increased in 8mg increments every 4 weeks. How many weeks will it take to increase them to the maximum daily dose of 32mg once?

8. A patient requires 1mg of bumetanide and you have a stock ampoule containing 2mg in 4mL. How much do you give?

9. Your patient has a GTN sublingual spray that has 400mcg per spray actuation. They can take 800mcg at a time for chest pain which can be repeated at 5-minute intervals up to a maximum of 3 doses before they should seek medical attention. How many sprays can they take before they should seek advice?

10. You have to calculate how many tablets to order for ward stock for a patient on isosorbide mononitrate 120mg daily for 7 days. The available tablets are 20mg in strength. How many do you order?

Multiple-choice questions

Try answering these multiple-choice questions to test what you have learned from reading this chapter. You can check your answers at the end of the book.

1. Flecainide acetate can be given to ...

a) Reduce blood pressure
b) Cardiovert the heart rhythm
c) Reduce cholesterol
d) Treat a myocardial infarction

2. Angina occurs with which of the following events?

a) Reduced blood pressure
b) Dilation of peripheral arteries
c) Narrowing of coronary arteries
d) Atrial fibrillation

3. Thrombolytic drugs used in MI aim to ...

a) Dissolve a blood clot
b) Reduce blood pressure
c) Increase heart rate
d) Reduce cholesterol

4. Heart failure symptoms can be ...

a) Cardiac in origin
b) Vascular in origin
c) Cardiac or vascular in origin
d) Neither cardiac or vascular in origin

5. Bendroflumethiazide acts by preventing the reabsorption of ...

a) Potassium
b) Calcium
c) Chloride
d) Sodium

6. Which drug group could be the step 1 management of hypertension?

a) Beta-adrenoreceptor antagonists
b) Diuretics
c) Calcium antagonists
d) ARBs

$\longrightarrow$

7. **What heart rate would we be aiming for in a patient on digoxin therapy?**

a) Less than 60bpm
b) 60–80bpm
c) 60–100bpm
d) Over 100bpm

8. **Which of the following drugs is a calcium channel blocker?**

a) Bendroflumethiazide
b) Captopril
c) Nifedipine
d) Prazosin

9. **Atenolol belongs to which class of drug?**

a) Beta blockers
b) Anti-arrythmics
c) Diuretics
d) ACE inhibitors

10. **GTN used in angina acts by …**

a) Blocking beta receptors
b) Dilating blood vessels
c) Having a diuretic effect
d) Increasing heart rate

Recommended further reading

British Heart Foundation (BHF) (2019) *Facts and Figures*. London: BHF. Available at: https://www.bhf.org.uk/what-we-do/news-from-the-bhf/contact-the-press-office/facts-and-figures.

Downie, G., Mackenzie, J. and Williams, A. (2007) *Pharmacology and Medicines Management for Nurses*, 4th edition. Edinburgh: Churchill Livingstone.

Greenstein, B. and Gould, D. (2008) *Trounce's Clinical Pharmacology for Nurses*, 18th edition. New York: Churchill Livingstone.

Karch, A.M. (2017) *Focus on Nursing Pharmacology*, 7th edition. Philadelphia, PA: Lippincott Williams & Wilkins.

Lapham, R. (2015) *Drug Calculations for Nurses: A Step-by-Step Approach*, 4th edition. London: Arnold.

NHS (2018) *Atrial fibrillation*. Available at: https://www.nhs.uk/conditions/atrial-fibrillation/.

National Institute for Health and Care Excellence (NICE) (2011) *Clinical Guideline CG126: Stable Angina: Management*. London: NICE. Last updated August 2016.

National Institute for Health and Care Excellence (NICE) (2014) *Clinical Guideline CG180: Atrial Fibrillations: Management*. London: NICE.

National Institute for Health and Care Excellence (NICE) (2019a) *Clinical Guideline NG136: Hypertension in Adults: Diagnosis and Management*. London: NICE.

National Institute for Health and Care Excellence (NICE) (2019b) *British National Formulary*. London: NICE. Available at: https://bnf.nice.org.uk.

Simonson, T., Aarbakke, J., Kay, I., Coleman, I., Sinnott, P. and Lyssa, R. (2006) *Illustrated Pharmacology for Nurses*. London: Hodder Arnold.

Drugs for Parkinson's disease and epilepsy

11

Chapter contents

Learning objectives – Parkinson's disease

After studying this chapter, you should be able to:

- Describe the basic pathology and diagnosis of Parkinson's disease.
- Explain the mode of action of medicines used in managing this condition and relate these to physiology.
- Demonstrate an understanding of the unwanted effects of medicines used in treating this condition.
- Demonstrate an understanding of the links between the pharmacology of therapies used in treating Parkinson's disease and the care given by the health practitioner.

Introduction

Epilepsy is a complex multifaceted condition which can affect anyone at any age, and therefore can be seen in all aspects of nursing. Parkinson's disease is largely a disease of old age. Both are conditions with neurological components.

Parkinson's disease

Parkinson's disease is a progressive disorder of movement. The pathological processes that lead to the development of the disease are not fully understood but some of the effects on functional anatomy have been identified. Neurones in the *substantia nigra* area of the brain are lost to degeneration. These neurones are dopamine producing and the effects of the reduction in this neurotransmitter are responsible for some of the symptoms and signs of the disease. These neurones project into other areas of the brain, which are collectively known as the basal ganglia. It is from these areas that the motor symptoms of the disease are manifest. The patient develops a persistent tremor, even at rest, and quite often there are head-nodding and pill-rolling movements of the fingers. Their posture becomes affected and they begin to bend forward and walk in small, shuffling steps. Textbooks used to describe the person's face as 'mask-like' because they acquire a stiff facial expression. There can be rigidity in other muscles and impaired balance. Finally, the patient has trouble in initiating and coordinating movement.

Parkinson's disease was first described by James Parkinson in 1817 in his *Essays on the Shaking Palsy*. It did not become known as Parkinson's disease until so named by the French neurologist Jean-Martin Charcot in 1888 (Goetz 1987). In 1960, Hornykiewicz demonstrated that the dopamine content of the substantia nigra in post-mortem examination of patients with the disease was extremely low – in some cases, 10% less than normal. This work was not published in full until much later (Ehringer and Hornykiewicz 1998). More sophisticated diagnostic tests have revealed similar findings and suggest the loss of dopamine occurs over several years. Symptoms only become apparent when the dopamine content of this area has fallen below between 20 and 40% of normal.

Drugs that are taken for this debilitating disease work by increasing dopamine in the brain in a number of ways; however, despite these pharmacological interventions, patients do *not* return to a normal state. In addition to the effects of the disease there are also side-effects to the medication (see Box 11.1). Drugs are prescribed following the recommendations of NICE guideline NG71 on Parkinson's disease in adults (NICE 2017), which categorizes treatment options into pharmacological interventions for motor symptoms, managing adverse effects of dopaminergic therapy, pharmacological management of non-motor symptoms and neuroprotective pharmacology.

Levodopa

Levodopa, a dopamine precursor, remains the first-line treatment for Parkinson's disease where motor symptoms decrease the patient's quality of life (NICE 2017, 2019). Dopamine alone is unable

Box 11.1   Drugs used in Parkinson's disease

Drug class	Generic name	Use
Dopamine precursor	Levodopa + benserazide / carbidopa / entacapone	Improves motor symptoms and activities of daily living. Some motor complications and few specified adverse events
Monoamine oxidase B inhibitors	Rasaligine Safinamide Selegiline	Less improvement in motor symptoms and activities of daily living but fewer motor complications and less specified adverse events
Catechol-O-methyl transferase inhibitors	Entacapone Tolcapone	Used when patients develop dyskinesia with levodopa
Dopamine receptor agonists	Amantadine Bromocriptine Cabergoline Pergolide Pramipexole Ropinirole Rotigotine	Less improvement in motor symptoms and activities of daily living but fewer motor complications and more specified adverse events
Antimuscarinics	Orphenadrine Procyclidine Trihexyphenidyl	Used for drug-induced extrapyramidal symptoms

Information taken from NICE (2017) and tabulated.
Specified adverse events include sleepiness, hallucinations and impulse control disorders (NICE 2019).

to cross the blood–brain barrier (BBB) and it is also destroyed quickly by enzymes in the peripheral tissues. Levodopa is a drug that can cross the BBB and then be converted by the central nervous system into dopamine. It is nearly always combined with another substance that stops peripheral enzymes breaking down dopamine. This means that more levodopa is available to the brain and a lower dose of dopamine can be given. Examples of medicines that are combined or given with levodopa are carbidopa, entacapone and benserazide.

When given levodopa, the initial response rates of patients are good and improvements in motor and non-motor symptoms are apparent. However, this improvement is often not sustained in the long term and the levodopa appears to become less effective. This loss of efficacy is probably due to the unrelenting course of the disease.

Two major side-effects are associated with levodopa. First, a condition called dyskinesia can develop, where the individual develops a series of jerky involuntary movements usually affecting the face and limbs. If the dose is lowered, the dyskinesia may recede but the symptom of rigidity it had improved returns. This requires the patient to be informed of this before prescription so that they can make an informed decision about the balance of the benefit of the medication and the potential for side-effects.

A second side-effect associated with this group of drugs is the 'on–off' effect. This is where, quite suddenly, the drug therapy seems to stop working. This can be quite distressing for the patient and can sometimes occur when they are in the middle of doing something. The reason for this fluctuation is not fully understood, but patients should be made aware of this when commencing treatment. Decisions on prescribing should be made based on the patient's individual circumstances and preference (NICE 2017, 2019).

The patient may also notice short-term side-effects from the dopamine precursors, although these are often transient. These include nausea, anorexia, anxiety, diarrhoea and postural hypotension. A small number of patients may develop delusions and hallucinations as the brain adjusts to the increase in dopamine. Part of the role of the nurse, together with the patient and their family, is to observe and monitor any side-effects as well as the therapeutic effects hoped for.

Selegiline

This medicine works by stopping the enzyme that breaks down dopamine in the synapses, therefore making more of the dopamine that is present in the synapse available for longer to activate post-synaptic receptors. The enzyme in question is monoamine oxidase-B (MAO-B) and appears in regions of the brain which are dopamine rich. This means that the drug only works in these areas of the brain, so limiting any side-effects or interactions. Giving this drug with levodopa seems to have better results than giving levodopa on its own. However, when levodopa is given in combination with either carbidopa or benserazide, there appears to be no difference than when giving selegiline alone.

Dopamine receptor agonists

This group of drugs works by mimicking the action of dopamine on dopamine receptors. Examples of this class are amantadine, bromocriptine, pramipexole and pergolide. Their duration of action is longer than that of levodopa, so they do not need to be given as often. The toxic effects of these drugs are similar to those of levodopa, although the hallucinations can be more severe. Sometimes these drugs are given in combination with levodopa to reduce overall side-effects or improve the patient's response.

Antimuscarinics

Antimuscarinics are used to combat the effects of the relative excess of central cholinergic activity that occurs as a result of the reduction in dopamine levels in some areas of the brain (NICE 2019).

Catechol-O-methyltransferase inhibitors

These drugs, of which entacapone is an example, act by preventing the breakdown of levodopa in the periphery, allowing more of it to cross the BBB to perform its central action. They are not used alone and are prescribed as adjunct medication to levodopa.

Epilepsy

Epilepsy is the most common chronic disabling condition of the nervous system. Epileptic seizures result from an imbalance of the excitatory and inhibitory mechanisms within the brain, whereby the nerve impulses generated from the neurones are abnormal and uncoordinated. The form of seizure that the person suffers usually depends on the part of the brain affected. Seizures can range from brief lapses in attention to full-blown convulsive fits which may last for several minutes. Epileptic seizures can be classified as follows:

- Focal onset seizures
- Generalized onset seizures
- Seizures of unknown onset

Seizures can also be classified by the level of awareness retained throughout the seizure. Sometimes the person will be completely aware of their surroundings and the fact that they are having a seizure, but that is not always the case. Information about types of seizure is provided by the UK Epilepsy Society (2018).

Focal onset seizures

Focal onset seizures occur in a localized areas of the brain. The symptoms depend on which region of the brain is discharging the abnormal impulses. Focal aware seizures are an example of this, where the person is alert and aware of the seizure activity, they may have a feeling of 'strangeness' but often cannot verbalize exactly how they felt. There may be visual disturbances, or smells or tastes that are experienced. There may be twitching or stiffness of part of the body. The exact signs will depend on the brain area involved.

Focal impaired awareness seizures affect a larger area of the brain but are usually restricted to one hemisphere. There may be a loss of consciousness or confusion. The person may have some awareness of their surroundings but may not respond to cues or commands. Aggression can occur in this type of seizure and it is frequently followed by a 'post ictal' period where confusion and aggression may persist, and the patient complains of tiredness and may have no memory of events.

Focal seizures can be a precursor of a generalised seizure.

Generalized onset seizures

This type of seizure involves the whole of the brain and affects areas responsible for consciousness and arousal. Abnormal impulses arise throughout both hemispheres. Two important categories are absence seizures and tonic clonic seizures.

Absence seizures are characterized by a brief alteration in consciousness that is sometimes very difficult to detect. This type of seizure occurs more in children and can be frequent in nature.

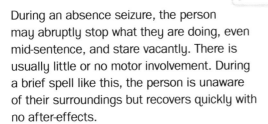

Clinical tip

During an absence seizure, the person may abruptly stop what they are doing, even mid-sentence, and stare vacantly. There is usually little or no motor involvement. During a brief spell like this, the person is unaware of their surroundings but recovers quickly with no after-effects.

Tonic clonic seizures consist of an initial strong contraction of the whole muscular system that causes a rigid spasm. Respiration is affected, the person may wet themselves, there may be increased salivation and they can bite their tongue. Skin colour can change and they may cry out. The person then begins to suffer a series of violent rhythmic jerking movements of the limbs which can last for a few minutes. The person is usually sleepy after the seizure (post ictal phase) and often cannot remember the event. They may be confused or complain of headache. Breathing quickly returns to normal.

Clinical tip

A condition known as *status epilepticus* can occur in some patients, where one tonic clonic seizure follows another. This may continue for a period of time and can become life-threatening. Medical treatment needs to be implemented urgently in such cases.

Treatment for epilepsy is aimed at eliminating seizures using the lowest possible dose of medication. If this cannot be achieved, then reducing seizures to a minimum must be the aim. A range of drugs, called *anticonvulsants* or *anti-epileptic drugs* (AEDs), is used (see Box 11.2). The choice of medication should be based on NICE guideline CG137: Epilepsies: Diagnosis and Management, which was updated in 2019.

AEDs are divided into three risk-based categories to help prescribers decide if the patient needs to be maintained on a specific manufacturer's product, as there can be differences in bioavailability across brands (see NICE 2019). The three categories are:

- Category 1: patients should be maintained on a specific manufacturer's product
  - Phenytoin, carbamazepine, phenobarbital and primidone
- Category 2: the need for continuing a particular manufacturer's product should be based on clinical judgement and review
  - Valproate, lamotrigine, perampanel, rufinamide, clobazam, clonazepam, oxcarbazepine, topiramate

- Category 3: it is usually not necessary to ensure patients are maintained on a specific manufacturer's product
  - Levetiracetam, lacosamide, tiagabine, gabapentin, pregabalin, ethosuximide, vigabatrin

AEDs modify neurotransmission through a number of different ion channels and receptor complexes. The majority have their effects at sodium or calcium channels or at the gamma aminobutyric acid (GABA) receptor, but some are known to have effects on glutamate transmission (White et al. 2007)

Box 11.2   Drugs used in the treatment of epilepsy

Seizure type	First-line AED	Adjuvant
Generalized tonic clonic	Carbamazepine Lamotrigine Oxcarbazepine Sodium valproate	Clobazam Lamotrigine Levetiracetam Sodium valproate Topiramate
Focal	Carbamazepine Lamotrigine Oxcarbazepine Sodium valproate Levetiracetam	Carbamazepine Clobazam Gabapentin Lamotrigine Levetiracetam Oxcarbazepine Sodium valproate Topiramate
Absence	Ethosuximide Lamotrigine Sodium valproate	Ethosuximide Lamotrigine Sodium valproate OR consider: Clobazam Clonazapam Levetiracetam Topiramate
Status epilepticus	Community Buccal midazolam Rectal diazepam IV lorazepam	In hospital Intravenous lorazepam Intravenous diazepam Buccal midazolam

Information taken from NICE (2012) and tabulated.

Inhibition of sodium channel function

In Chapter 4, we discussed the firing of a neurone and the importance of the passage of sodium into the neurone. If sodium movement across membranes is inhibited, then neurones are less likely to fire. Sodium-inhibiting drugs do not block all sodium channels but are selective to channels that allow high-frequency impulses to take place. In other words, they dampen down the excitability in neurones without switching them off. Examples of common drugs in this class are phenytoin, carbamazepine, lamotrigine, oxcarbazepine, rufinamide, lacosamide and eslicarbazepine acetate. They all have similar efficacy and have similar dose profiles and side-effects (Brodie 2017).

Phenytoin

This drug was first used clinically as an AED in the 1930s. It blocks the high-frequency sodium channels in neurones in many parts of the brain. It is the oldest known drug in this class and is thus the forerunner of drugs that have similar actions. It interacts with many other medications due to its induction effect on liver drug metabolizing enzymes. It has many side-effects, including gingival hyperplasia, which can be distressing, even at therapeutic doses and is toxic in overdose; its use therefore is now limited.

Phenytoin works to its full potential at specific concentrations in the blood. If the range exceeds this, the patient gets more toxic side-effects without any further protection from seizures. Regular blood monitoring is required while on this therapy, which is not the case with many of the newer AEDs.

Phenytoin is also associated with teratogenic effects and its use in women of childbearing potential should be avoided. If it is used, then the dose will need to be adjusted owing to changes in plasma protein concentrations in pregnant woman (Brodie 2017).

Lamotrigine

This AED is well tolerated and has a broad range of effect across seizure types. Although newer than phenytoin, it is well established as an AED and is a first-line drug in treating focal and generalized

seizures (NICE 2012, 2019; Brodie 2017). It is deemed safer in pregnancy, though like phenytoin, the dose needs to be adjusted. It can be used by breastfeeding women, as little of it is passed to the infant. One notable side-effect that seems to be specific to this drug in this class is that of insomnia or disordered sleep. If this is a problem, then patients can be switched to another drug in this class, which usually resolves the problem. The drug should not, however, be withdrawn abruptly but instead tapered over 2 weeks (NICE 2019).

Carbamazepine

Like phenytoin, carbamazepine is an AED of long standing and it is also a known inducer of hepatic metabolizing enzymes. With the range of drugs now available, it is not often the first drug of choice in newly diagnosed cases of epilepsy (Brodie 2017). It is also one of the AEDs associated with a hypersensitivity syndrome that is a rare but potentially fatal consequence of using this drug. If signs of hypersensitivity occur (fever, rash and lymphadenopathy), it should be withdrawn immediately and a new AED found (NICE 2019).

Inhibition of calcium channels

Some of the anticonvulsant drugs are thought to have minor involvement in blocking calcium channels.

Ethosuximide

This is the first-line management drug when it comes to treatment for absence seizures. It has little or no effect in other types of epilepsy and can sometimes actually increase the risk of seizures. The drug works on T-type calcium channels. Its side-effects are relatively minor and include nausea, anorexia and sometimes lethargy and dizziness. Very rarely the drug can cause severe hypersensitivity reactions.

Zonisamide

This drug is thought to act on T-type calcium and sodium channels and is often used to treat focal onset seizures. It may also have some neuroprotective effects independent of its AED action (Biton 2007).

175

Enhancement of GABA action

Sodium valproate

It is not entirely clear exactly how valproate works, as it does several things in the brain. First, the chemical messenger (or neurotransmitter) GABA is 'inhibitory' on the brain, i.e. it reduces neuronal cell firing. After its effect it is broken down and activity stops. Increasing the amount of GABA or potentiating its action can enhance this neuro-inhibitory effect and this is anticonvulsant.

Second, it may inhibit 'repetitive firing' of neurones. When a message is passed, there is a short refractory period or gap (about one-thousandth of a second) before the next message can be passed, during which time the nerve ending resets itself. Valproate may increase this refractory period, or time, by a small amount. Under normal circumstances, this will make no difference at all, but if the brain is overactive and lots of messages are being passed in quick succession, the valproate will reduce the number of messages back to the normal level.

Sodium valproate has a number of side-effects, but the main reason for its reduction in use as an AED is its link to teratogenicity. In 2018, the Medicines and Healthcare Products Regulatory Agency issued guidance contraindicating its use in women and girls of childbearing potential unless the conditions of their pregnancy prevention programme are met (NICE 2019). The most serious side-effect is hepatotoxicity. For the first 6 months of treatment, the patient will need regular blood tests to check that the drug is not affecting their liver. The patient may also need to have blood tests from time to time to make sure that the dose of valproate is neither too much nor too little.

Gabapentin

Gabapentin and an associated drug, pregabalin, were initially licensed as AEDs whose main effect was augmentation of GABA neurotransmission, which has an inhibitory effect on neuronal cell firing. Gabapentin is thought to do this by increasing the synthesis of the neurotransmitter (Taylor 1997). More recently, it has been used as a neuropathic analgesic and little or no recent evidence about its exact AED mechanism has been published. Nevertheless, it remains a very useful AED in focal seizures.

Modification of glutamate transmission

Unlike GABA transmission in the brain, which is inhibitory, glutamate transmission is excitatory. Drugs which can suppress the excitatory effects of glutamate have been found to be effective AEDs. Glutamate transmission is calcium dependent, so in addition to the effects on sodium channel opening, many of the AEDs in this category also reduce glutamate transmission. The exact mechanisms behind managing the balance between excitation in the brain and inhibition of neuronal firing is therefore very complex (Barker-Halinski and White 2015).

Topiramate

Topiramate is known to modify glutamate transmission through suppression in the hippocampus (Barker-Halinski and White 2015). It is used in the treatment of focal and general onset seizures but tends to be second line or adjunct. Like other drugs in this area of pharmacology, care must be taken in pregnancy, as congenital malformations and growth effects have been seen; it should also be avoided in breastfeeding (NICE 2019).

Case studies

① Eric Vardey is a 55-year-old man who has recently been diagnosed with early Parkinson's disease. He has been quite upset and depressed about the diagnosis and has lost interest in his usual activities and hobbies. His wife reports that his tremors, slowness in

→

movement, rigidity and postural instability have worsened over the past 12 months. He has been taking the following medications for 6 months: carbidopa/levodopa (CD/LD) 25mg/100mg four times a day. The doctor has now increased it to carbidopa 25mg/levodopa 250mg.

With reference to Eric's changed medicines, outline the mode of action of levodopa and suggest what the main side-effects of this medicine might be for Eric.

② Younis Khan is a 45-year-old Type I diabetic patient who has recently been diagnosed with epilepsy that requires control with medication. His insulin regime is maintaining his blood sugars nicely. His current medication is:

- insulin glargine once daily;
- fluvastatin 40mg once daily;
- aspirin 75mg once daily.

The neurologist has started Younis on anticonvulsant medication of phenytoin 500mg daily.

Look in Appendix 1 of the BNF and review the interactions of phenytoin with Younis's current medication.

Reflect on the risk of balancing possible interactions and side-effects with the need for the epilepsy medication.

Key learning points

Parkinson's disease

▶ Progressive disorder of movement due to lack of the neurotransmitter dopamine.
▶ Persistent tremor, head nodding and pill-rolling are examples of movement disorder.
▶ Drugs used in the treatment process include levodopa, selegiline and dopamine receptor agonists.
▶ Drugs do not offer a cure but manage the symptoms that reduce quality of life.

Epilepsy

▶ Common disabling neurological condition.
▶ Classified into partial seizures and generalized seizures.
▶ Drugs used inhibit sodium and calcium channels in the neuronal membrane and also increase the amount of GABA.
▶ Phenytoin is an anticonvulsant drug which is highly protein bound.
▶ Phenytoin can have unpleasant side-effects such as ataxia and vertigo.
▶ Ethosuximide is used only in absence seizures.
▶ Sodium valproate increases GABA.
▶ Need to check blood levels of patients taking anticonvulsants.
▶ Vigabatrin is a new drug which raises the level of GABA.

Calculations

1. A patient requires oral co-beneldopa which contains benserazide and levodopa, 100mg 3 times daily. The dose is expressed by the levodopa content. Your stock is benserazide 12.5mg/levodopa 50mg. How many tablets are required for a 7-day supply?

2. Sodium valproate suspension 200mg is prescribed for an individual. You only have 125mg in 5mL. How many mL would you give?

3. Orphenadrine 150mg is prescribed orally to be given in 3 divided doses over the day. Your stock solution is 10mg/mL. How many mL would you give for each individual dose?

4. Your mentor asks you to check a dose of medication for oral administration. The patient requires amantadine 100mg and the drug comes as 50mg in 5mL. How much should be dispensed?

5. Sodium valproate suspension 50mg is prescribed for an individual. You only have 200mg in 5mL. How many mL would you give?

6. A child requires 50mg of phenobarbitone. If the stock ampoules contain 200mg in 2mL, how much will you draw up?

7. A patient requires 1mg of cabergoline daily for 7 days, then 1.5mg daily for 7 days, and finally 2mg daily for 14 days. You have none in stock and need to order 500mcg tablets from the pharmacy. How many do you order for a 28-day period?

8. Carbamazipine 0.25g is needed and the suspension you have contains 100mg in 5mL. How much would you administer?

9. Pramipexole dosing in the BNF is stated by amount of pramipexole base but there is an equivalence by amount of pramipexole salt for immediate-release preparations. The equivalence is 88mcg of base to 125mcg of salt. The doctor has prescribed 88mcg 3 times per day. What is the equivalent in salt of this for the whole day?

10. Sodium valproate suspension 90mg is approximately equivalent to 100mg capsules or tablets. You have a patient with swallowing difficulties. How many mL of suspension (30mg in 5mL) should you give for a dose of 300mg capsules?

Multiple-choice questions

Try answering these multiple-choice questions to test what you have learned from reading this chapter. You can check your answers at the end of the book.

1. **Which of the following drugs is used in status epilepticus?**

a) Lamotrigine
b) Diazepam

←

c)   Topiramate
d)   Sodium valproate

2.   **Which of these drugs is a dopamine precursor?**

a)   Levodopa
b)   Ropinirol
c)   Procyclidine
d)   Cabergoline

3.   **Which part of the brain shows dopamine neurone depletion in Parkinson's disease?**

a)   The cortex
b)   The mesencephalon
c)   The substantia nigra
d)   The cerebellum

4.   **Which of the following is a side-effect of increased dopamine in the treatment of Parkinson's disease?**

a)   Tremor
b)   Muscle rigidity
c)   Hallucinations
d)   All of the above

5.   **Which of the following drugs inhibits MAO-B?**

a)   Selegiline
b)   Levodopa
c)   Pramipexole
d)   Entacapone

6.   **Catechol-*O*-methyltransferase inhibitors stop the breakdown of levodopa where?**

a)   The blood–brain barrier
b)   The periphery
c)   The synapse
d)   The receptors

7.   **Levodopa is often given with which other drug in the treatment of Parkinson's disease?**

a)   Pergolide
b)   Carbidopa
c)   Selegiline
d)   All of the above

→

←

8. Parkinson's disease is caused by a lack of which substance?

a) Acetylcholine
b) Dopamine
c) Serotonin
d) Noradrenaline

9. The drug of choice in treating absence seizures is …

a) Ethosuximide
b) Gabapentin
c) Phenytoin
d) Sodium valproate

10. Which of the following neurotransmitters has an inhibitory function?

a) Noradrenaline
b) Acetylcholine
c) Gamma aminobutyric acid
d) Serotonin

Recommended further reading

Barker-Halinski, M. and White, H.S. (2015) Glutamatergic mechanisms associated with seizures and epilepsy, *Cold Spring Harbor Perspectives in Medicine*, 5 (8): a022863. Available at: https://doi.org/10.1101/cshperspect.a022863.

Biton, V. (2007) Clinical pharmacology and mechanism of action of zonisamide, *Clinical Neuropharmacology*, 30 (4): 230–240.

Brodie, M.J. (2017) Sodium channel blockers in the treatment of epilepsy, *CNS Drugs*, 31 (7): 527–534. Available at: https://doi.org/10.1007/s40263-017-0441-0.

Ehringer, H. and Hornykiewicz, O. (1998) Distribution of noradrenaline and dopamine (3-hydroxytyramine) in the human brain and their behavior in diseases of the extrapyramidal system, *Parkinsonism and Related Disorders*, 4 (2): 53–57.

Goetz, C.G. (1987) Excerpts from nine case presentations on general neurology delivered at the Salpetriere Hospital in 1887–8, in J.M. Charcot (ed.) *The Tuesday Lessons*. New York: Raven Press.

Greenstein, B. and Gould, D. (2008) *Trounce's Clinical Pharmacology for Nurses*, 18th edition. New York: Churchill Livingstone.

Karch, A.M. (2017) *Focus on Nursing Pharmacology*, 7th edition. Philadelphia, PA: Lippincott Williams & Wilkins.

Lapham, R. (2015) *Drug Calculations for Nurses: A Step-by-Step Approach*, 4th edition. London: Arnold.

NHS (2019) *Sodium valproate*. Available at: https://www.nhs.uk/medicines/sodium-valproate/.

National Institute for Health and Care Excellence (NICE) (2012) *Clinical Guideline CG137: Epilepsies: Diagnosis and Management*. London: NICE. Last updated October 2019.

National Institute for Health and Care Excellence (NICE) (2017) *NICE Guideline NG71: Parkinson's Disease in Adults*. London: NICE.

National Institute for Health and Care Excellence (NICE) (2019) *British National Formulary*. London: NICE. Available at: https://bnf.nice.org.uk.

Parkinson J. (1817) *Essay on the Shaking Palsy*. London: Sherwood, Neely, and Jones.

Simonson, T., Aarbakke, J., Kay, I., Coleman, I., Sinnott, P. and Lyssa, R. (2006) *Illustrated Pharmacology for Nurses*. London: Hodder Arnold.

Taylor, C.P. (1997) Mechanisms of action of gabapentin, *Revue Neurologique*, 153 (suppl. 1): S39–S45.

UK Epilepsy Society (2018) *Seizure types*. Available at: https://www.epilepsysociety.org.uk/seizure-types#.XOU8j25KiUl.

White, H.S., Smith, M.D. and Wilcox, K.S. (2007) Mechanisms of action of antiepileptic drugs, *International Review of Neurobiology*, 81: 85–110.

Drugs used in mental health

12

Chapter contents

Learning objectives

After studying this chapter, you should be able to:

- Provide an overview of the incidence of mental health problems in the UK.
- Define the term 'pathological anxiety'.
- List three major classifications of anxiety disorder.
- Explain how defence and behavioural systems contribute to anxiety.
- List two neurotransmitters thought to be implicated in anxiety.
- Explain in simple terms how benzodiazepines work.
- Outline the biological basis of depression.
- Give three examples of different groups of antidepressant drugs.

- Outline the mode of action of selective serotonin re-uptake inhibitors (SSRIs).
- Name two drugs used in bipolar depressive illness.
- Explain simply the biological basis of schizophrenia.
- List the positive and negative symptoms of schizophrenia.
- Give reasons why there are differences between typical and atypical antipsychotics.
- Give examples of typical and atypical antipsychotic drugs.
- Give reasons for the difference in side-effects between typical and atypical antipsychotics.

Introduction

The aim of this chapter is to introduce you to drugs used in common mental health problems. The chapter examines three key areas of mental health intervention:

- anxiety;
- depression;
- psychosis.

Mental health issues extend into all aspects of nursing and an appreciation of the range of medications and how they work is essential for all nurses. One in four adults in the UK experience at least one diagnosable mental health problem in any one year, and one in six experience this at any given time (Office for National Statistics 2001). It is estimated that approximately 450 million people worldwide have a mental health problem (World Health Organization 2001).

The Nursing and Midwifery Council's Standards for Pre-Registration Nursing Programmes published in May 2018 state that education must:

ensure that field-specific content in relation to the law, safeguarding, consent, pharmacology and medicines administration and optimisation is included for entry to the register in one or more fields of nursing practice

Although this could be interpreted as only relating to mental health students, Platform 3 of the Proficiencies from the NMC also states:

3.3 demonstrate and apply knowledge of all commonly encountered mental, physical,

behavioural and cognitive health conditions, medication usage and treatments when undertaking full and accurate assessments of nursing care needs and when developing, prioritising and reviewing person-centred care plans

The main mental health conditions encountered are as follows.

Anxiety

Anxiety is a common, normal and usually self-limiting emotion, with which we are all familiar. For some people, however, feelings of anxiety can be intolerable and can become disabling. This level of anxiety is pathological and requires prompt diagnosis and active treatment to help the sufferer regain and maintain their previously normal lifestyle. At this level, anxiety can manifest with wide and varied symptoms, both physical and psychological.

Anxiety is not simply one illness, but a group of disorders characterized by psychological symptoms such as diffuse, unpleasant and vague feelings of apprehension, often accompanied by physical symptoms of autonomic arousal such as palpitations, light-headedness, perspiration, 'butterflies' and, in some patients, restlessness.

According to the *International Statistical Classification of Diseases and Related Health Problems* (ICD-10; WHO 2016), there are six main classifications of anxiety disorders:

1. panic disorder;
2. social phobia;
3. generalized anxiety disorder;

4 obsessive-compulsive disorder (OCD);

5 post-traumatic stress disorder (PTSD);

6 mixed anxiety and depressive disorder.

An understanding of the physiological mechanisms thought to be involved in the development of pathological anxiety is vital to ensure appropriate treatment of anxiety disorders. First, it is important to understand that two brain systems appear to be involved in the generation of anxiety.

The defence system

The defence system controls our responses to danger. It receives stimuli related to the threat of danger and the brain interprets these stimuli and responds as required. The defence system is responsible for the so-called 'fear, fight or flight' responses. It can be a protective mechanism, whereby we can respond to threats or perceived threats and prepare the body to defend itself or to flee from the danger. It can also be activated by things which are not real threats but are *perceived* to be real by the anxiety sufferer and can become pathological.

The behavioural inhibition system

This system prevents a person from getting into danger and is responsible for *avoidance behaviour*. It is also involved in learning not to do dangerous things, thereby allowing future avoidance of anxiety-provoking situations. This can lead to anxiety sufferers withdrawing from real-life situations because of the fear of being placed in danger, leading to agoraphobia, claustrophobia and social isolation.

Neurotransmitters in anxiety

The brain is a complex organ and with respect to anxiety many different neurotransmitters are involved. These include the following monoamines:

■ noradrenaline (NA);

■ 5-hydroxytryptamine (5-HT) or serotonin;

■ gamma-aminobutyric acid (GABA).

The exact role these neurotransmitters play in anxiety is not fully elucidated but using drugs that act on these systems can be beneficial in the management of anxiety.

Medicine management of anxiety

Although the various anxiety disorders share some characteristics, they each need to be evaluated and treated in their own way. Anxiety management can be broken down into the following categories:

■ **non-pharmacological:** psychological;

■ **pharmacological:** single and combined psychotropic and non-psychotropic treatments;

■ **combinations** of pharmacological and non-pharmacological treatments.

Much treatment for anxiety involves a pharmacological component. Anxiolytic treatment should ideally be effective and rapid for the relief of disabling symptoms. The treatment should not be too sedative, as this can be as detrimental as the anxiety itself. This is achievable in the current pharmacological climate but can often come at a price. The following drugs have all been used to treat the symptoms of anxiety, many of which are still in use today:

■ barbiturates;

■ benzodiazepines;

■ beta-adrenergic blockers;

■ azaspirodecanediones;

■ antipsychotics;

■ antidepressants.

Barbiturates

Barbiturates are potentiators of the GABA$_A$ receptor, which has a *pentameric structure*. It consists of five sub-units that surround an ion channel which conducts chloride (Cl⁻) ions (see Figure 12.1). It is the major inhibitory neurotransmitter in the brain and central nervous system. Therefore, potentiation of an inhibitory transmitter channel leads to increased inhibition, or reduced activity at the receptors the chloride ion acts on. This causes a 'dampening down' of neuronal activity. When the chloride ion channel is opened up by GABA,

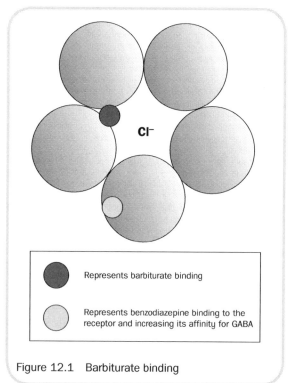

Cl⁻

■ Represents barbiturate binding

○ Represents benzodiazepine binding to the
receptor and increasing its affinity for GABA

Figure 12.1   Barbiturate binding

Benzodiazepines

For many years, the most common first-line pharmacological treatment for anxiety disorders was a benzodiazepine drug. More recently, however, benzodiazepines such as diazepam and temazepam have become associated with problems of addiction and dependence, and the potential for abuse. And because the use of benzodiazepines has been related to significant long-term problems, they should be used in the short term only for the management of anxiety-related conditions. NICE clinical guideline CG113 (2011) on the management of generalized anxiety disorder and panic disorder in adults suggests:

1 – Benzodiazepines should not be offered except as a short-term measure during crisis. This applies to primary and secondary care settings.
2 – The use of benzodiazepines is associated with a less good outcome long term and should not be prescribed in panic disorder.

Despite the above, benzodiazepines are still an effective treatment for acute, transient anxiety. Like barbiturates, these drugs potentiate the effects of GABA but do so by a different mechanism. They bind to a specific benzodiazepine binding site (or receptor) situated on one of the sub-units of the GABA$_A$ receptor. Their mechanism of action is to increase the affinity of GABA, which increases the ability of and frequency with which GABA can open the chloride ion channel. Unlike barbiturates, benzodiazepines need GABA to be present all the time the channel is open, not just at activation, for them to have their effect. This makes them safer than barbiturates because they have a wider therapeutic index, so there is less chance of toxicity and accidental overdose.

For use in anxiety, the dose tends to be low, with higher doses being reserved for use with insomniacs. This means that the side-effect of sedation should occur less often, although for some people drowsiness is a problem.

Another major side-effect of benzodiazepines is respiratory depression, and this should be monitored on initiation of therapy.

the barbiturate drug molecule enters the channel and causes it to remain open for longer than GABA on its own can. This allows for more chloride from outside the neurone to enter, so reducing the likelihood of an action potential being generated. This means that the barbiturate drug causes a potentiation of GABA transmission and a reduction in neuronal activity.

There are downsides to using barbiturate drugs such as amobarbital (formerly amylobarbitone) because they have a narrow therapeutic index, which means that the dose of the drug needed for a beneficial effect is very close to that considered toxic. Thus it is easy to take too little and have no effect, or too much and result in an overdose. They also have addictive properties and patients can easily become dependent on them. The effects of barbiturates can also be magnified when taken with alcohol. For these reasons, they are rarely used in the management of anxiety today.

Clinical tip

When a patient starts taking a benzo-diazepine, it is very important that you warn them of the possible sedative effects and discuss the dangers of driving or operating heavy machinery. This is a requirement of legislation amending the Road Traffic Act to incorporate 'The Drug Driving (Specified Limits) (England & Wales) (Amendment) Regulations 2015'.

Beta-adrenergic blockers

These drugs are used not to treat the central nervous system transmitters thought to be involved in anxiety, but to treat the *physical* symptoms that are manifest in anxiety such as palpitations, tremors, sweating and shortness of breath. They do not have an effect on the psychological aspects of anxiety, so the patient will still feel anxious.

There are many beta-blocking drugs, but only propranolol and oxprenolol are licensed for use in the management of anxiety. These drugs may help people with mild anxiety to function in everyday situations where before their symptoms would have proved problematic.

Clinical tip

If a patient also suffers from diabetes, do not forget to warn them that taking a beta blocker may inhibit the normal signs and symptoms of a hypoglycaemic attack.

Azaspirodecanediones

Buspirone is the only member of this class of drugs available for the treatment and management of anxiety symptoms. Its mechanism of action is not fully elucidated but it is known to affect the serotonergic receptors, inhibiting serotonergic transmission. This effect develops quickly but the anxiolytic effect does not typically occur for 2–3

weeks. This can be problematic in the treatment of anxiety, as patients often cannot tolerate the delayed onset of action.

Buspirone is not associated with addiction or dependence. Although usually licensed for short-term use only, it can be used for several months under specialist supervision. In practice, this drug is not used alone but in combination with other medication and can be a useful adjunct.

Antipsychotics

There is evidence that certain antipsychotic drugs have a positive effect in the treatment and management of anxiety. The method by which they relieve anxiety is not known, but these drugs are associated with emotional changes and the relief of symptoms such as agitation. In the management of anxiety, they are used in doses much lower than would be required to induce their antipsychotic effects. Drugs such as haloperidol, flupentixol and tri-fluoperazine can be used as anxiolytics and have a rapid onset. They are especially useful if the patient has a diagnosis of psychosis, as their anxiety may be related to this.

Like barbiturates and benzodiazepines, some of the side-effects of antipsychotic drugs can be compounded by alcohol. This makes the prescription of these drugs less likely.

Antidepressants

The tricyclic antidepressants (TCAs) have a positive effect in generalized anxiety disorder and panic disorder, although many of these drugs are not licensed for such indications. The TCAs were used in the past for mixed anxiety/depressive disorders but they do not appear to have any specific anxiolytic activity. It may be that their anxiolytic effect is related to their sedative properties. It takes 2–3 weeks for the anxiolytic and antidepressant effects to develop, suggesting that the mechanisms for these effects may be related.

Another type of antidepressant, the selective serotonin re-uptake inhibitors (SSRIs), can appropriately be used in chronic anxiety of more than 4 weeks' duration. Their mechanism of action is fully explained in the section on depression. Their anxiolytic action takes 2–3 weeks to develop, which is consistent with the onset of their antidepressant effect, again suggesting that the mechanisms are related. Some SSRIs are associated with increased anxiety until the antidepressant effect kicks in, and for this reason concomitant use of a benzodiazepine for the first 2–3 weeks is often recommended, with a low starting dose that can be increased as tolerated.

Treatment is usually long term and often the doses prescribed are at the higher end of the scale for full effect. The SSRIs commonly use for anxiety include:

- fluoxetine and sertraline, licensed to treat anxiety symptoms with depression and for OCD and PTSD;
- fluvoxamine, licensed for the treatment of OCD;
- citalopram, licensed for the treatment of panic disorder;
- paroxetine, licensed for the treatment of social phobia, panic disorder, OCD and mixed anxiety and depression.

Depression

Depression is a common serious psychiatric illness. Depressive or affective disorders involve disturbances of mood or affect (cognitive and emotional symptoms), which are frequently associated with changes in behaviour, energy levels, appetite and sleep patterns (biological and physiological symptoms). People who suffer from depression report a poor quality of life. This often extends to their carers, and can be detrimental to their close relationships. Depression is associated with a high incidence of suicidal tendency and thus mortality. Depression can be either:

- **Unipolar** – where the mood or affect is always low. This is characterized by misery, malaise, despair, guilt, apathy, indecisiveness, low energy and fatigue, changes in sleep patterns, loss of appetite and thoughts of suicide. It can be either reactive or endogenous. *Reactive* depression implies that the cause of the illness

is brought about by severe stress. *Endogenous* depression, on the other hand, occurs when no obvious external causative factor can be identified; or

- **Bipolar** – where the mood or affect and behaviour swing between depression and mania. This type of depression has a greater tendency to include an inherited component.

For a diagnosis of depression to be applied, the patient must display certain key symptoms and also exhibit some ancillary symptoms. This assists the diagnosis and categorization of the depression.

Key symptoms

- depressed mood;
- an inability to experience pleasure from normally pleasurable life events such as sex (anhedonia);
- a lack of energy.

Ancillary symptoms

- changes in weight and appetite;
- sleep disturbance;
- low self-esteem;
- psychomotor agitation or retardation;
- guilt or self-reproach;
- difficulty concentrating;
- suicidal thoughts.

The National Institute for Health and Care Excellence (NICE) base their definition of the severity of depression on the *Diagnostic and Statistical Manual of Mental Disorders IV* (DSM-IV; APA 1994) and ICD-10 (WHO 2016). This gives the following classifications of depression for treatment and management purposes:

- *Sub-threshold depressive symptoms*, where the patient has fewer than five of the above symptoms of depression (can be called reactive sadness and may be in response to a life event).
- *Mild depression*, where the patient has more than five of the symptoms of depression but displays only a mild functional impairment.

- *Moderate depression*, or the stage between mild and severe depression where more than five symptoms are displayed.
- *Severe depression*, where the patient has most of the symptoms of depression and also shows a marked functional impairment. Although psychotic features will always indicate severe depression, they are not necessary for a diagnosis of severe depression to be made.

The aetiology of depression is still unclear. The biological theories relating to the disease would suggest that there are many factors in the development of depressive disorders, including psychological, genetic, biological and neurochemical.

Psychological factors

These are known to play a part in the development of many types of depression and can be categorized as follows:

- Childhood and developmental experiences that are seen as negative, such as abuse, whether it be physical, mental or sexual; separation from one or both parents, with maternal separation being particularly traumatic; breakdown of the relationship between parents and/or problems with the parent-child relationship.
- An unusually high number of what are termed 'significant life events'. These are often ranked according to their perceived impact, with bereavement, especially of a spouse, at the top of the list. Surprisingly, 'positive' life events such as getting married or the birth of a baby can also have a significant negative impact. This may be due to a major change in lifestyle.
- Stress that can be deemed unusual or continual, such as stress at work or in a relationship.
- The absence of a secure or confiding relationship. This can be particularly relevant to the elderly and those who have lost a loved one, and may also explain why those who live alone have a higher tendency to become clinically depressed.

Genetic factors

Genetic factors are implicated in many areas of mental and physical health. Although no individual gene has been identified in depressive disease, there is a strong suggestion from family and twin studies that there is a genetic basis for vulnerability to depression. A number of genes may be related to the function of known neurotransmitters and receptors, suggesting a biological effect. Other genes may be involved in influencing how a person perceives and responds to a certain kind of event or stressor, which may lead to depression in certain people but not in others.

Biological factors

Biological factors are a major focus for research into depression and antidepressant drugs. Much of this research has concentrated on:

- hormonal influences; or
- the monoamine hypothesis.

Hormonal influences

Cortisol, a corticosteroid, is known as the 'stress hormone' and has been linked to depression. Many people go on to develop depression if they are subjected to repeated and prolonged stress. Ongoing research is linking corticosteroids with monoamines to try to complete the picture.

The monoamine hypothesis

Many monoamines have been implicated in depression. Monoamines are, as their name suggests, organic compounds with a single (mono) amine group. They have the biological function of being neurotransmitters and neuromodulators and exert their effects at receptors located predominantly on neurones. They were first implicated as having a role in depression in the 1960s. This was because the main antidepressant drugs used at that time (the TCAs and monoamine oxidase inhibitors, MAOIs) both have chemical actions on monoamines. It was suggested that reduced levels of monoamines could be a causative factor in depressive illness, although a case can be made both for and against this claim. Hence the monoamine hypothesis could explain why:

- drugs that deplete levels of monoamines are depressant in nature (e.g. reserpine, methyldopa);
- drugs that increase the availability of monoamines *can* improve mood in depressed patients (e.g. TCAs and MAOIs);
- the concentration of some monoamines is notably reduced in the cerebrospinal fluid (CSF) of depressed patients.

But equally the hypothesis does not explain why:

- drugs that increase the availability of monoamines have *no effect* on mood in depressed patients (e.g. amphetamines, cocaine);
- some of the older antidepressants have no effect on monoamine systems (e.g. iprindole);
- there is a therapeutic delay of 2 weeks for the full effects of monoamine antidepressants to be seen.

Medicine management of depression

The BNF (NICE 2019) describes the main antidepressant drugs as shown in Box 12.1.

Tricyclic antidepressants

Tricyclic antidepressants (TCAs) are powerful drugs which block the reuptake of two major monoamines, noradrenaline and serotonin, also known as 5-HT. This means that there is more of the monoamine available to the receptors and this has an antidepressant effect. However, drugs in this class, such as amitriptyline, act at other receptors. which can lead to side-effects such as:

- **Sedation**, which can be useful if the drug is taken at night and insomnia is a problem. However, the sedation can be amplified if the drugs are taken with alcohol, which can be serious.
- **Cardiac rhythm problems**, which can be severe in overdose.
- **Anticholinergic effects** – action at muscarinic receptors, such as urinary retention and constipation.
- **More seizures** in epileptic patients.

These side-effects and the advent of newer, safer medications for depression mean that TCAs are not prescribed as first-line treatment for depression.

> **Clinical tip**
>
> Remember to reassure the patient that side-effects of TCAs such as a dry mouth, blurred vision and becoming dizzy on standing (postural hypotension) are common. However, if the patient finds these intolerable, they should make an appointment to discuss other drug options.

Monoamine oxidase inhibitors

Monoamine oxidase (MAO) exists in two forms, MAO-A and MAO-B, both of which are responsible for chemically breaking down monoamines to render them inactive. The monoamine oxidase inhibitors (MAOIs), of which phenelzine is an example, block this breakdown. This increases the availability of the monoamines, which, as with the TCAs, leads to an antidepressant effect.

The MAOIs are used infrequently due to the high risk of drug interactions, especially with other antidepressants. They also interact negatively with some foodstuffs that contain tyramine and dopamine (e.g. some cheeses, red wine, pickled herring), which can cause blood pressure to increase to a dangerous level and patients on these medications are warned to avoid such foods.

Although most MAOIs bind irreversibly, moclobemide is reversible.

> **Clinical tip**
>
> Rarely will you encounter the use of MAOIs in clinical practice. However, if you do, remember that the patient will require a treatment card. This will have information about diet, the taking of other medicines and alcohol consumption. The patient should carry this card at all times and show it to any doctor or dentist treating them.

Box 12.1 Antidepressants

Group	Abbreviation	Example
Tricyclic antidepressants	TCAs	Amitriptyline
Antidepressants related to TCAs		Trazodone
Monoamine oxidase inhibitors	MAOIs	Phenelzine
Reversible inhibitor of monoamine oxidase-A	RIMA	Moclobemide
Selective serotonin re-uptake inhibitors	SSRIs	Citalopram
		Sertraline
Other drugs	NARIs	Reboxetine
	SNRIs	Venlafaxine
	AAAs	Mirtazapine

Selective serotonin re-uptake inhibitors

This class of drugs act selectively at serotonin (5-HT) neurones to produce their antidepressant effect. They have very similar drug profiles, the main differences between them being their drug interactions and times to take effect.

5-HT is released from the neurone into the synapses where it activates receptors (see Figure 12.2). After release, it is taken back up into the neurone that released it by a transporter located in the neuronal membrane. Selective serotonin re-uptake inhibitors (SSRIs) inhibit the re-uptake of 5-HT from the synapses after it has been released. This increases the amount of 5-HT in the synapses available to activate receptors which respond to 5-HT, thus having an antidepressant effect (see Figure 12.3).

The SSRIs have far fewer side-effects than other antidepressants and are safe in the case of an overdose. This makes them a good choice of first-line drug for treating most types of depression.

The main drugs prescribed in this class are fluoxetine and citalopram. The main reported side-effects include nausea and diarrhoea, loss of sexual desire and libido, some anxiety during initiation of treatment and, occasionally, sleep disturbances.

The effects of SSRIs take 14–21 days to fully develop and this should be explained to patients when treatment commences. The NICE guideline on the management of depression (2009) recommends the use of SSRIs. There is some evidence to suggest that, particularly in adolescence, SSRIs can increase the risk of suicide and self-harm. Any such risks should be balanced against the effectiveness of using these drugs in treating a patient's depression.

Clinical tip

When prescribing SSRIs, doctors, nurses and pharmacists should warn patients of the possible risks of suicidal behaviour and monitor them closely in the early stages of treatment.

Other drugs

There are some other drugs that are useful in the treatment of depression (see Box 12.2). They include:

- **Flupentixol:** an antipsychotic drug that can be used to treat mild-to-moderate depression.
- **Mirtazapine:** an alpha adrenoceptor antagonist which is a relatively sedating antidepressant.

- **Reboxetine:** a noradrenaline specific re-uptake inhibitor.
- **Venlafaxine:** a noradrenaline and 5-HT specific re-uptake inhibitor which may have a quicker onset of action than noradrenaline or SSRIs alone.
- **Tryptophan:** a naturally occurring precursor to 5-HT which is obtained from our diet but can

be given in its pure form. It is believed that if more of the precursor is available, the body will make more 5-HT, prompting an antidepressant effect. It can be used as an adjunct therapy with MAOIs and TCAs.

For bipolar depression, the treatment options are limited to lithium and some anticonvulsant drugs. Lithium treatment has been used for many years to prevent and treat bipolar depression. It is referred to as a 'mood stabilizer', as it helps to

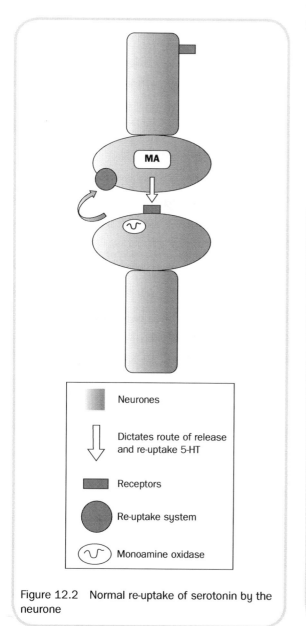

Figure 12.2   Normal re-uptake of serotonin by the neurone

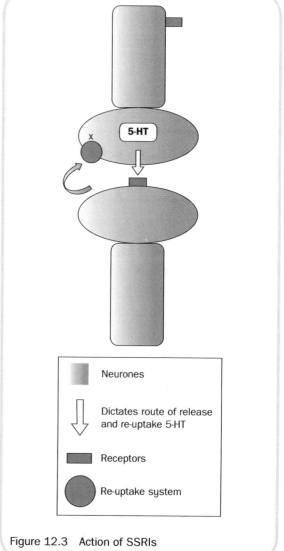

Figure 12.3   Action of SSRIs

Box 12.2 Other drugs used in the treatment of depression

Drug class	Example
TCAs	Amitriptyline
MAOIs	Phenelzine
SSRIs	Fluoxetine
NARIs (noradrenaline re-uptake inhibitors)	Reboxetine
SSRI/NARI	Venlafaxine

prevent the swings of mood (from depression to mania) typical of this illness. Lithium is a naturally occurring metallic element. Its action in the management of bipolar depression is poorly understood but is thought to be linked to its actions on monoamine neurotransmission. However, it is unclear how its actions relate to its therapeutic effects. It is a drug with a narrow therapeutic index and a long half-life, so requires careful monitoring as there is a high risk of toxicity in overdose which can be fatal.

Clinical tip

It is important that every patient taking lithium be provided with a treatment card detailing the correct dose, blood test details and advice on drinking alcohol, taking other medicines and the effects of toxicity. When caring for someone who is taking lithium, you should be aware of the need to monitor the patient's fluid intake and also the implications of sickness and diarrhoea. It is important that the patient avoids dehydration, as this will increase the risk of lithium toxicity.

Some anticonvulsant medicines such as sodium valproate and carbamazepine have been found to have beneficial effects in bipolar depression. They are thought to be safer than lithium but are still associated with serious side-effects.

St. John's wort (Hypericum perforatum)

Although not prescribed for depression in the UK, St. John's wort is a popular herbal remedy, readily available for the management of mild forms of depression and used by many people. However, it can induce drug metabolizing enzymes in the liver, which can lead to changes in how the body metabolizes other medications, causing interactions and side-effects. For this reason, the use of St. John's wort is not recommended alongside many other medications. Appendix 1 of the British National Formulary (NICE 2019) should be consulted to ascertain the risk of a patient taking St. John's wort alongside other medicines. Interestingly, many of the drugs affected are conventional antidepressants. The concentration of active ingredients in St. John's wort varies from preparation to preparation, making monitoring difficult.

When patients cease taking St. John's wort, there are concomitant changes in drug metabolizing enzyme performance, and therefore a risk of drug toxicity. MIND (2017), a UK mental health charity, provides useful information on its website for patients who are taking or are considering taking St. John's Wort.

Psychosis

Schizophrenia is one of the main psychotic mental health disorders because of its prevalence, its young age of onset (15–45 years) and its chronic and disabling nature. Its pathophysiology is not completely understood but several theories have been proposed, including one linking the condition to dopamine. This is supported by the fact that many drugs that are effective in schizophrenia act as dopamine receptors.

Schizophrenia is a disorder of thought and thought processes, perception, emotion and volition. Its symptoms fall into two main categories, either positive or negative in character. The *positive* symptoms include:

- delusions;
- hallucinations;
- disordered thought;

while the *negative* symptoms include:

- poverty of speech;
- flattened affect;
- social withdrawal;
- anhedonia (inability to experience pleasure);
- apathy;
- attention deficit.

The distinction between positive and negative symptoms is important, as the main drug treatments tend to have most effect on the positive symptoms, whereas the negative symptoms are very hard to treat.

Other psychotic illnesses include:

- schizoaffective disorder;
- delusional disorders;
- some depressive and manic disorders.

Neuroleptic or antipsychotic medications, which act on the dopaminergic system and receptors, are the mainstay of antipsychotic intervention. These drugs, which are associated with a number of side-effects, may take several weeks to have their full effect. The antipsychotic actions and extra-pyramidal side-effects of neuroleptic drugs are strongly correlated with their ability to block central dopaminergic transmission. The extra-pyramidal system is a neural network located in the brain that is part of the motor system involved in the coordination of movement. By blocking dopamine receptors, antipsychotic drugs can trigger a variety of movement disorders owing to their effect on the extra-pyramidal system. This means that, to

obtain full control of the symptoms of schizophrenia, the doses used can often intensify side-effects. The ability of certain drugs to act on dopaminergic transmission and relieve the symptoms of psychosis was the basis of the dopamine hypothesis of schizophrenia first postulated in the 1960s.

Antipsychotic drugs are classified as typical or atypical in their actions. Many dopamine receptors and other types of receptor are acted on by these drugs. Most typical antipsychotics act at D_2 receptors, while most atypical antipsychotics act at D_1 and D_4 receptors. Having said this, most of these drugs have actions at other receptors as well, especially at higher doses and this is often what causes the side-effects.

A particular problem with taking antipsychotic medications daily is that certain patients may not see the need to continue taking them. Quite often the patient has little understanding of their problem and as a result they may feel well and therefore reduce intake. Certain antipsychotic drugs are therefore given as what is known as a *depot injection*. This is an injection of a drug, usually given via the IM route, which releases its active compound in a consistent way over a long period of time. Depot injections are usually either solid or oil based. The advantages of using a long-acting depot injection include increased medication compliance and a more consistent serum concentration. However, one significant disadvantage is that the drug is not immediately reversible since it is released slowly.

Clinical tip

When giving a depot injection, you should use a 'Z track' injection method. This seals the medication deeply within the muscle and allows no exit path into the subcutaneous tissue and skin. This is accomplished by moving the skin and subcutaneous tissues by 2.5–3.75cm laterally, prior to the injection, and immediately releasing the same tissues after the injection.

Box 12.3   Drugs used in the treatment of psychosis

Typical	Atypical
Chlorpromazine	Sulpiride
Promazine	Clozapine
Flupentixol	Olanzapine
Haloperidol	Quetiapine
Trifluoperazine	Risperidone

Examples of typical and atypical antipsychotic drugs are listed in Box 12.3.

Typical antipsychotics

Typical antipsychotics are associated with more side-effects despite their good antipsychotic action, due to their activity at the D_2 receptors. They are structurally similar and chemically related. The actions at D_2 receptors can be viewed in terms of the three main pathways they influence (see Figure 12.4):

① the mesolimbic pathway;

② the tuberoinfundibular pathway;

③ the nigrostriatal pathway.

Mesolimbic pathway

This pathway is associated with the psychological effects of antipsychotics:

- antipsychotic effects;
- sedation;
- impaired performance.

Tuberoinfundibular pathway

This pathway is associated with the neuroendocrine effects of antipsychotics:

- **Hyperprolactinaemia:** this involves a high circulating level of prolactin from the pituitary gland, which can have an adverse effect on the production of breast milk as well as menstrual/erectile problems.
- **Amenorrhoea:** the absence of periods in a woman of reproductive age.
- **Galactorrhoea:** the spontaneous flow of milk from the breast.
- **Gynaecomastia:** the enlargement of male breast tissue.
- **Infertility:** the biological inability of a man or a woman to contribute to conception.

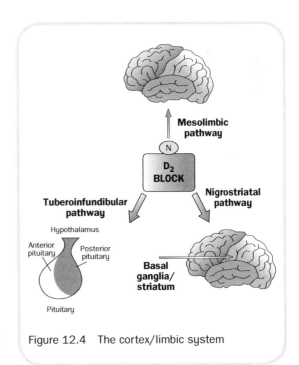

Figure 12.4   The cortex/limbic system

Nigrostriatal pathway

This pathway is associated with movement disorders produced by antipsychotics:

- **Parkinsonism:** characterized by a lack or slowness of movement, muscular rigidity and tremor.
- **Dystonia:** characterized by sustained muscle contractions resulting in twisting or repetitive movements, or the adoption of abnormal postures.
- **Akathisia:** characterized by restlessness and unease.
- **Tardive dyskinesia:** characterized by abnormal involuntary movements of the face.

Clinical tip

As a nurse, it is important that you act as advocate on behalf of the patient. This means reporting any signs and symptoms of any medication to senior colleagues or the medical staff. This will ensure side-effects can be dealt with early.

Atypical antipsychotics

These drugs, unlike the typical antipsychotics, share very little in terms of structure or chemistry.

- **Clozapine** is a dibenzodiazepine neuroleptic and exerts its effect via dopamine receptors but also acts at muscarinic and 5-HT receptors.
- **Sulpiride** is a dopamine and 5-HT blocker and is effective in the treatment of schizophrenia. It is suggested that sulpiride has is more active at mesolimbic dopamine receptors.
- **Risperidone** has a higher affinity for 5-HT than dopamine and a lower incidence of sedation and extra-pyramidal side-effects at low doses than other neuroleptics.

Clinical tip

Clozapine carries the risk of lowering the agranular white blood cell count (agranulocytosis); thus monitoring of blood levels of neutrophils is a mandatory condition of treatment. As these blood cells protect us from infection, it is important that the level does not drop significantly. You should be aware of patients on this medication that complain of relatively minor ailments such as recurring sores.

Side-effects

The side-effects of typical antipsychotics occur because of their action at a variety of receptors, including the dopamine receptors, which are responsible for their beneficial effects. Antipsychotics are associated with many side-effects, some of which can be quite severe and are commonly referred to as extra-pyramidal side-effects. Examples include:

- **Dopaminergic side-effects:** acute neurological effects (dystonia, Parkinsonism) and chronic neurological effects (tardive dyskinesia, tardive dystonia).
- **Neuroendocrine side-effects:** amenorrhoea, galactorrhoea and infertility.
- **Idiosyncratic side-effects:** neuroleptic malignant syndrome. This is a life-threatening reaction that some people have to antipsychotic medicines.

Clinical tip

Often the first sign of neuroleptic malignant syndrome is a fever. Therefore, you should be observant and report any changes in the temperature of an individual who has just commenced antipsychotic medication. If treated early, this condition does not have to be fatal.

- **Cholinergic side-effects:** dry mouth, blurred vision, constipation, urinary retention and ejaculatory failure.
- **Histaminergic side-effects:** sedation.
- **Adrenergic side-effects:** hypotension and arrhythmia.
- **Miscellaneous side-effects:** photosensitivity, heat sensitivity, cholestatic jaundice and retinal pigmentation.

It is often necessary to prescribe other drugs to mitigate the side-effects of antipsychotics. These drugs can be grouped as follows:

- **Anticholinergics:** used for motor side-effects (e.g. benzhexol, procyclidine).
- **Psychostimulants:** used in demotivation.
- **Benzodiazepines:** used for akathisia (e.g. lorazepam).

- **Beta blockers and antihistamines:** occasionally used for akathisia.

Atypical antipsychotics in general have a much better side-effect profile and are generally better tolerated and safer to use than typical antipsychotics.

Clinical tip

Atypical antipsychotics are far from being free of side-effects. You should warn patients that on certain drugs weight gain can be a significant problem. Also, secondary type II diabetes is an emerging problem associated with taking atypical antipsychotics and you may be involved in screening patients by urine testing or carrying out random blood glucose measurements.

Case studies

① Debbie Butcher is a well-educated 37-year-old woman with two previous episodes of depression in the last 10 years, both of which were treated. The first (post-natal depression) was treated with fluoxetine for one year and the second (as a result of her ninth miscarriage) with citalopram for 2 years. The doctor has prescribed her another SSRI and she asks you to explain how it works. How would you describe the mechanism of action of SSRIs, with particular reference to their onset of action and the monoamines involved?

② Anil Khan is a 53-year-old man who has been diagnosed with schizophrenia since the age of 23. He has been cared for in a number of institutions and has recently been admitted to an independent mental health hospital. For many years he has been treated with a variety of typical antipsychotics, and the medical staff suggest he is drug resistant and are trying him on the newer atypical therapy.

- How would you describe to a junior nurse the actions of such drugs on the individual?
- How would you explain the differences between the two types of antipsychotic medication?

③ Rona McKenzie is a successful architect but has recently been experiencing the symptoms of extreme anxiety when presenting to clients. She finds that her palms and underarms sweat profusely, her hands shake and she has 'butterflies'. Discuss the pros and cons of medication for Rona and suggest which class of antidepressant would be most suitable for her anxiety disorder.

←

④ Lisa Ryman is 19 years old and has autism spectrum disorder and a degree of learning disability. She suffers from anxiety and is finding she panics as she arrives at college and does not want to enter. Her mother has asked you about benzodiazepines to help 'calm Lisa down' so she doesn't miss out on her education. How would you explain to Lisa and her mother that benzodiazepines are not a long-term option?

Key learning points

Introduction

▶ One in four adults in the UK experiences at least one diagnosable mental health problem in any one year.
▶ There are some 450 million people worldwide with a mental health problem.

Anxiety

▶ Anxiety can become intolerable for some people and is therefore considered to be pathological.
▶ It is a group of disorders characterized by both physical and psychological symptoms.
▶ There are six main classifications.
▶ Our defence mechanism can become stimulated by perceived threats.
▶ Avoidance behaviour can be initiated.
▶ A number of neurotransmitters are involved (e.g. noradrenaline).
▶ Anxiolytic treatment should be effective and quick-acting.

Medicine management of anxiety

▶ Barbiturates potentiate GABA.
▶ They have a low therapeutic index.
▶ They have addictive properties.
▶ They are rarely used in anxiety management.
▶ Benzodiazepines are still one of the most effective treatments for acute and transient anxiety.
▶ They also potentiate the effects of GABA.
▶ These drugs have a wider therapeutic index and are therefore less toxic than barbiturates.
▶ Beta-adrenergic blockers are used to treat the physical symptoms of anxiety.
▶ They may help people with mild anxiety to function in certain situations.
▶ Buspirone is the only azaspirodecanedione in its class used for the treatment of anxiety.
▶ Some evidence exists to suggest that antipsychotics may have a positive benefit in the treatment of anxiety.
▶ How they relieve anxiety is not known and they are only used in low doses.
▶ Drugs such as haloperidol and flupentixol may be used.

→

- Antidepressants such as tricyclic compounds seem to have an effect in generalized anxiety disorder.
- SSRIs can appropriately be used in chronic anxiety (e.g. fluoxetine).

Depression

- Depression is the most common serious psychiatric illness.
- It is associated with high morbidity.
- Unipolar depression is characterized by a continuous lowering of mood.
- Bipolar disorder is characterized by the swinging of mood between depression and mania.
- Depression is characterized by certain key symptoms such as lowering of mood, sleep disturbance and changes in weight and appetite.
- The aetiology is still unclear but is thought to include psychological factors, genetic factors and biological factors.
- A variety of neurotransmitters (monoamines) have been implicated in the causation of depression.

Medicine management of depression

- TCAs affect the re-uptake of noradrenaline and serotonin.
- Side-effects include sedation, anticholinergic effects and cardiac dysrhythmias.
- MAOIs work by stopping the body breaking down neurotransmitters such as serotonin.
- These drugs are now rarely used due to the high risk of drug interactions.
- SSRIs act selectively at serotonin neurones.
- Serotonin is increased at the synapses.
- SSRIs have fewer side-effects and are safer in overdose than other antidepressants.
- Venlafaxine is a drug that has a quick onset and raises the levels of noradrenaline and serotonin available to the body.
- Bipolar depression is treated with lithium or certain anticonvulsant drugs.
- Lithium needs careful monitoring as it can cause toxicity.
- Drugs such as sodium valproate and carbamazepine have also been found to be beneficial in the treatment of bipolar disorder.

Psychosis

- Schizophrenia is the main psychotic mental health disorder.
- Positive symptoms include delusions, hallucinations and disordered thought.
- Negative symptoms include social withdrawal, flattened affect and apathy.
- Drugs used in the treatment of schizophrenia block the actions of dopamine in the brain.
- Typical antipsychotics are associated with more side-effects.
- Typical antipsychotics block the three main dopamine pathways.
- Typical antipsychotics produce side-effects which are often described as being extra-pyramidal.
- Atypical antipsychotics include clozapine, sulpiride and risperidone.
- Atypical antipsychotics in general have less severe side-effects, are tolerated better and are safer to use.

Calculations

1. A client is prescribed 50mg of amitriptyline and 25mg tablets are available. How many tablets will you give?
2. A client is prescribed 300mg of promazine and 100mg tablets are available. How many tablets will you give?
3. A client is prescribed 100mg of promazine and 25mg tablets are available. How many tablets will you give?
4. A client is prescribed 1.25mg of clonazepam and 0.5mg tablets are available. How many tablets will you give?
5. A client is prescribed 20mg of haloperidol decanoate by intramuscular injection and 50mg in 1mL of liquid for IM injection is available. How many mL will you administer?
6. A client is prescribed 5mg of flupenthixol decanoate by intramuscular injection and 40 mg in 2mL of liquid for IM injection is available. How many mL will you administer?
7. A client is prescribed 5mg of haloperidol orally and 2mg in 1mL of syrup is available. How many mL will you administer?
8. A client is prescribed 10mg of promazine orally and 50mg in 5mL suspension is available. How many mL will you administer?
9. A client is prescribed 4g of trifluoperazine orally and 5g in 5mL liquid forte is available. How many mL will you administer?
10. A client is prescribed 2.5mg of promethazine hydrochloride orally and 5mg in 5mL of elixir is available. How many mL will you administer?

Multiple-choice questions

Try answering these multiple-choice questions to test what you have learned from reading this chapter. You can check your answers at the end of the book.

1. Depression can be described as …

a) Unipolar and multipolar
b) Multipolar and oligopolar
c) Oligopolar and bipolar
d) Bipolar and unipolar

2. SSRI drugs act on which monoamine?

a) Adrenaline
b) Dopamine
c) Serotonin
d) Noradrenaline

→

←

3.   Benzodiazepines bind to which receptor complex?

a)   NA
b)   DA
c)   BZD
d)   GABA

4.   Neuroleptic medications are used for ...

a)   Psychosis
b)   Neurosis
c)   Epilepsy
d)   Parkinson's disease

5.   Lithium can be described as ...

a)   A mood enhancer
b)   A mood reflector
c)   A mood inducer
d)   A mood stabilizer

6.   5-hydroxytryptamine is also known as ...

a)   Buscopan
b)   Serotonin
c)   Adrenaline
d)   5-BC

7.   Amylobarbitone is an example of ...

a)   A barbiturate
b)   A benzodiazepine
c)   A tricyclic
d)   An SSRI

8.   Which of the following is a benzodiazepine?

a)   Benzopine
b)   Tazepam
c)   Diazepam
d)   Lazypram

9.   How long does it take until SSRI antidepressants begin to have a therapeutic effect?

a)   The same day
b)   2–3 weeks
c)   One month
d)   6 days

→

10. Psychotic symptoms can be …

a)   Positive and additive

b)   Negative and additive

c)   Positive and negative

d)   Negative and cumulative

Recommended further reading

American Psychiatric Association (APA) (1994) *Diagnostic and Statistical Manual of Mental Disorders IV (DSM-IV)*. Washington, DC: APA.

Beckwith, S. and Franklin, P. (2007) *Oxford Handbook of Nurse Prescribing*. Oxford: Oxford University Press.

Coben, D. and Atere-Roberts, E. (2005) *Calculations for Nursing and Healthcare*, 2nd edition. Basingstoke: Palgrave Macmillan.

Downie, G., Mackenzie, J. and Williams, A. (2007) *Pharmacology and Medicines Management for Nurses*, 4th edition. Edinburgh: Churchill Livingstone.

Greenstein, B. and Gould, D. (2008) *Trounce's Clinical Pharmacology for Nurses*, 18th edition. New York: Churchill Livingstone.

Karch, A.M. (2017) *Focus on Nursing Pharmacology*, 7th edition. Philadelphia, PA: Lippincott Williams & Wilkins.

Lapham, R. (2015) *Drug Calculations for Nurses: A Step-by-Step Approach*, 4th edition. London: Arnold.

MIND (2017) *St. John's Wort – Hypericum perforatum*. Available at: https://www.mind.org.uk/information-support/drugs-and-treatments/st-johns-wort/#.XNveg25KiUk.

National Institute for Health and Care Excellence (NICE) (2009) *Clinical Guideline CG90: Depression in Adults: Recognition and Management*. London: NICE. Last updated 2018.

National Institute for Health and Care Excellence (NICE) (2011) *Clinical Guideline CG113: Generalised Anxiety Disorder and Panic Disorder in Adults: Management*. London: NICE. Last updated July 2019.

National Institute for Health and Care Excellence (NICE) (2019) *British National Formulary*. London: NICE. Available at: https://bnf.nice.org.uk.

Nursing and Midwifery Council (NMC) (2018) *Standards of Proficiency for Registered Nurses*. London: NMC.

Robertson, D. (2016) *Essentials of Medicines Management for Mental Health Nurses*. London: Open University Press.

Simonson, T., Aarbakke, J., Kay, I., Coleman, I., Sinnott, P. and Lyssa, R. (2006) *Illustrated Pharmacology for Nurses*. London: Hodder Arnold.

UK Government (2015) *The Drug Driving (Specified Limits) (England & Wales) (Amendment) Regulations*. Retrieved from: https://www.legislation.gov.uk/ukdsi/2015/9780111128824.

World Health Organization (WHO) (2001) *The World Health Report 2001: Mental Disorders Affect One in Four People*. Press release WHO/42, 28 September. Geneva: WHO.

World Health Organization (WHO) (2016) *ICD-10: International Statistical Classification of Diseases and Related Health Problems*, 10th revision. Geneva: WHO.

Cancer chemotherapy and symptom management

13

Chapter contents

Learning objectives

After studying this chapter, you should be able to:

- Identify the main groups of drugs used as antibody responsive or cytotoxic agents in malignancy and their mode of action.
- Discuss the general side-effects that cytotoxic drugs have on individuals and how these can be managed.
- Demonstrate knowledge of the use of steroid drugs in cancer therapy.
- Demonstrate an understanding of the drugs used to treat nausea and vomiting in cytotoxic chemotherapy.
- Correctly solve a number of drug calculations with regard to cancer treatment and antiemetics.

Introduction

The body is made up of many types of cells. These cells grow and divide in a controlled way to produce more cells in order to keep the body healthy. When cells become old or damaged, they die and are replaced with new cells. However, sometimes this orderly process goes wrong. The genetic material deoxyribonucleic acid (DNA) of a cell can become damaged or changed, producing mutations that affect normal cell growth and division. When this happens, cells do not die when they should, and new cells form when the body does not need them. The extra cells may form a mass of tissue called a *tumour*.

A tumour can be either benign or malignant. Benign tumours are non-cancerous and are rarely life-threatening. They do not spread (metastasise) to other parts of the body. Malignant tumours are cancerous and can spread to other parts of the body. When a malignant tumour spreads, the malignant cells break off and travel through the blood lymph system to other parts of the body to settle and multiply; or metastasise, resulting in a secondary tumour, or metastasis. The name given to the cancer, however, is reflective of the origin of the cancer, even if it has spread to other areas of the body. For example, if prostate cancer has spread to the liver, it is called metastatic prostate cancer.

Cancer

There is no single cause for cancer, so several areas require consideration. First, there are substances referred to as carcinogens. Carcinogens are a group of substances that are thought to be directly responsible for damaging DNA and causing cancer. Tobacco, asbestos, arsenic, radiation such as gamma and X rays, the sun and compounds in car exhaust fumes are all examples of carcinogens. When our bodies are exposed to carcinogens, free radicals are formed that try to steal electrons from other molecules in the body. These free radicals damage cells and affect their ability to function normally.

Cancer can also be the result of a genetic predisposition that can be inherited. In addition, as we

age, there is an increase in the number of possible cancer-causing mutations in our DNA. This makes age an important risk factor for cancer.

Finally, several viruses have also been linked to cancer, such as the human papillomavirus (a cause of cervical cancer). In the UK, girls in year 8 at school (aged 12–13) are offered the human papillomavirus vaccine, which has seen a reduction in the incidence of cervical cancer.

Other important viruses to consider in relation to cancer are hepatitis B and hepatitis C, which can cause liver cancer; Epstein-Barr virus, a cause of some childhood cancers; the human immunodeficiency virus (HIV) – plus anything else that suppresses or weakens the immune system or inhibits the body's ability to fight infections and therefore increases the chance of developing cancer.

Cancer symptoms

Cancer symptoms can be quite varied and depend on where the cancer is located, where it has spread, and how big the tumour is. Some cancers are more obvious than others. For example, some can be felt or seen through the skin – a lump on the breast or testicle can be an indicator of cancer in those locations. Skin cancer (melanoma) is often noted by a change in pigmentation or a wart or mole on the skin. Some oral cancers present as white patches inside the mouth or white spots on the tongue.

Other cancers have symptoms that are less physically apparent. Brain tumours, for example, tend to present symptoms early in the disease, but rather than being physically apparent the person may show changes in cognitive or affective functions. Pancreatic cancers are often too small to cause symptoms until they cause pain by pushing against nearby nerves or interfere with liver function to cause jaundice. Pancreatic tumours may well cause an imbalance in the blood sugar levels. This can make diagnosis difficult in the early stages of the disease.

Other symptoms arise when a tumour grows and pushes against organs and blood vessels. For example, colon cancers lead to symptoms such as constipation, diarrhoea, and changes in stool size and colour. Bladder or prostate cancers cause changes in bladder function such as polyuria or oliguria.

As cancer cells use the body's energy and interfere with normal cellular function, symptoms such as fever, fatigue, excessive sweating, anaemia and unexplained weight loss are common.

When a cancer spreads, or metastasises, additional symptoms can present in the newly affected area. Swollen or enlarged lymph nodes are common and likely to be present early. A cancer cell can be carried to a lymph gland and can become a secondary tumour. Some cancer cells enter the bloodstream and are carried to other parts of the body where they grow to become a secondary tumour. If cancer spreads to the brain, patients may experience vertigo, headaches or seizures. Spread to the lungs may cause coughing and shortness of breath. The liver may become enlarged and cause jaundice and bones can become painful, brittle and break easily. Symptoms of metastasis ultimately depend on the location to which the cancer has spread.

Cancer classification

Cancers can be grouped under five major headings. These headings are based on the type of tissue from which the cancer originates:

- Carcinomas are cancers that arise from epithelial tissue. Epithelial tissue covers the outside of the body and lines organs and cavities. Examples of this type of cancer include lung, breast and colon cancer.
- Sarcomas are cancers that arise from cells that are in bone, cartilage, fat, connective tissue, muscle and other supportive tissues.
- Lymphomas are cancers that begin in the lymph nodes and immune system tissues.
- Leukaemias are cancers that begin in the bone marrow and often accumulate in the bloodstream.
- Adenomas are cancers that arise in glandular tissue such as in the thyroid, pituitary or adrenal gland.

Cancers are also often labelled according to the cell type where the disease originated, plus a term such as -sarcoma, -carcinoma or just -oma. For example, haemangio, which relates to the blood vessels, followed by the suffix '-oma' gives us haemangioma, a cancer arising from the blood vessels.

Staging and grading of cancer

The stage of a cancer is a measure of how much the cancer has grown and spread. Some cancers are also graded based on histology. The stage and grade of a cancer assist us in knowing how 'advanced' that cancer is, and how well it may respond to treatment. As a general guide, the earlier the stage and the lower the grade of a cancer, the better the prognosis.

Several different staging classifications are used for various cancers. The simplest classifications are those the NHS uses to give information to patients and which we should refer to when discussing with patients their cancers to ensure continuity and understanding. The following is the most common used by the NHS in the UK:

- Stage 0 – indicates that the cancer remains where it started (in situ) and hasn't spread;
- Stage I – the cancer is small and hasn't spread anywhere else;
- Stage II – the cancer has grown, but hasn't spread;
- Stage III – the cancer is larger and may have spread to the surrounding tissues and/or the lymph nodes (part of the lymphatic system);
- Stage IV – the cancer has spread from where it started to at least one other body organ; this is also known as 'secondary' or 'metastatic' cancer.

Cancers can also be graded if a biopsy is taken and the cells are viewed under a microscope. The simplest form used by the NHS is as follows:

- Grade I – cancer cells that resemble normal cells and aren't growing rapidly;
- Grade II – cancer cells that don't look like normal cells and are growing faster than normal cells;
- Grade III – cancer cells that look abnormal and may grow or spread more aggressively.

Other grading systems are available for certain cancers and if you are involved in the care of patients where a specific classification is employed, then you should familiarize yourself with it. Cancer Research UK (2017) provides information on cancer grading in a readable and accessible format.

There are a range of management options for cancer, including chemotherapy, radiation therapy, surgery, immunotherapy, monoclonal antibody therapy, as well as other treatments. Which is chosen will depend on the location and grade of the tumour and the stage of the disease, as well as the general state of the individual's health.

Cancer treatments

The word chemotherapy, which means drug treatment, has almost exclusively become linked to the treatment of cancer. The treatment of cancer is complex and is a field of medicine in its own right, known as oncology. You will encounter cancer patients who are young, old, have mental health problems or suffer from a learning disability, so the treatment of cancer will arise irrespective of which field of nursing you practise in. A basic understanding of the pharmacology underpinning the treatment of cancer is thus imperative.

The drugs used in chemotherapy largely have their effect by acting on cells that are in the process of splitting into two, a process that is more common in tumour cells than most normal cells. Many of the drugs given in the management of cancer are called cytotoxic drugs. This name is not used lightly and means deadly to cells. So although these drugs do have anti-cancer activity, they can also destroy healthy tissue. Chemotherapy is not always given as a cure, but sometimes to palliate the disease process. This may prolong a person's life or help with other problems caused by the tumour.

Chemotherapy is often given in combination with other treatments. For example, it may be used to shrink the size of a tumour prior to radiotherapy or surgery. Similarly, it is also used if there is a high chance of metastasis following surgery or radiotherapy.

The BNF classifies drugs used in malignant disease under the following headings based on malignancy (NICE 2019):

- antibody responsive malignancy;
- carcinoid syndrome;
- cytotoxic responsive malignancy;
- hormone responsive malignancy;
- immunotherapy responsive malignancy;
- photodynamic therapy responsive malignancy;
- targeted therapy responsive malignancy.

We will now consider some of the more widely used drugs in each of these categories.

Antibody responsive malignancy

The drugs within this category are called monoclonal antibodies and act as anti-neoplastic drugs. Their primary function is to bind to cells or ligands and help reactivate the body's immunes system as a defence against certain tumours. Others can activate cell death processes in the tumour cells themselves or prevent the over-proliferation of tumour cells, meaning tumour growth can be slowed or stopped. Many of these drugs are tumour specific. An example of a drug in this class is atezolizumab, which can be used in the treatment of bladder or urinary cancers and some non-small cell lung cancers. It is given as a course intravenously and can be used as monotherapy or in combination with other drugs.

Carcinoid syndrome

The drug in this group acts as an enzyme inhibitor to reduce the production of serotonin to alleviate the symptoms of carcinoid syndrome, which is a collection of symptoms patients experience secondary to neuroendocrine tumours. The drug telotristat ethyl is given orally under specialist supervision and reviewed after 12 weeks of treatment to monitor response. If no benefit is seen in that time, the drug is stopped.

Cytotoxic responsive malignancy

This category includes the cytotoxic drugs, the most widely used in chemotherapy. They can be used alone or in combination dependent on the tumour, location and spread. Specific drug-handling guidelines are in place for these drugs of which you should make yourself aware, and training is required before handling or administering these medications. They are prone to many of the side-effects that patients associate with chemotherapy and we will discuss these later in the chapter. This group can be further subdivided into alkylating agents, anthracyclines, vinca alkaloids and antimetabolites.

Cyclophosphamide is a widely used alkylating agent that can be given orally or intravenously. It is used in the treatment of a wide range of malignancies and usually as part of combination therapy. Chlorambucil and busulfan are other drugs in this category. As these drugs have been around for many years, there is vast experience and knowledge of using them, their effects and side-effects. They act by causing damage to DNA and interfering in the rapid cell replication seen in tumour proliferation.

The anthracyclines and related agents are in widespread use and often termed cytotoxic antibiotics. Doxorubicin hydrochloride, for example, is used in acute leukaemia and in Hodgkin's and non-Hodgkin's lymphomas. Anthracyclines work by interacting with DNA strands and inhibiting DNA production and function.

Vincristine and vinblastine sulphate are well-known cytotoxic medications. Used to treat a variety of malignancies, they are administered by the IV route only. They act by binding to a protein called tubulin, preventing the next stage in cell division and stopping chromosomes from replicating. This leads to cell death of the rapidly dividing cells seen in many cancers.

Antimetabolite drugs such as capecitabine and fluorouracil are also common cytotoxic drugs. These drugs, which are able to incorporated themselves into the new nuclear material of dividing cells or combine with intracellular enzymes, disrupt cellular division. These drugs can be used in advanced carcinoma and in the treatment of many solid tumours.

Hormone responsive malignancy
Drugs within this class are used to treat breast and prostate cancer. Breast cancer is the most common malignancy in women, especially in the over-50 age group. There are established risk factors for this malignancy that are hormone related, such as early onset of menses, late menopause, older age at first complete pregnancy and family history. Oral contraceptive use and hormone replacement therapy are also linked to an increased risk. Screening programmes in the UK are aimed at women over 50 to improve early detection and treatment.

Prostate cancer is the most common malignancy in men, especially in the over-65s. It is often slow-growing and asymptomatic. Screening programmes have been put in place because if detected early, this is a very curable condition.

The treatment of these two conditions involves surgery and often chemotherapy and radiotherapy.

Tamoxifen is a well-known drug in the treatment of breast cancer. It is an anti-oestrogen and works by preventing oestrogen from binding to oestrogen receptors. This prevents the oestrogen from further stimulating tumour growth. Tamoxifen is generally well tolerated compared with other medications in this chapter, although its side-effects include oedema, changes to the menstrual cycle, nausea, vomiting and fatigue. Tamoxifen is given as a daily dose and is typically taken for 5–10 years post diagnosis and surgery.

Diethylstilbestrol is an oestrogen drug that can be used in post-menopausal women with breast cancer or in men with prostate cancer. It is taken orally but must be used with caution in patients with cardiovascular disease. Flutamide is an anti-androgen drug used in the treatment of prostate cancer. It works in a similar way to tamoxifen but instead of acting on oestrogen, it inhibits testosterone-fuelled tumour cell growth. It can be given orally but patients require their liver function to be monitored due to possible adverse effects on the liver.

Immunotherapy responsive malignancy and photodynamic therapy responsive malignancy
The immunotherapy agent interferon-alpha is used to treat leukaemia and some other tumours such as lymphoma and some solid tumours. Thalidomide has an immunomodulatory and

anti-inflammatory effect and can be used in multiple myeloma. Porfimer sodium and temoporfin drugs accumulate in malignant cells and are activated by laser light to produce their cytotoxic effects. They are used in lung and oesophageal cancer as well as in head and neck cancers unresponsive to other therapies.

Targeted therapy responsive malignancy

These drugs include proteasome inhibitors, protein kinase inhibitors and vascular endothelial growth factor inhibitors. There are many drugs in this category, most of which are tumour or target specific. These are very specialist therapies that we cannot address here. You may wish to consult *A Beginner's Guide to Targeted Cancer Treatments* (2018) by Elaine Vickers for more information.

General side-effects of cytotoxic drugs

Cytotoxic drugs are powerful drugs that often cause unwanted side-effects. Cytotoxic drugs work by destroying cells in the process of dividing and so some normal cells are also damaged. However, side-effects vary from drug to drug and some people develop more severe side-effects than others to the same drug. Sometimes, if side-effects are particularly severe, change to a different drug might be an option.

> **Clinical tip**
>
> It is important that the doctor or chemotherapy nurse inform the patient of any possible side-effects of the drugs, as they are best placed to provide appropriate and evidence-based information and support.

Mouth problems

A painful mouth is common during chemotherapy and is referred to as mucositis, a condition caused by a number of drugs, including fluorouracil. This side-effect is best avoided if possible, as once it becomes established it is very difficult to treat. The key, here, is good oral care both by the patient and nurse.

> **Clinical tip**
>
> The basic principle to be followed here is effective brushing of the teeth. This should be done twice a day with a soft toothbrush and fluoride-containing toothpaste. The patient should also rinse their mouth both after meals and at night. This is best done with water or 0.9% sodium chloride solution (saline or salt water). Fresh sodium chloride solution for each rinse can be made by dissolving half a teaspoon of salt in 250mL fresh water. Cool or warm water can be used, whatever the patient prefers. It is not necessary that they use anti-septic or anti-inflammatory mouthwashes, as there is little evidence that they are any more effective. If the person has dentures, they ought to continue cleaning them as normal.

Nausea and vomiting

These side-effects cause a great deal of distress for some individuals. Sometimes the nausea and vomiting may be so distressing that the individual refuses any further treatment. Some groups of patients seem to suffer from these side-effects more than others, including females, those over 50, patients who are anxious and those who tend to suffer from motion sickness. Some patients find that their nausea and vomiting increase as their treatment progresses. Some drugs can cause more nausea and vomiting than others (emetogenic). Fluorouracil, for example, induces mild nausea and vomiting, whereas doxorubicin is highly emetogenic.

Antiemetic medication will usually help and is commonly taken at the same time as, or just before, a cycle of chemotherapy. There are different types of antiemetic medications, so if fails to work, changing to a different one may improve the outcome.

Drugs used to treat nausea and vomiting as a result of cytotoxic chemotherapy

The acute phase of emesis in chemotherapy responds well to 5HT$_3$ antagonists like ondansetron. However, emesis in cytotoxic chemotherapy has what is known as a delayed phase (vomiting 2–5 days after commencing treatment) and this remains difficult to control. The development of neurokinin (NK1) receptor antagonists has helped. These elicit an antiemetic effect in both the acute and delayed, but especially delayed phases of emesis. This group of drugs blocks the actions at neurokinin receptors in both the chemotactic trigger zone and the vomiting centre. The drug aprepitant belongs to this class and is given in combination with a 5HT$_3$ antagonist such as ondansetron and a corticosteroid in the treatment of nausea and vomiting induced by cytotoxic drugs.

Aprepitant is prescribed as a capsule by mouth. To prevent nausea and vomiting caused by cancer chemotherapy, aprepitant is usually taken once daily, with or without food, during the first few days of treatment. The capsules come in two different strengths. The doctor may prescribe both strengths to be taken at different times. The patient must be advised to take the right strength at the right time as directed by the doctor. When used to prevent nausea and vomiting during cancer chemotherapy, aprepitant is usually used only during the first 3 days of the treatment cycle.

Clinical tip

Aprepitant is normally given 1 hour before the first dose of chemotherapy, and then each morning for the next 2 days.

Fosaprepitant is an intravenous (IV) form of the drug that is converted into aprepitant once it is in the body. As an IV infusion, the drug is

Clinical tip

It is important not to take this medicine alongside some other drugs. For example, aprepitant should not be prescribed if the patient is taking pimozide.

administered over 15 minutes, starting about 30 minutes before chemotherapy, together with a serotonin (5HT$_3$) receptor antagonist and a steroid such as dexamethasone.

Aprepitant may reduce the contraceptive effect in women taking the oral contraceptive. Alternative contraception should be used during treatment and for one month after the last dose of this drug. Furthermore, co-administration of aprepitant with warfarin may result in a reduction of the anticoagulation activity of warfarin.

Clinical tip

If the patient is taking warfarin, their international normalized ratio should be checked frequently. The patient should also be made aware of the possible effect of aprepitant on warfarin.

As with most drugs, side-effects do occur and these range from fatigue and feeling listless, constipation, loss of appetite and pain at the injection site to more serious side-effects such as allergic reactions.

Hair loss

As already noted, cytotoxic therapy tends to affect cells that divide rapidly or uncontrollably, particularly hair follicles. Thus it is not surprising that one of its side-effects is for the patient's hair to fall out, a condition known as alopecia. This usually occurs 2–3 weeks after a course of treatment starts. In addition to scalp hair, the patient may lose their body hair and eyelashes. After their treatment has finished, their hair will usually grow back within 4–12 months.

Chemotherapy-induced temporary hair loss is one of the most common and distressing side-effects of cancer therapy. If the patient finds the thought of losing their hair very upsetting, their doctor may be able to suggest a treatment that is less likely to cause hair loss. Sometimes there is a choice of drugs that the patient can be prescribed.

However, the doctor will want to give the treatment that is likely to work best in treating the patient's cancer.

> **Clinical tip**
>
> Some people are affected by hair loss more than others. The patient may wish to cut their hair short before starting chemotherapy so that any changes are less dramatic. Some people like to wear a wig; others prefer to wear a hat or scarf. In particular, the patient should be reminded to cover their head or wear high protection sun screen when out in the sun. If their eyelashes fall out, they can wear glasses or sunglasses to protect their eyes on windy days.

Bone marrow suppression

All cytotoxic drugs except vincristine and bleomycin cause bone marrow suppression. This normally occurs 7–10 days after administration of the drug. The bone marrow is where red blood cells, white blood cells and platelets are made. The patient may experience problems due to depletion of these blood cells.

The patient may become anaemic and complain of tiredness and look pale, they may need a blood transfusion to correct the cell count, and they may become more prone to infection due to a drop in their white blood cell count (leucopenia). Important symptoms to be on the lookout for are any signs of infection such as fever or a sore throat, as the patient may need to receive IV antibiotics if

they develop an infection. Finally, bleeding problems can occur. Platelets (thrombocytes) help the blood to clot. If the number of platelets in the patient's blood drops, they may bruise easily and bleed for longer than usual after a cut. They might require a platelet transfusion if the platelet level drops significantly.

Prior to each cycle of treatment, it is usual for the patient to have a blood test to ascertain their blood cell counts: red blood cells, white blood cells and platelets. If any of these counts is too low, then a treatment cycle may be delayed, the choice of drugs may be altered, or they may be given treatment to boost the levels of these blood constituents.

Reproductive function

Most of the cytotoxic groups of medicines are teratogenic and they should not be administered during pregnancy, especially in the first trimester. Advice regarding contraception should also be offered where appropriate before any therapy commences and should continue throughout treatment and beyond.

Some chemotherapy drugs can affect fertility in both men and women – sometimes temporarily, sometimes permanently. Treatment regimens that do not involve alkylating agents have less of an effect on fertility than those that do involve these agents. If this is a concern, one option may be for men to store sperm or women to store ova (eggs) before their chemotherapy treatment begins. These can be frozen and may be able to be used in the future if the patient wishes to try for a child. Some women develop an early menopause when taking some cytotoxic drugs.

> **Case studies**
>
> ① Elizabeth Green is a 56-year-old nurse who has been diagnosed with breast cancer. She has undergone routine mammography since the age of 40, as her mother and grandmother had breast cancer. The patient has undergone lumpectomy and axillary node dissection. She is currently undergoing cycles of chemotherapy with cyclophosphamide, doxorubicin and
>
>

fluorouracil. She wants to know the difference between each of the chemotherapeutic drugs being used. What information do you give her?

② You are a senior student working on a surgical ward; a student from your group has just started their allocation and approaches you. They say they do not understand much about antiemetic drugs and ask you to tell them about aprepitant. What can you tell them?

Key learning points

Introduction

▶ Cells do not die when they should, and new cells form when the body does not need them. The extra cells may form a mass of tissue called a tumour.

Cancer

▶ Carcinogens are a group of substances that are thought to be directly responsible for damaging DNA.
▶ Cancer can also result as a genetic predisposition.

Cancer symptoms

▶ Cancer symptoms can be quite varied and depend on where the cancer is located, where it has spread, and how big the tumour is.

Cancer classification

▶ Cancers can be grouped under five major headings: carcinomas, sarcomas, lymphomas, leukaemias and adenomas.

Staging and grading of cancer

▶ Staging is a measure of cancer size and spread.
▶ Grading is done after biopsy and microscopic analysis.

Cancer treatments

▶ Drug treatments are used dependant on the type and advance of the malignancy.
▶ Chemotherapy is often done in combination with surgery and/or radiotherapy.
▶ Side-effects from chemotherapy often need pharmacological management.

Calculations

1. A patient weighs 50kg and has been commenced on busulfan 60mcg per kg. What should be the daily dose in mg be, based on the patient's weight?

2. A patient has been prescribed doxorubicin intravenously over a 4-week treatment cycle. They have been prescribed a dose of 40mg/m^2; the patient's body surface area has been calculated as 1.15m^2. What is the required dose?

3. The paediatric consultant has prescribed vincristine 1.75mg/m^2. The child has a body surface area of 0.40m^2. What dose would be required?

4. A patient is receiving 1 litre of chemotherapy via a pump at a rate of 400mL per hour. How long will it take to complete the dose?

5. A patient has been prescribed ondansetron 8mg every 12 hours for 5 days. It comes as 4mg dispersible tablets. How many will the patient need to complete the course?

6. Aprepitant should be given as 125mg as an initial dose and then 80mg daily for 2 days. How many mg in total will the patient receive?

7. Your patient is prescribed diethylstilbestrol 3mg daily for prostate cancer. They have been told that their treatment is expensive and want to know more about cost. A pack of 28 tablets costs £117.85. How much is this per tablet (round to nearest whole penny)?

8. Your patient requires their tamoxifen dose in a liquid format. They are prescribed 20mg per day. The solution is 2mg/mL strength and comes in a bottle size of 150mL. How many doses does the bottle contain?

9. Thalidomide is to be given at a dose of 200mg daily for 6 weeks. It is available in a 50mg capsule in boxes of 28. How many boxes are required for the treatment cycle?

10. The cost per box of the thalidomide in question (9) is £298.48. How much will it cost for the 6-week treatment cycle?

Multiple-choice questions

Try answering these multiple-choice questions to test what you have learned from reading this chapter. You can check your answers at the end of the book.

1. Aprepitant works by blocking ...

a) D_4 receptors
b) H_1 receptors
c) $5HT_3$ receptors
d) NK_1 receptors

$\longrightarrow$

←

2. Grade III cancer cells ...

a) Look like normal cells
b) Look like normal cells and are not rapidly dividing
c) Don't look like normal cells and are not rapidly dividing
d) Don't look like normal cells and are growing and spreading

3. The BNF classifies chemotherapy how?

a) In relation to malignancy
b) In relation to side-effects
c) In relation to grade
d) In relation to state of advance

4. What are the symptoms of carcinoid syndrome?

a) Patients have many symptoms
b) Patients have many symptoms related to neuroendocrine tumours
c) Patients have one symptom related to neuroendocrine tumours
d) Patients have multiple tumours causing differing symptoms

5. Cyclophosphamide belongs to which class of cytotoxic drugs?

a) Anthracyclines
b) Alkylating agents
c) Vinca alkaloids
d) Antimetabolites

6. Tamoxifen is mostly used in which type of cancer?

a) Prostate cancer
b) Lung cancer
c) Breast cancer
d) Colon cancer

7. Porfimer sodium becomes active on exposure to ...

a) Laser light
b) Sunlight
c) X-rays
d) Proton beams

8. Mouth problems in cancer therapy are often called ...

a) Mucolytic
b) Mucositis
c) Orocystic
d) Orositis

→

9. **Aprepitant is effective in …**

a) Acute stage emesis
b) Acute and end stage emesis
c) Acute and delayed stage emesis
d) Delayed stage emesis

10. **Ondansetron acts at which receptors?**

a) NK_1
b) $GABA_A$
c) Dopamine
d) $5HT_3$

Recommended further reading

Cancer Research UK (2017) *Cancer grading*. Available at: https://www.cancerresearchuk.org/about-cancer/what-is-cancer/cancer-grading.

Downie, G., Mackenzie, J. and Williams, A. (2007) *Pharmacology and Medicines Management for Nurses*, 4th edition. Edinburgh: Churchill Livingstone.

Greenstein, B. and Gould, D. (2008) *Trounce's Clinical Pharmacology for Nurses*, 18th edition. New York: Churchill Livingstone.

Karch, A.M. (2017) *Focus on Nursing Pharmacology*, 7th edition. Philadelphia, PA: Lippincott Williams & Wilkins.

Lapham, R. (2015) *Drug Calculations for Nurses: A Step-by-Step Approach*, 4th edition. London: Arnold.

National Institute for Health and Care Excellence (NICE) (2019) *British National Formulary*. London: NICE. Available at: https://bnf.nice.org.uk.

National Institute for Health and Care Excellence (NICE) (undated) *NICE Guidance on Cancer*. London: NICE. Available at: https://www.nice.org.uk/guidance/conditions-and-diseases/cancer.

Simonson, T., Aarbakke, J., Kay, I., Coleman, I., Sinnott, P. and Lyssa, R. (2006) *Illustrated Pharmacology for Nurses*. London: Hodder Arnold.

Vickers, E. (2018) *A Beginner's Guide to Targeted Cancer Treatments*. Oxford: Wiley-Blackwell.

Patient concordance

14

Learning objectives

After studying this chapter, you should be able to:

■ Articulate the meaning of adherence, compliance and concordance with regard to the taking of medication.
■ Discuss the factors that influence effective medicine use and concordance.
■ Outline the salient points a nurse must consider in assessing, planning, implementing and evaluating patient education about medicines.
■ Describe how a patient with a chronic disease may be empowered to manage their medication.
■ Explain how patients may become partners in medicine management.

Introduction

Medicines that are prescribed but not taken by patients represent a large financial loss, in terms of the price paid for them and health professionals' (pharmacists, GPs, etc.) time. In 2018, the King's Fund estimated that about £300 million is wasted each year on medications dispensed but returned to pharmacies or otherwise disposed of. The aim of this chapter is to introduce the reader to the concepts of adherence, compliance and concordance with respect to medicine management. Nurses need to have an understanding of pharmacology at a level that will allow them to inform and educate the patients in their care. Without effective information and education, patients might not understand the need for them to take their medications as prescribed to ensure optimum drug performance.

Adherence, compliance and concordance

Often, the terms *adherence, compliance* and *concordance* are used interchangeably, when in fact they each have quite different and specific meanings.

Adherence has a dictionary definition that suggests sticking to something. For a patient to adhere to their medication regimen, they need specific information from the prescribing physician. At a consultation with the medical practitioner, they present with a problem or symptom. The medical practitioner makes a diagnosis, prescribes the medication and the patient is issued with a prescription to take to the pharmacist. Information needs to be given verbally to the patient about how to take their medication, and printed instructions are issued when the medication is dispensed. The patient needs to adhere to these instructions and follow the prescriber's guidance. The information given to the patient should make the reasons for adherence clear. However, the prescriber also needs to consider any aspect of the medication regimen that may make adherence difficult for the patient and factor that into any decision-making. Although it would be easy to consider adherence a foregone conclusion, patients frequently, and for many reasons, do not take their medication in accordance with the instructions they are issued with. Non-adherence to medication regimens can have serious consequences, depending on the medication being prescribed. Failure to adhere is, not surprisingly, a particularly serious problem in the management of chronic illnesses, especially when the patient does not 'feel' ill. Some of the drug therapies for conditions covered in this book, such as asthma, diabetes and hypertension, incur especially high levels of non-adherence, and it is common for patients to alter the way in which they take – or abandon completely – the drugs they have been prescribed.

Compliance with a medication regimen is not the same as simple adherence. By complying with the prescriber's instructions, the patient automatically adheres to the medication regimen. But compliance suggests that information is provided to allow the patient to make the *choice* to comply. So the patient is involved to some extent in discussing the medication regimen, but compliance relies largely on the patient following the prescriber's recommendations. Some patients do not like the term 'compliant', as it suggests that if they diverge from the regimen they are likely be seen as non-compliant, and thus viewed in a negative light. 'Non-compliant' is a term that you will hear, though it is not the best way to describe a person's medication-taking behaviour.

Concordance is where the relationship between patient and medical practitioner is seen to be more equal and there is an ongoing initiative to involve patients in the treatment process and so improve their compliance and adherence. This requires active participation on the part of the patient, and a confident and self-aware prescriber or medicines educator. Concordance involves the sharing of knowledge, understanding and beliefs.

The prescriber shares their knowledge and expertise of the condition to be treated and the range (if appropriate) of treatments available, be they pharmacological or non-pharmacological. The prescriber then provides information about the medicines to be considered, including any cautions, contraindications and side-effects. This gives the patient an *informed choice*. Patients, in contrast, are able to share with the prescriber information about their lifestyle and practices. This may include work patterns, social, religious and cultural aspects, and practicalities, such as an inability to open medicine bottles. This can help the prescriber to reduce the range of options available. Through good knowledge-sharing and communication, a decision about the most appropriate medicine to be prescribed can more easily be reached, which is likely to improve both concordance and compliance.

It could be argued that all of this should be part of the adherence model, and for many patients it is. The goal is ultimately for the patient to take their prescribed medicine in the most effective way so that their condition improves. In 2009, NICE published guidance on medicines adherence and how to enable patients to make informed choices by involving and supporting them in decisions about prescribed medicines. This guideline is still pertinent today and, after a review in 2015, shows the impact of medication-taking behaviour on favourable patient outcomes.

Factors influencing effective medicine use and concordance

Many factors can influence a patient's medicine-taking behaviour. Non-compliance or non-adherence may be an intentional act on behalf of the patient, or it may be an involuntary act of which they might not even be aware. Either way, the reason may be associated with the amount and quality of education and information provided to them by the prescriber, dispenser and administrator of medicines at the time treatment is initiated. It may be that the patient finds the impact of the medication regimen on their daily routine intolerable. They may not be able to take the medication as prescribed or even attend to the filling of their prescription. It may equally be that they feel that by taking the medication in a way other than prescribed by the doctor, they are exerting control over the means to improve, in their minds, the final outcome.

The main factors to consider can be summarized as follows:

- patient awareness of the need for medication;
- patient awareness of the consequences of *not* taking medication;
- time of dosing;
- side-effects;
- product formulation;
- product packaging;
- interactions with other medication;
- ability to obtain prescription;
- confusion or agitation states, including memory impairment.

Patient awareness of the need for medication

It is important that patients are made fully aware of the need for them to take their medication. Although the importance of adherence might seem obvious, some patients, if not fully cognisant of the need for their medication, might not comply. This is especially true of patients who have received a diagnosis when they had not been feeling unwell, such as when a condition is picked up on routine screening (e.g. raised blood pressure). The importance of taking antihypertensive medication should be made explicit to the patient, including the consequences of failing to adhere.

Patient awareness of the consequences of not taking medication

This is perhaps more important than the reasons *for* taking medication. Patients' perceptions of the benefits and risks of taking medication have been shown to influence compliance. Using the example of high blood pressure, there are many consequences of not taking antihypertensive medication. A continuous raised blood pressure increases the patient's risk of stroke and heart attack, both of which can lead to premature death. It cannot therefore be understated how important good information and education are.

Time of dosing

Time of dosing is very important to some patients. A good example is antibiotic prescriptions. Some schools will not administer medications to children during school hours, and insist on a parent attending to do so. For a child who is prescribed antibiotics three or four times a day and who is well enough to attend school, thus necessitating dosing during school hours, this can be a problem.

It could be that the child is kept off school, the parent misses work or the antibiotics are taken in an inappropriate way. It may be prudent therefore to consider prescribing an antibiotic that can be taken once or twice daily that can be appropriately administered out of school hours.

Side-effects

Intolerable side-effects are one of the main reasons for non-compliance with medicine regimens. No drug is completely free from side-effects. Some side-effects are tolerable for some patients but not for others. Information and education about potential side-effects is vital in medicines management. If a patient experiences a side-effect, it may lead to them stopping the medication and possibly not seeking advice from the prescriber. A good example of this is citalopram, an antidepressant medication which can cause nausea as a side-effect. This nausea is usually transient and will pass after about 2 weeks, hence it is important to educate the patient about this, as most people can put up with a mild side-effect for a short period if they know it will pass, and they will continue with their medication.

Some side-effects can be severe and may even become life-threatening for the patient if left unchecked. It is very important to stress to patients that if they experience any side-effects, they should seek advice at once.

Product formulation

In some cases, the simple formulation of the medication makes adhering to the regimen difficult if not impossible. Children are important in this respect. Many children under the age of 10 have great difficulty swallowing tablets, so liquid medicine is the preferred choice. Some children, especially the younger ones, also dislike the taste of their medicine. If this is an analgesic, it is worth the parent trying different brands, as they may well find one with a different flavour that is more palatable to the child.

In inflammatory bowel disease, the use of rectal medications can make patients anxious because of their route of administration. Even with a clear educational plan of action, it is unrealistic to expect patients to willingly take their medication in such circumstances. This issue should be thoroughly explored with the patient before any medication is prescribed.

Product packaging

The elderly and people with manual dexterity problems often have trouble with product packaging. The main problem is child-proof caps on medicine bottles, but some blister packs can also prove difficult to get into. However, dispensing pharmacies are happy to help. For example, tablets can be supplied in bottles with normal caps on request or in easy-to-open packs.

Interactions with other medications

Although patients may be taking a certain medication as prescribed, it is important to consider other medications and any specific instructions on timing of dosing. For example, some drugs are not fully absorbed from the stomach if they are taken at the same time as an antacid preparation. Also, some medications should be taken with food, others after food and still others before food, so it is important that the patient takes their medication(s) exactly as prescribed to ensure optimum effect.

Ability to obtain prescription

For some elderly or infirm patients, this could be a hurdle to medication adherence. If the patient cannot physically get to the pharmacy to collect their prescription, it follows that they cannot take that medication. This has become much less of a problem because of initiatives by some pharmacies to collect prescriptions, issue the medication and deliver it to the patient's home. There is now in many areas an online repeat prescription service available to patients, where pharmacies can electronically request repeat prescriptions, dispense and deliver. Many community pharmacies offer this service and will collect repeat prescriptions direct from the doctor's surgery or electronically. It is important that patients are made aware of this service where it is available.

Another problem for some patients is ability to pay. Not everyone who requires medications receives help in paying for them. Some people in employment who have to pay for their prescriptions ration themselves to those medications that they perceive to be the most important or most obviously efficacious. The 'lesser' medications (in the patient's eyes) may not be purchased.

Confusion or agitation states, including memory impairment

If patients who suffer from agitation states and/or memory impairment are on several different medications, the condition itself can cause problems in terms of adherence and compliance. Multi-dose boxes and dated boxes are available that can be made up by pharmacies to cover all the medicines needed by a patient. These boxes contain a strip for each day, with time to take the medication highlighted. This allows patients to see whether they have taken their medication. In more srious cases, patients may need family or carers to administer their medicines.

Forgetfulness is a major cause of non-compliance. Patients should be taught behaviour strategies such as reminders, self-monitoring tools, cues and reinforcements. Such aids as a dosette box should not be viewed as being for older people only – they will also be useful to anyone who has an unstructured or hectic lifestyle, including young adults.

Patient empowerment in chronic disease management

Patients who suffer from long-term or chronic diseases usually wish to be empowered in the management of their condition, and this can include the choice and modification of any medications prescribed. They can feel despondent about having to take medication for life, and naturally want the medication used to treat their condition to have minimal impact on their lifestyle and daily routine. More and more patients want to be involved and to feel in control of their disease, rather than the disease controlling them.

Education and information are key to patient empowerment, as they bolster the patient's knowledge and understanding of their condition. A wealth of information is now available to patients, including via internet search facilities. However, some people have problems accessing the internet, such as those living in deprived areas. For patients not able to access the internet, information can be provided in leaflet format, or by attending one of the many 'help' groups set up for sufferers of chronic diseases.

One caveat about the internet is that not all the information posted there is reliable, and patients need to be selective in the websites they consult. At the end of the day, there is no substitute for the quality information provided by health care professionals.

Patient education

Patient education should be tailored to the individual and is an important component of nursing care. Patients should have an individualized medication programme as part of their discharge plan. The nurse should provide the patient with any relevant leaflets to promote recall of the details of any medication guidance given to them. The nurse should plan in advance what such guidance aims to achieve as well as what the preferred outcomes are. When developing a teaching plan such as this, nurses should allocate time to discuss with patients what they would like to know about their medication. Remember, some patients are very knowledgeable about their condition and the medicines that they take. Therefore, it is important not to be patronizing and to determine in advance what the patient's level of understanding is. This is a good example of why it is so important that nurses keep abreast of new developments in pharmacology

Once a patient leaves hospital, other members of the primary care team have a duty to put in place a long-term education plan about their medicines. Primary care specialists, GPs and pharmacists should continue to provide information to the patient and monitor their level of concordance. This is especially important with the elderly, as their medication regimens often tend to be complex.

Patients as partners in decision-making

Except when patients are in hospital, it is they who have to manage their own medications. Ironically, patients often remain passive when it comes to consulting with health care professionals about their medicine management and behavioural changes. Considering the patient as a partner in any decision-making process about the management of their care is a relatively new concept, let alone bringing medication into the equation. This is, however, one of the most important considerations in promoting concordance and why health care professionals should always involve the patient at all stages of the consultation. Patient trust and cooperation can enhance the information obtained by the health care professional, leading to a better outcome.

Many patients want to be an active partner in decision-making and this should be encouraged. People are more likely to be concordant if they feel they were able to negotiate on their own behalf. Therefore, asking patients' views, listening and helping them think the problem through and decide, is more effective than simply telling them what to do.

Listening skills are important in information exchange so that each party can think about and reflect on the other's viewpoint. The nurse needs to be aware of verbal and non-verbal cues which may indicate that the patient is becoming reluctant or defensive. Such a reaction usually means that the approach taken by the nurse is having the effect of making the patient feel uncomfortable. Thus the nurse must develop an increased level of sensitivity and understanding of the interaction taking place.

It is however essential that the partnership is *functional*. Some patients believe that because this is *their* disease, *they* ought to make the decisions about their care. This can lead to an imbalance in the partnership with the health care professional and may even be detrimental, to the extent that their knowledge and expertise fails to be acknowledged.

Some patients, on the other hand, do *not* want to be active partners in decision-making, and their wishes should not be ignored either. Many patients visit their doctor with a symptom or problem, and want the doctor to make a diagnosis and decide on treatment. They respect the doctor's knowledge and expertise believing that 'doctor knows best'. This attitude requires more skill on behalf of the doctor who, in order to most appropriately prescribe, requires information about lifestyle and practices that will enable them to make a more informed decision.

Relapse is common, so the need for an open discussion is extremely important. All nurses need to acknowledge that it is possible that a patient may want to stop or change their medication.

Several psychological models have been developed in order to understand health behaviours relevant to compliance. The most popular model is the Health Belief Model (Becker 1974), which proposes that health-related behaviours or the seeking of health interventions depend on four factors:

1. **perceived susceptibility** – the person's assessment of their risk of getting an illness;

2. **perceived severity** – the person's assessment of the seriousness of the illness, and what this could mean for them;

3. **perceived barriers** – the person's assessment of the influences that may discourage the adoption of health-related behaviours; and

4. **perceived benefits** – the person's assessment of the beneficial outcomes of adopting a health-related behaviour.

Another popular model is the Theory of Planned Behaviour (Ajzen 1991). This model focuses on the attitudes and intentions of the patient in relation to performing certain health behaviours within expected norms. The theory suggests that the intention of the person to perform a compliant act depends on their attitude, subjective pressure and perception of being controlled by others.

Often these models are adopted by nurses and others in an attempt to empathize with the patient and to ensure a positive outcome to health education. Both models rely on what psychologists call the *locus of control*. This refers to a patient's belief about what causes the positive or negative outcomes in their lives, especially in relation to such things as health. Some people have what is known as an *internal locus of control*, which means that they believe that they have the ability to control change in their lives. The opposite to this is an *external locus of control*, where people believe that they have little or no control and that their life circumstances are dictated by factors external to them.

As we have discussed, how patients perceive themselves is important in planning care and treatment options. Concordance with medication is more likely, therefore, if there is some understanding on the part of the nurse and other medical staff of why a patient may or may not adopt a given behaviour. We must seek to see the patient's perspective and understand what taking medications means to them. Without this knowledge, any attempt at promoting concordance will be at best transitory and superficial.

The role of the carer

In today's complex care system, both in and out of hospital, family members, friends or paid employees are having to perform the role of carer for patients that we might see on a regular basis. The carer can be anyone in the patient's life who provides any aspect of care, but the following are the most common:

- parents of children of any age requiring health care;
- spouses;
- children (of any age) whose parents have care needs;
- other relatives with moral or legal responsibility;
- close friends or neighbours;
- paid carers.

Although it is important to consider the role of the carer, you should never forget that your primary responsibility is to your patient.

Carers often want to help in any way they can, and this should be considered when caring for your patient. It is often as important to involve the carer as to involve the patient in discussion around the patient's care and well-being, sometimes more so (in the case of a parent of a young child). This also should extend to and include medication need, use and administration.

The nurse should include an assessment of the role of the carer in aspects of activities of daily living when planning care. Starting to involve the carer at this point can often prevent misunderstandings later.

Many carers adopt the role of medication administrator for the person in their care. This may extend to the management of the whole of the person's medication needs, including organizing and collecting prescriptions as well as administering the correct dose and drug at the correct times. It is therefore important that you educate the carer as you would the patient about the following aspects of the medication:

- the indication for each medication;
- the time each dose should be taken;
- the side-effects to look out for;
- the risks associated with not giving the medication;
- safe storage and disposal.

Acting on this information, the carer will be in a position to administer the medication in the most appropriate way, taking over responsibility from the patient who may no longer be able to manage their medication independently.

It is important that the carer is able to understand these important issues, as an inability to do so (for example, in the case of a child performing caring duties for a parent) may require nursing intervention to maintain medication management.

Case studies

① Kubi Garise is a 75-year-old woman who suffers from rheumatoid arthritis and hypertension, and has the early symptoms of dementia, in particular memory problems. She is on medication for her arthritis and hypertension, but also takes aspirin daily and a drug to protect her stomach. She lives alone and is only mobile around her house and garden. Her family are worried that she may not be taking her medication properly. Can you suggest strategies to improve her compliance?

② Ella Jenkins is 4 years old and needs antibiotics for an ear infection. Her mother is struggling to get her to take the medicine the doctor has prescribed, as she does not like the taste. Mrs Jenkins has decided not to give the medicine to Ella, as she does not like upsetting her.

- How would you go about educating Mrs Jenkins as to the importance of complying with the medication?
- What would you suggest to the prescriber to help improve the likelihood of Ella taking her antibiotics?

③ Oliver Paresi is an 80-year-old man with moderate dementia living at home with his wife, who is also his carer. He also has high blood pressure for which he takes medication and statins to reduce his cholesterol. He is becoming increasingly muddled as to when to take his tablets.

- How would you involve Oliver's wife – his carer – in his medication regime?
- What might you suggest to help Oliver remember to take his medication?

Key learning points

Introduction

▶ Nurses need a sound knowledge of pharmacology to inform health promotion.

Adherence, compliance and concordance

▶ Adherence to a medication regimen is sticking to the prescribed instructions for the taking of medication.
▶ Compliance involves the patient making some choices based on information given by the prescriber.
▶ Concordance involves the sharing of knowledge, understanding and beliefs between the prescriber and the person taking the medicine.

Factors influencing effective medicine use and concordance

▶ Non-compliance and non-adherence may be intentional or unintentional on the part of the patient.
▶ It is important that patients are fully aware of the need to take their medication.

←

▶ The patient must be aware of the consequences of not taking their medication.
▶ Lifestyle and the timing of a dose are important.
▶ Considering the side-effects a medicine has on a person is of paramount importance.
▶ How the product is formulated may have an impact on whether a person will take the medicine or not.
▶ Product packaging can be troublesome for people with limited dexterity.
▶ Other medications that the person is taking need to be assessed to ensure drug interactions are prevented.
▶ Even the ability of a person to obtain the prescription itself can be an obstacle.
▶ People who suffer from confusion or other cognitive impairments have special requirements.

Patient empowerment in chronic disease management

▶ Include the patient in choosing medication and any modifications to their medicines.
▶ Enable the patient through internet access and self-help groups.
▶ Each patient should have an individual plan.
▶ Use educational leaflets to reinforce the knowledge base of the patient.
▶ Draw up learning objectives and consider how you will evaluate what has been taught.
▶ Good consultation skills should always include the patient.
▶ Problems in the patient–prescriber relationship lead to poor decision-making.

The role of the carer

▶ Include the carer in all aspects of the patient's care, especially around medication where appropriate.
▶ Remember your main responsibility is to the patient.
▶ Educate and involve the carer with regard to medication.

Calculations

1. A doctor has prescribed 0.25mg of digoxin. You have 125mcg tablets. How many should you give?

2. How many grams are in 2.5kg?

3. You have a vial of actrapid containing 100 units per mL. How much do you need to give 12 units?

4. How many micrograms are in 1.25g?

5. You have a bottle of amoxicillin syrup containing 250mg in 5mL. How many mL do you need to give 125mg?

6. You have a vial of gentamycin containing 80mg in 2mL. How much do you need to administer 100mg?

7. A patient is being given an IV infusion, and is to receive 1 litre of fluid over 5 hours. What volume of fluid in mL will they receive each hour?

8. How many milligrams are in 0.1kg?

9. Given that w/v (weight to volume) = number of grams in 100mL, you have a solution of glucose 50% w/v. How many grams of glucose will you have in 50mL?

10. Given that w/v (weight to volume) = number of grams in 100mL, you have a solution of sodium 30% w/v. How many grams of sodium would be in 1000mL?

Multiple-choice questions

Try answering these multiple-choice questions to test what you have learned from reading this chapter. You can check your answers at the end of the book.

1. Adherence in drug therapy is defined as ...

a) Sticking to a medicines regimen with information given
b) Commencing a medicines regimen
c) Stopping a medicines regimen
d) Monitoring a medicines regimen

2. One should aim for concordance ...

a) In patients on four or more medicines
b) In chronic disease management
c) In all patients prescribed medicines
d) Only in patients who have prescription-only drugs

3. Patient partnership in prescribing ...

a) Can only work in patients with a health care background
b) Helps promote concordance
c) Can only be achieved in hospital settings
d) Is inappropriate with children

4. Concordance is best achieved when ...

a) The doctor makes the prescribing decisions
b) The nurse makes the prescribing decisions
c) The patient makes the prescribing decisions
d) All of the above are involved

←

5. Concordance can be affected by …

a) The drugs prescribed for the patient
b) The patient's understanding of the medicines
c) The cost of the medications
d) How often the patient attends the surgery

6. Providing patients with information on their medicines …

a) Is the main responsibility of the prescriber and the pharmacist
b) Is the responsibility of the patient and the nurse
c) Is the responsibility of the prescriber only
d) None of the above

7. What route of administration of drugs is likely to result in the best compliance?

a) IV
b) IM
c) Rectal
d) Oral

8. Non-compliant patients should always …

a) Be advised to find a new doctor
b) Have their medicines changed
c) Be given help and information regarding their medicines
d) Have their medicines given by another route

9. The best way to promote concordance is through …

a) Information and cheaper drugs
b) Education and free prescriptions
c) Cheaper drugs and easier medicines regimens
d) Easier medicine regimens and education

10. Non-compliance with medicines regimens is …

a) Restricted to the elderly
b) A potential problem for all prescribers
c) Not a problem in children
d) Avoidable only in well-educated patients

Recommended further reading

Ajzen, I. (1991) The theory of planned behaviour, *Organizational Behavior and Human Decision Processes*, 50 (2): 179–211.

Badger, F. and Nolan, P. (2006) Concordance with antidepressant medication in primary care, *Nursing Standard*, 20 (52): 35–40.

Banning, M. (2004) Enhancing older people's concordance with taking their medication, *British Journal of Nursing*, 13 (11): 669–674.

Becker, M.H. (1974) The Health Belief Model and personal health behaviour, *Health Education Monographs*, 2: 324–508.

Beckwith, S. and Franklin, P. (2011) *Oxford Handbook of Prescribing for Nurses and Allied Health Professionals*, 2nd edition. Oxford: Oxford University Press.

Coben, D. and Atere-Roberts, E. (2005) *Calculations for Nursing and Healthcare*, 2nd edition. Basingstoke: Palgrave Macmillan.

Downie, G., Mackenzie, J. and Williams, A. (2007) *Pharmacology and Medicines Management for Nurses*, 4th edition. Edinburgh: Churchill Livingstone.

Ekman, I., Schaufelberger, M., Kjellgren, K., Swedberg, K. and Granger, B. (2007) Standard medication information is not enough: poor concordance of patient and nurse perceptions, *Journal of Advanced Nursing*, 60 (2): 181–186.

Gatford, J.D. and Phillips, N. (2006) *Nursing Calculations*, 7th edition. Edinburgh: Churchill Livingstone Elsevier.

Greenstein, B. and Gould, D. (2008) *Trounce's Clinical Pharmacology for Nurses*, 18th edition. New York: Churchill Livingstone.

Karch, A.M. (2017) *Focus on Nursing Pharmacology*, 7th edition. Philadelphia, PA: Lippincott Williams & Wilkins.

King's Fund (2018) *The Rising Cost of Medicines to the NHS: What's the Story?* London: King's Fund. Available at: https://www.kingsfund.org.uk/sites/default/files/2018-04/Rising-cost-of-medicines.pdf.

Lapham, R. (2015) *Drug Calculations for Nurses: A Step-by-Step Approach*, 4th edition. London: Arnold.

Matthews, E. (2004) Reflective practice: concordance with pain medication, reflection on an adverse incident, *British Journal of Nursing*, 13 (9): 551–555.

Newell, K. (2006) Concordance with asthma medication: the nurse's role, *Nursing Standard*, 20 (26): 31–33.

National Institute for Health and Care Excellence (NICE) (2009) *Clinical Guideline CG76: Medicines Adherence: Involving Patients in Decisions about Prescribed Medicines and Supporting Adherence*. London: NICE.

Simonson, T., Aarbakke, J., Kay, I., Coleman, I., Sinnott, P. and Lyssa, R. (2006) *Illustrated Pharmacology for Nurses*. London: Hodder Arnold.

Willis, J. (2000) Patient compliance, *Nursing Times*, 96 (35): 36–37.

Legal and professional issues

15

Chapter contents

Learning objectives
Introduction
The correct patient
The correct medicine
The correct dose
The correct site and method of
  administration
Covert administration of medicines
Mental capacity and competence in
  consent

Alteration of medicines
Reporting of drug errors
Controlled drugs
Supply and administration of medicines
Prescribing law and non-medical prescribing
  Unlicensed and off license prescribing
Case studies
Key learning points
Multiple-choice questions
Recommended further reading

Learning objectives

After studying this chapter, you should be able to:

■ Discuss the importance of identifying the correct patient as part of administering a medication.
■ List the issues that are important in giving a patient the correct medicine.
■ Describe the steps you would take to accurately calculate a drug dosage.
■ Outline why it is important to recognize the correct route of administration when giving a drug.
■ Discuss legal and professional dilemmas concerning giving a medicine in a covert manner.
■ Explore the issues relating to a nurse crushing or tampering with a drug prior to its administration.
■ Describe why it is important that nurses report any errors in the giving of medication.
■ Describe the procedure a nurse must undertake when giving a controlled drug.
■ Demonstrate an understanding if what is meant by the term 'patient group directions'.
■ Discuss the history of nurse prescribing.
■ List the Acts of Parliament that have led to nurse prescribing.
■ Describe what is meant by the terms 'supplementary' and 'independent' prescriber.

Introduction

The aim of this chapter is to introduce you to the legal and professional issues faced by nurses in medicines management. Nurses are bound by the Code of Conduct laid out by the Nursing and Midwifery Council (NMC 2015). They specify standards for administration of medication that nurses must adhere to.

The NMC's Standards for Pre-Registration Nursing Programmes published in May 2018 states that a nurse's education must

ensure that field-specific content in relation to the law, safeguarding, consent, pharmacology and medicines administration and optimisation is included for entry to the register in one or more fields of nursing practice

Administration of medicines is a skill that you will be exposed to during your pre-registration education. To become confident and competent as a practitioner, you need to be assertive on your placements in requesting to be involved in the administration of medicines because qualified nurses perform this task without necessarily involving students.

Medicines are used for their therapeutic effects, so their careful administration is paramount. As a result, several legislative and professional standards are in place to mitigate the chances of errors occurring, including the NMC Code (2015). Guidance highlights the importance of identifying the correct patient, the correct drug, the correct dose, the correct site and method of administration, and the correct procedure. This chapter will explore the legal and professional issues that may arise during your initial education. The chapter will conclude by exploring the future of the nurse's role in medicine management.

The correct patient

It is essential that you are aware of the relevant details of the person you are about to give a medicine to. For example, you need to have some knowledge of their background even before correctly identifying them. The first question that you might ask yourself is whether the individual has the capacity to consent (this is dealt with later in the chapter). You also need to consider the individual's diagnosis and physical capabilities, as well as the question of hypersensitivity and allergies. There may also be special instructions that are important to remember such as whether the patient is to be kept nil by mouth.

At some point you will be working in a busy acute setting where there is a high turnover of patients. In this environment it is unlikely that you will get to know patients very well and the safest way to identify an individual patient before giving them a medicine is by checking their identity verbally where possible and confirming this with their wristband (identity band). This band should carry accurate details that correctly identify the wearer.

In 2018, NHS Improvement published recommendations based on National Patient Safety Agency (NPSA) alerts that remain relevant to the 'never events' list of that year. It identified that wristbands for hospital inpatients improved safety and that *all* patients should be issued on admission with a wristband with accurate details that correctly identifies them. They also highlight a 2007 safer practice notice regarding standardization of wristbands. It states the following core patient identifiers only should appear in black text on a white wristband:

- Last name
- First name
- Date of birth
- NHS number

In long-term settings, you may also find that photographs of patients are provided on their charts to help ensure that the chance of misidentification is substantially reduced. When working in the community, you will mostly be in patients' homes and will be relying on their verbal confirmation, or that of their carer, to establish identity.

The correct medicine

Most medicines have two names, the generic approved name (e.g. diazepam) and the proprietary or manufacturer's brand name (e.g. Valium). As a student, one of your first tasks is to learn both the generic and proprietary (brand) names. On placement you will find that most health care professionals refer to drugs by their generic name whereas patients often do so by their brand name. The fact that drugs have more than one name makes the potential for error greater.

Prescription charts must be written up using the drug's generic name, so limiting the chance for error, unless there is a specific reason to prescribe by brand, such as to ensure consistency of supply of a particular drug. However, stocks of drugs on the wards and patients' individual drug boxes often carry *both* names. You must make sure that when you are checking a drug you are satisfied it is the drug that is named on the prescription sheet. Most nurses would probably agree that medication packaging can be quite misleading and the names that are given to medicines can look and sound very similar. If in doubt – ask!

You must ensure you can read the name of the drug clearly, both on the prescription chart and on the packaging it is being dispensed from. You must *never* transfer drugs from one container to another, or be tempted to agree to a drug being dispensed from a container that has had the label defaced or altered in some way.

When administering medicines to a patient, it is also part of the nurse's responsibility to ensure that the drug is *appropriate* for that patient. Knowledge of the patient's medical history and their medical diagnosis is the means of determining this, together with discussion with the prescriber and the patient. A patient should only be prescribed a medicine where there is a clinical need, and where non-pharmacological methods have proved ineffective.

Some medicines may be prescribed to a patient for a reason not under the drugs licensing remit. This is not abnormal and discussion with the prescriber can reassure the nurse prior to administration that the drug is appropriate. A good example is that of amitriptyline. This drug is well known for treating depression but today is often prescribed in low doses to alleviate chronic back pain.

The correct dose

Another reason why drug errors occur relates to the potential for over- or under-dosing the prescribed medicine. As a nurse, it is not enough for you to be able to give a drug but you should also have some understanding of *what* you are giving. Administering a medicine should not be a case of mechanically following a set of instructions but instead an intellectual event that is carried out thoughtfully. When you are involved in the procedure of medicine administration, it is good practice to understand the drug's actions, interactions and side-effects. It is no defence to simply agree with the giving of the medicine because you trust the doctor or the nurse. You must consult the BNF if you are in any way uncertain. All care settings that dispense drugs must have a copy of the BNF on hand as a reference for all staff members. Find out where it is kept and make use of it during your placements. Make use of Appendix 1 of the BNF (NICE 2019), which covers drug interactions. Some patients are prescribed many medications for multiple conditions, so it is important to be aware of any interactions between prescribed and over the counter (OTC) medicines, for example. Many combinations of drugs may involve interactions that are of little or no clinical relevance, but others may involve interactions that have potentially serious or hazardous consequences. The ultimate responsibility lies with the prescriber, but the pharmacist involved in dispensing the medicines and the nurse who administers them also have a role to play in identifying potential interactions to ensure patient safety.

Our advice to you is to learn about a small number of drug groups which you will come across regularly on your placement. If you do this on all the placements you visit over your three years of training, you will build up a comprehensive portfolio of information and knowledge.

In promoting safe practice, some nurses have called for the more widespread use of calculators in practice settings to improve the accuracy of the drug calculations required before administering some drugs. However, there is a counter-argument that we should use calculators *less* in practice, the thinking being that calculators are a substitute for nurses using basic arithmetic. As a student nurse, we're sure you will get your fair share of theoretical sessions on numeracy in nursing as part of your pre-registration education. The testing of basic levels of numeracy has now become part of the criteria for entry onto nurse education programmes. If you have not engaged with the calculation exercises in this book, then you are missing out on a critical area of knowledge. Most of the questions we have posed are basic in nature and are only included to provide you with a foundation. However, it is important that we all start somewhere, and the self-testing element of the book is an opportunity for you to get it wrong without undue criticism or pressure.

In practice, we suggest that when involved in working out drug calculations you should do as follows:

- Take *time* to work out your calculations.
- Always *recheck* your answers.
- Do not be rushed by colleagues or be embarrassed to tell them that you have arrived at a different answer; answers that look wrong probably are wrong and it might be useful to make an initial logical estimate to base your final calculation on.
- If you are unsure do *not* be tempted to avoid losing face by simply agreeing for agreeing sake – this is dangerous.
- Always use a 'common sense' check – if you arrive at an answer of 17 litres for infusion, your common sense should tell you this is way too high.

The correct site and method of administration

You should be aware of which route the medicine is to be given by. To simply ask for a medicine to be given by injection is not specific enough. As you will be aware, there are three ways in which a drug can be injected: SC, IM or IV. The exact route of administration should be stated on the prescription chart and should not be deviated from.

Medicines are designed and formulated to be absorbed according to the route of delivery; therefore, getting the route of a drug right is of paramount importance.

Covert administration of medicines

The covert administration of medicines is a highly contentious issue in nursing. For example, to administer a medicine covertly to a capable adult would, in law, be considered a case of *trespass*, since the person receiving the medicine would not have provided their consent. The Human Rights Act 1998 describes the need for nursing care to be given with respect and to be proportionate to the needs of the patient.

For a person to provide consent, they need to have the mental capacity to understand what is being explained to them, to be able to make some form of choice and to be able to communicate. Every person with mental capacity has a right to refuse medication if they so wish.

In exceptional circumstances, the law accepts that the giving of medicine to a patient who is not able to provide consent is acceptable provided that their carer is acting in the best interests of the patient and that the care given is of a reasonable standard. Courts have also accepted that doctors may treat patients without their consent if it is seen to be in the best interests of the patient. And there are other circumstances in which it is permissible for consent to be given by someone other than the patient, as in the case of parental responsibility, where a parent has the right to consent on behalf of their child.

Where a patient lacks capacity, the law in England does not currently allow others, for example relatives, to give consent on their behalf without legal intervention. When dealing with somebody who does not have the capacity to provide consent, professionals must rely on the principle of *necessity and best interests*. This means that treatment should only be given when it is necessary for the patient's health and well-being *and* is in their best interests. However, relatives and carers are likely to have a detailed understanding of the patient's circumstances and can offer insights into what their best interests are. Therefore, the nurse should work in partnership with relatives and partners to provide the best care for the patient.

Despite the legal and professional debate, you may still come across patients being given medicines in their food or drink, something that is especially prevalent in nursing homes. As a student nurse and future professional, you should not engage in giving medications covertly except under exceptional circumstances and where the patient has been deemed to lack capacity to consent and the medicine prescribed is in the patient's best interests.

Mental capacity and competence in consent

For those deemed unable to provide consent due to lack of mental capacity, prior legal recourse can give relatives or carers the ability, in law, to act in the best interests of the patient under power of attorney and power of welfare.

The Mental Capacity Act 2005 was designed to protect those who cannot make decisions for themselves or lack the mental capacity to do so. The Act's purpose is:

- to allow adults to make as many decisions as they can for themselves;
- to enable adults to make advance decisions about whether they would like future medical treatment;
- to allow adults to appoint, in advance of losing mental capacity, another person to make decisions about personal welfare or property on their behalf at a future date;
- to allow decisions concerning personal welfare or property and affairs to be made in the best interests of adults when they have not made any future plans and cannot make a decision at this time;
- to ensure an NHS body or local authority will appoint an independent mental capacity advocate to support someone who cannot make a decision about serious medical treatment, or about hospital, care home or residential accommodation, when there are no family or friends to be consulted;
- to provide protection against legal liability for carers who have honestly and reasonably sought to act in the person's best interests;

- to provide clarity and safeguards concerning research in relation to those who lack capacity.

The Act should only be used when the patient is unable to provide consent for themselves and has been judged by a medical professional to be lacking in capacity. The medical professional should ascertain three things:

1. Can the person understand the information given to them?
2. Can they retain this information?
3. Can they use this information to come to a decision?

In relation to children and young adults, it is lawful for doctors to provide advice and treatment without parental consent providing certain criteria are met. These criteria, known as the Fraser Guidelines, but often referred to as Gillick Competencies, require the medical professional to be satisfied that:

- the young person will understand the professional's advice;
- the young person cannot be persuaded to inform their parents;
- the young person is likely to begin, or to continue having, sexual intercourse with or without contraceptive treatment;
- unless the young person receives contraceptive treatment, their physical or mental health, or both, are likely to suffer;
- the young person's best interests require them to receive contraceptive advice or treatment with or without parental consent.

Gillick v West Norfolk &
Wisbech Area Health Authority [1986] AC 112

Although these criteria specifically refer to contraception, the principles are deemed to apply to other treatments. Although the judgment in the House of Lords that produced these criteria referred specifically to doctors, it is considered to apply to other health professionals, including nurses.

If a person under the age of 18 refuses to consent to treatment, it is possible in some cases for their parents or the courts to overrule them. However, this right can be exercised only on the basis that the welfare of the young person is paramount.

In 2015, attention was once more drawn to the issue of informed consent. The ruling of the Supreme Court established that rather it being a matter of clinical judgement for the health care professional to decide what information a patient requires, a patient should be told whatever they want to know, not what the medical professional 'thinks' they need to know, including alternative options (*Montgomery v Lanarkshire Health Board* [2015] UKSC 11, [2015] 1 AC 1430). For nurses, this means we need to heed what the patient tells us they want in relation to information about their medicines prior to them agreeing to take them.

Alteration of medicines

Drugs are only licensed to be administered in the form in which they are packaged, because crushing tablets or separating capsules can alter the delivery system. This in turn will affect the pharmacokinetics and dynamics of the medicine, resulting in changes in the speed of absorption and therapeutic efficacy.

A nurse who administers a medicine in a way that falls outside the product licence is to some extent liable for any adverse effects caused by that maladministration. The nurse can take steps to reduce personal liability when giving a drug outside its product licence. One reasonable step would be to obtain the medication in an alternative form, say a liquid. For example, if a patient is struggling to take medication in tablet or capsule form, you should inform the nurse in charge so that they can speak to the medical staff and get the prescription changed to a liquid version of the drug (some companies specialize in the manufacture of drugs in liquid form). Another precaution would be to discuss the crushing of a drug in tablet form with the pharmacist and get written approval from them that the practice is appropriate.

The issue of tampering with or crushing tablets is a dilemma when giving drugs enterally. Enteral feeding refers to the delivery of a complete nutritional feed directly into the stomach, duodenum or jejunum. This type of feeding is usually adopted with malnourished patients, or patients at risk of malnutrition who have a functional GI tract but are unable to maintain an adequate or safe oral intake. On your placement, you may come across a variety of methods for giving enteral feeds, such as nasogastric (NG) and percutaneous endoscopic gastrotomy (PEG).

While tampering with or crushing medications is not a usual means of drug administration, it is likely that this will need to be done when giving drugs enterally, especially if they are not available in liquid form. The nurse may crush or separate capsules if the doctor is aware that the drugs are to be given by this route – that is, the doctor will prescribe the drugs enterally, therefore making administration lawful. The problem with this type of administration arises when the prescriber is not informed that tampering has taken place. Some clinical settings have developed separate protocols for enteral administration of medicines. When working in a hospital setting, informing the pharmacy regarding this route of administration is usually enough – they will then facilitate the drugs being available in an appropriate form. You will find that all hospitals have their own medicines policy, which usually contains information on crushing or tampering with medicines. You need to become familiar with this document when on placement.

Reporting of drug errors

In its advice to nurses, the NMC highlights the importance of an *open culture* in practice settings as regards reporting of drug errors. This needs to be fostered to encourage the immediate reporting of errors or incidents in the administration of medicines. Unfortunately, as we work in an increasingly litigious society, drug errors are often not viewed on a case-by-case basis and disciplinary action is frequently taken against nurses for any mistake they make. It could be argued that by taking this approach, all that is achieved is to make nurses reluctant to report such incidents.

As a student nurse, if you make a mistake you are not always deemed culpable in law. However, you need to learn from your mistakes. Therefore, if you make a drug error you may be asked to complete a *critical incident analysis* of what went on. Using this as a reflective tool, you can identify risk management issues that you should have developed to minimize the likelihood of the error occurring again. The reflective analysis allows you to revisit the situation and to explore your reasons for the course of action you took. This can then be compared with the medicines policy to educate you of the importance of adhering to such documentation.

The adoption of a no-blame culture is more conducive to the reporting of drug errors. It is a duty of care to the patient that you report any errors to the person in charge of your placement setting. If you have observed an error being made, you *must* report it. This can be very difficult as a student nurse because you will want to fit into the team, and reporting an error will likely leave you open to being viewed as a 'whistle-blower'. However, to ignore the incident is a breach of the legal duty of care that you owe to the patient. You would also be failing to follow the standards set by the NMC for raising concerns (NMC 2018b).

Controlled drugs

There is a great deal of legislation surrounding the prescription, supply, storage and administration of medications. The Misuse of Drugs Act 1971 regulates activities in relation to controlled drugs in terms of manufacture, supply and possession. The Act outlines three classes into which the medications it controls fall: class A (e.g. morphine), class B (e.g. codeine) and class C (e.g. buprenorphine).

The Misuse of Drugs Regulations 2001 define the classes of person who are authorized to supply and possess controlled drugs in a professional capacity and under set conditions. The activities governed are import and export, production, supply, possession, prescribing and record-keeping. The Regulations lay out five schedules defining the drugs covered (see Table 15.1).

The Controlled Drugs (Supervision of Management and Use) Regulations 2013 require trusts and hospitals to appoint a Controlled Drugs Accountable Officer (CDAO) who has full responsibility for all aspects of controlled drugs within their organization. This person must be a senior manager in the organization and not routinely involved in handling controlled drugs as part of their normal duties.

You will find that controlled drugs are stored in a separate locked cupboard, often within a second locked cupboard. The keys for the controlled drugs cupboard should be kept separate from other keys and the nurse in charge should keep these on their person at all times while on duty. When working on a hospital ward, you will find a warning light affixed to the outer cupboard. This indicates to staff whether the cupboard has been left open. No other items should be placed in the controlled drugs cupboard.

When giving a controlled drug kept in this cupboard, a separate drug register will need to be updated. This register not only keeps a tally of the drugs used but also lists the patients that the drugs have been administered to, along with the dates and times of administration; this is a requirement of certain schedules of drugs (see Table 15.1).

When giving a controlled drug in schedule 2, procedure must be followed. This involves two people, one of whom must be a qualified nurse or doctor. Some Trusts ask that in the case of two nurses, *both* ought to be qualified. Nevertheless, try to get involved in the administration of this category of medicines to gain a full understanding of the procedure and the nurse's role.

Before administering a controlled drug, it must be checked against the stock last entered in the controlled drugs register. Once you have removed the drug from the controlled drug cupboard, you must lock the cupboard and prepare the drug for administration. Once the drug has been administered, you must detail in the controlled drug register the date, time, patient name, amount of drug given, who gave the drug, who witnessed the drug being given, and finally the new balance of stock. You may also be involved in checking the stock of controlled drugs at a ward level, which is carried out on a regular basis. It is good practice to involve yourself in this aspect of medicines management.

The ordering of a controlled drug is carried out using a specially designed order book. Controlled

Schedule	Example drug	Conditions
1	LSD	Possession and supply prohibited unless under Home Office rule, deemed to have no medicinal use
2	Morphine	Full controlled drug restriction, register required
3	Barbiturates	Special prescription requirements
4	Benzodiazepines	Minimal control, no safe custody, records required
5	Codeine	Minimal control, no safe custody, record-keeping less stringent than schedule 4

Table 15.1 Misuse of Drugs Regulations 2001: The five schedules

drugs can only be ordered by the nurse in charge. The pharmacy will have a copy of that person's signature, which helps them to decide to dispense the drug or not.

Finally, when controlled drugs are delivered to the setting, they are usually contained in a locked box and/or delivered by a designated person, who will have had to sign for the drugs when collecting them from the pharmacy. Then someone has to sign to confirm the drugs have been received in the clinical setting. On receipt, the drugs are checked by two nurses, one of whom must be qualified, and signed for. The newly ordered drugs are then entered onto the controlled drugs register by both nurses and the stock of drugs updated accordingly.

These checks are also in place in community settings, where nurses sign in medications and do so again on administration. Storage advice should be given to patients in the community to maintain safe and appropriate home storage.

Supply and administration of medicines

In the past, nurses were only involved in administering medications. However, under certain circumstances, they now take part in the supply and administration of medications, usually under a Patient Group Direction (PGD). PGDs are written instructions for the supply or administration of medicines to homogeneous groups of patients who require the same treatment. PGDs are used when there is an advantage to patient care without compromising safety. In 1998, a report on the supply and administration of medicines under group protocols was published by the Department

of Health. This provided the legal framework for PGDs.

The PGD must be signed by the senior doctor or senior pharmacist involved in developing the direction. The legislation specifies that each PGD must contain the following information (see MHRA 2017):

- the name of the business to which the direction applies;
- the date the direction comes into force and the date it expires;
- a description of the medicine(s) to which the direction applies;
- class of health professional who may supply or administer the medicine;
- signature of a doctor or dentist, as appropriate, and a pharmacist;
- signature by an appropriate organization;
- the clinical condition or situation to which the direction applies;
- a description of those patients excluded from treatment under the direction;
- a description of the circumstances in which further advice should be sought from a doctor (or dentist, as appropriate) and arrangements for referral;
- details of appropriate dosage and maximum total dosage, quantity, pharmaceutical form and strength, route and frequency of administration, and minimum or maximum period over which the medicine should be administered;
- relevant warnings, including potential adverse reactions;

- details of any necessary follow-up action and the circumstances;
- a statement of the records to be kept for audit purposes.

Prescribing law and non-medical prescribing

Traditionally, doctors prescribed, pharmacists dispensed, and nurses administered medication. Changes in legislation and the extension of health professionals' roles has seen this alter in recent years. The idea of prescribing other than by a doctor was first suggested in 1986 following a review of community nursing services, leading to a report by Baroness Julia Cumberlege. In this report, *Neighbourhood Nursing: A Focus for Care* (DHSS 1986), it was concluded that much of a district nurse's time was being wasted in obtaining prescriptions for basic dressings and appliances required for patient care. The report also detailed the frustration of some nurses involved in palliative care at not being able to vary timing and dosage of prescribed analgesics as dictated by the patient's condition.

A further review by June Crown (DH 1989) and her advisory group began the revolution in prescribing practice. Her initial suggestions included:

- 'initial prescribing' from a restricted formulary;
- supply within an agreed clinical protocol;
- amendment of timing and dosage of medicines prescribed previously within a patient-specific protocol.

It was a further 5 years before the first nurse began prescribing. The Medicinal Products: Prescription by Nurses etc. Act was passed in 1992 and nurse prescribing was made legal in 1994 when secondary legislation came into force. Thus, suitably qualified district nurses were able to prescribe from a limited formulary for specific clinical conditions.

For nurses, however, these changes did not go far enough in addressing their need to prescribe for their patients. They found the formulary restrictive and in some cases were not able to prescribe

appropriately for the patients in their care. The Review of Prescribing, Supply and Administration of Medicines (DH 1999) took nurse prescribing further and described two different groups of prescribers: the *dependent prescriber*, now known as the *supplementary prescriber* and the *independent prescriber*, who was a doctor or a dentist.

It was suggested that the dependent prescriber would be able to prescribe certain medications following initial assessment and diagnosis of the patient by the independent prescriber and the development of an agreed clinical management plan (CMP). This allowed nurses access to many more medications if stated on the CMP.

By now, other allied health professionals were in roles that would benefit from them being able to prescribe. The Health and Social Care Act 2001 (Section 63) allowed the extension of prescribing rights and privileges to certain health care professionals. Changes to the 'Prescription Only Medicines Order' and NHS regulations gave suitably qualified nurses and pharmacists supplementary prescribing rights in April 2003 (DH 2005).

These rights were also extended to chiropodists/podiatrists, radiographers, physiotherapists and optometrists in May 2005 and allowed the government to help meet targets set in the *NHS Plan* (DH 2000). It led to increasing flexibility among multidisciplinary teams by empowering staff and providing efficient and timely access to medicines and increased patient choice. This flexibility was further increased when in 2013 physiotherapists and podiatrists gained independent prescribing rights. Subsequent amendments have seen the introduction of prescribing rights for dieticians (supplementary prescribing training commenced in 2017), the extension of independent prescribing rights to therapeutic radiographers in 2017 and, most recently, independent prescribing for paramedics in 2018.

Further reviews by the Department of Health enabled nurses and pharmacists to prescribe independently from 2006. These autonomous practitioners are responsible for the assessment, diagnosis and treatment of patients for whom their clinical conditions fall within that area of competence. They can prescribe from the whole BNF, with only some restrictions surrounding controlled drugs. These restrictions as outlined by the Home Office relate to prescriptions in addiction.

Nurse prescribers must have an identified prescribing role within their area of practice, be at least one year post-registration and have successfully completed an approved programme of training. This allows additional registration with the NMC as a nurse prescriber, with the nurse following guidelines and standards laid out by their governing body.

Further developments in the field of nurse prescribing have occurred more recently with independent prescribing of unlicensed medications in 2009 and the ability to prescribe controlled drugs on an independent basis, with the exception of drugs in addiction granted in 2012. It is important to be aware that although it is not expected that student nurses will become prescribers, they must be aware of who can prescribe to safely participate in medicines management as part of their role.

Unlicensed and off license prescribing

The term 'unlicensed' medicine is used when a drug that has been prescribed does not have a product licence for its use in the UK, or use with a particular patient group in the UK. Common areas where medicines have no UK product licence are covered by the guidelines we will now outline.

Unlicensed medicines should only be prescribed where there is no suitable licensed alternative. In such cases, the prescriber must take responsibility for the assessment of the patient and the need for the unlicensed medicine.

The General Medical Council (GMC) provides very specific guidelines to doctors when prescribing unlicensed medicines to patients. They outline the areas where unlicensed prescribing is permissible and appropriate. These include:

- where no suitable licensed medication meets the patient's needs (this can include prescribing for children);
- the patient needs an unlicensed medication when the licensed alternative is not available (this may be due to supply issues or may cover specially prepared liquid formulations);
- prescribing as part of a clinical trial;
- prescribing an imported drug.

More information can be obtained from the GMC (2013).

When an unlicensed medicine is prescribed, the patient (and/or their carers) must be given appropriate and comprehensive information (where it exists) about that medication to allow them to make an informed choice about whether or not to use it. In the prescribing of medicines for children, for example, this is commonly done outside of licence and is often seen as custom and practice and may even be referred to as 'off-licence' or 'off-label' use rather than unlicensed. Also, in an emergency situation where an unlicensed drug may be life-saving, the best interests of the patient would apply.

The term 'off-licence' medicine refers to a medicine which does have a UK product licence but is being used outside the terms of that product licence but on the basis of best available evidence. Examples of this would be:

- use of a medicine for an illness different to that stated in the product licence (such as the drug amitriptyline, licensed for depression but used in back pain);
- use of a medicine in an age group outside that stated in the licence (children or elderly);
- use of a medicine at a dose not stated in the licence (such as high doses in palliative care).

Case studies

① As a student nurse, you are accompanying the staff nurse on a drug round. Mr Ajani has been prescribed paracetamol but the drug prescription chart has not been signed by a doctor. The staff nurse asks you to give the medicine to the patient, saying she will get it signed later. Look at the NMC Code and review the implications for yourself and the staff nurse if you administer this medication.

② You are accompanying a district nurse on a patient home visit. The nurse is a prescriber and can prescribe paracetamol for Mrs Simpson (age 66) under a clinical management plan (CMP).

- Using supporting literature from the internet, what conditions must the nurse have satisfied to become a prescriber?
- Reflect on and compare the holistic care of Mrs Simpson with the nurse being a prescriber and what she would receive if the nurse were not able to prescribe.

③ You are visiting a patient in their home with a district nurse. She does not check the patient's identity before proceeding to dress a leg wound. Discuss the reasons for this and how you ensure that the correct patient has been given the correct treatment.

④ Josep Bosko is an elderly patient left with swallowing difficulties after a stroke. His mental function is unimpaired. He requires a medication that has no licensed oral liquid form. What are the alternatives available to the doctor who must prescribe this essential medication?

⑤ Max Jones is 19 years old and living in a community integrated care setting where he has 24-hour carer support. Max has Angelman's syndrome and as part of his condition has severe epilepsy requiring regular medication. You notice in the morning that his carer hides his medicine in his porridge before feeding him. You recognize this as covert administration and wonder about the legality of this measure. Reviewing information around capacity and consent and the best interests priniciple, what sort of circumstances would mean this is an acceptable practice?

Key learning points

Introduction

▶ Medicines are used for their therapeutic effects and careful administration of these is paramount.
▶ The NMC has set out guidance for the administration of medicines.
▶ There are legal and ethical principles to consider when administering a medicine.

The correct patient

▶ Capacity to consent is an important issue.
▶ Checking for allergies is also important.
▶ You need to ensure you have identified the correct patient before administering any medicine.

The correct medicine

▶ Drugs generally have at least two names: the generic name and brand name.
▶ Prescription charts are written using the generic name.
▶ Being able to read clearly the name of the medicine on the prescription chart and on the packaging is important.

The correct dose

▶ Over- and under-dosing of patients is a very important consideration.
▶ Using the BNF is imperative in drug administration.
▶ Nurses' basic arithmetic has been criticized for drug errors.
▶ Practise calculating medicine doses when you are on placement.

The correct site and method of administration

▶ Drugs can be given by a number of routes.
▶ It is important that you use the correct route.
▶ Drugs are designed to be delivered by the correct route.

Covert administration of medicines

▶ Covert administration of a medicine to a capable adult is seen as a trespass in law.
▶ Consent is an important area of drug administration.

Mental capacity and competence in consent

▶ Mental capacity to consent is an issue for children and vulnerable adults.

Alteration of medicines

▶ Drugs must not be crushed or tampered with.
▶ Altering the delivery system of a medicine is outside its licence.
▶ Alteration of a drug will affect its pharmacokinetics and dynamics.
▶ You will not be able to predict side-effects if you alter a drug.
▶ Involve the pharmacy department if a patient is having problems taking the medication in its prescribed format.
▶ Giving a medicine in an unlicensed manner is unlawful.

Reporting of drug errors

▶ An open no-blame culture is important in the reporting of drug errors.
▶ Student nurses are not culpable in law for errors.
▶ If you are involved in a drug error or if you see a drug error being made, you must report it.
▶ If you make a drug error you should work through a reflective critical incident analysis in order to learn from your mistake.

←

Controlled drugs

▶ The Misuse of Drugs Act 1971 prohibits certain activities in relation to controlled drugs.
▶ The Misuse of Drugs Regulations 2001 define the classes of person authorized to supply and possess controlled drugs.
▶ Controlled drugs are normally stored in a locked cupboard within a second locked cupboard.
▶ There are special procedures for giving controlled drugs.
▶ Only the nurse in charge of the ward can order a controlled drug.
▶ Controlled drugs are ordered and catalogued in separate books and registers.

Supply and administration of medicines

▶ Nurses can now be involved in the supply and administration of medicines under PGD.
▶ The Department of Health (1998) lays down specific criteria that must be adhered to.

Prescribing law and non-medical prescribing

▶ Nurses and pharmacists can now prescribe medicines and medicinal products.
▶ Nurses can now be supplementary prescribers provided they follow agreed clinical management plans.
▶ Changes have enabled nurses and pharmacists and other allied health professionals to take a further step and prescribe independently or to an agreed clinical management plan.
▶ Patients may be prescribed unlicensed or off-licence medications and the nurse should be aware of these.

Multiple-choice questions

Try answering these multiple-choice questions to test what you have learned from reading this chapter. You can check your answers at the end of the book.

1. The Misuse of Drugs Act was published in which year?

a) 1975
b) 1971
c) 1970
d) 2001

2. Which class of drug does morphine belong to?

a) A
b) B
c) C
d) D

→

←

3. Which schedule does cannabis belong to?

a) 5
b) 3
c) 2
d) 1

4. What does PGD stand for?

a) Patient Group Direction
b) Prescribing Good Drugs
c) Public Grouped Decisions
d) Patient Generated Directions

5. Most drugs have two names. What are they?

a) General and specific
b) Pharmacological and popular
c) Generic and brand
d) Hospital and manufacturer

6. If you gave a drug covertly to a capable adult in law, you would have committed what?

a) A slander
b) A defamation
c) A trespass
d) A libel

7. If an adult lacks the capacity to consent, can another person consent on their behalf?

a) Yes
b) No
c) Only in an emergency
d) Only under a CMP

8. Which of the following allied health professionals cannot prescribe?

a) Occupational therapist
b) Pharmacist
c) Nurse
d) Physiotherapist

9. What is the most important factor in facilitating the reporting of drug errors?

a) Reading the NMC's guidelines
b) Weekly drug audit meetings

→

c) A robust drugs policy

d) A no-blame culture

10. Tampering or crushing of a medicine is unlawful because …

a) It affects the pharmacokinetics and dynamics

b) It invalidates the product licence

c) It means that you cannot predict the side-effects

d) It does not involve a pharmacist

Recommended further reading

Beckwith, S. and Franklin, P. (2007) *Oxford Handbook of Nurse Prescribing.* Oxford: Oxford University Press.

Brenner, G.M. and Stevens, C.W. (2017) *Pharmacology,* 5th edition. Philadelphia, PA: Elsevier.

Coben, D. and Atere-Roberts, E. (2005) *Calculations for Nursing and Healthcare,* 2nd edition. Basingstoke: Palgrave Macmillan.

Department of Health (DH) (1989) *Report of the Advisory Group on Nurse Prescribing* (the Crown Report). London: DH.

Department of Health (DH) (1998) *Review of Prescribing, Supply and Administration of Medicines: A Report on the Supply and Administration of Medicines Under Group Protocols.* London: DH.

Department of Health (DH) (1999) *Review of Prescribing, Supply and Administration of Medicines –Final Report* (the Crown Report 2). London: DH.

Department of Health (DH) (2000) *NHS Plan: A Plan for Investment, a Plan for Reform.* London: DH.

Department of Health (DH) (2005) *Supplementary Prescribing by Nurses, Pharmacists, Chiropodists/ Podiatrists, Physiotherapists and Radiographers within the NHS in England: A Guide for Implementation.* London: DH.

Department of Health and Social Security (DHSS) (1986) *Neighbourhood Nursing: A Focus for Care* (the Cumberlege Report). London: HMSO.

Downie, G., Mackenzie, J. and Williams, A. (2007) *Pharmacology and Medicines Management for Nurses,* 4th edition. Edinburgh: Churchill Livingstone.

Gatford, J.D. and Phillips, N. (2006) *Nursing Calculations,* 7th edition. Edinburgh: Churchill Livingstone Elsevier.

Gillick v West Norfolk & Wisbech Area Health Authority [1986] AC 112.

Greenstein, B. and Gould, D. (2008) *Trounce's Clinical Pharmacology for Nurses,* 18th edition. New York: Churchill Livingstone.

Karch, A.M. (2017) *Focus on Nursing Pharmacology,* 7th edition. Philadelphia, PA: Lippincott Williams & Wilkins.

Lapham, R. (2015) *Drug Calculations for Nurses: A Step-by-Step Approach,* 4th edition. London: Arnold.

Medicines and Healthcare Products Regulatory Agency (MHRA) (2017) *Patient Group Directions: Who Can Use Them.* Available at: https://www.gov.uk/government/publications/patient-group-directions-pgds/patient-group-directions-who-can-use-them.

Montgomery v Lanarkshire Health Board [2015] UKSC 11 [2015], 1 AC 1430.

National Institute for Health and Care Excellence (NICE) (2019) *British National Formulary.* London: NICE. Available at: https://bnf.nice.org.uk.

NHS Improvement (2018) *Recommendations from National Patient Safety Agency Alerts that Remain Relevant to the Never Events list 2018.* London: NHS Improvement. Available at: https://improvement.nhs.uk/documents/2267/Recommendations_from_NPSA_alerts_that_remain_relevant_to_NEs_FINAL.pdf.

NHS UK (2005) Managing someone's legal affairs, www.nhs.uk/CarersDirect/moneyandlegal/legal/Pages/MentalCapacityAct.aspx.

Nursing and Midwifery Council (NMC) (2015) *The Code: Professional Standards of Practice and Behaviour for Nurses, Midwives and Nursing Associates.* London: NMC. Updated 2018.

Nursing and Midwifery Council (NMC) (2018a) *Standards of Proficiency for Registered Nurses.* London: NMC.

Nursing and Midwifery Council (NMC) (2018b) *Raising Concerns; Guidance for Nurses, Midwives and Nursing Associates.* London: NMC. Last updated 2019.

Simonson, T., Aarbakke, J., Kay, I., Coleman, I., Sinnott, P. and Lyssa, R. (2006) *Illustrated Pharmacology for Nurses.* London: Hodder Arnold.

UK Government (1971) The Misuse of Drugs Act.

UK Government (1992) The Medicinal Products: Prescription by Nurses etc. Act.

UK Government (1998) The Human Rights Act.

UK Government (2001) The Misuse of Drugs Regulations.

UK Government (2005) The Mental Capacity Act.

UK Government (2013) Controlled Drugs (Supervision of Management and Use) Regulations.

Conclusion

To administer medicines safely and become competent in the education of patients about their medication, the nurse must have knowledge of basic pharmacology, physiology and pathophysiology. Also, in the interests of patient safety, they must be able to complete simple drug calculations. This book has introduced you to the knowledge necessary when engaging in these skills.

The focus of your career is nursing and so the clinical tips in this book have been designed to give you an insight into the importance of pharmacology and its relevance to the profession of nursing. It is also important in your role in medicines administration that you have a good understanding of pharmacology and safe drug calculation. The first three chapters introduced topics and concepts that we hope will provide a basis for reading the rest of the book.

Chapters 4–13 address pharmacology in detail and demonstrate how important it is that nurses have a good understanding of medicines, their actions and contraindications. The links to physiology are intended to aid your understanding of drugs and the conditions they are used to treat. We hope that the breadth and depth of the discussion will encourage you to read around the areas you work in – this is, after all, an essentials text and by no means comprehensive in its coverage,

and there are a range of books and resources that provide more detail and cover a wider range of medicines.

Chapter 14 provides an insight into the patient's role and responsibility about their medicine management. Nurses generally are well placed to help patients understand the need to adhere to instructions and advice. Often the nurse is the one provider of continuity in care during the patient's journey, so we hope you have gained some insight into the importance of your role as a health educator.

The accuracy of drug calculation is central to nurse training and this has resulted in changes taking place at a pre-registration education level. We hope that the questions at the end of most chapters are realistic enough and help you to practise your calculations in relation to drug dosages.

Medicines management is fraught with potential pitfalls. Calculating the correct dose is obviously important, but there are areas of law and professional standards that also need to be adhered to if you are to become a safe practitioner, and these are addressed in Chapter 15.

Overall, we hope this book has given you the motivation and interest to want to improve your knowledge of pharmacology in nursing. For other texts that will aid you in your journey, see our suggestions for further reading at the end of each chapter.

Glossary

A

absorption: process by which a drug reaches the general circulation and becomes biologically available

acetylcholine: chemical transmitter released by certain nerve endings

adrenaline: hormone produced by adrenal medulla to prepare the body for fight or flight

alopecia: hair loss

angiotensin: a hormone involved in the renin–angiotensin system which is a target for blood pressure lowering medication

antidote: a remedy which counteracts the action of a chemical

anti-emetic: a drug given to stop nausea and vomiting

anti-epileptic drugs (AEDs): drugs used primarily in the management of epilepsy and convulsive disorders

aperient: a drug given to help loosen the bowels

arachidonic acid: substance liberated from the cell enabling the cyclo-oxygenase pathway

B

basophil: a granular white cell that contains heparin and histamine

benign: a tumour that is not cancerous

bioavailability: the extent and rate of a drug that becomes available to its target receptor following administration

blood–brain barrier (BBB): the membranes between the circulating blood and the brain

bradykinin: powerful pain-producing substance

bronchoconstriction: the narrowing of the bronchial passages in the lungs

C

carcinogen: cancer-causing substances

chemotaxis: the movement of white cells towards an area of inflammation

chemotherapy:
any drug treatment but commonly used to refer to cancer therapy

collagen: an essential protein that helps make up many tissues in the body

complement proteins: a group of proteins that are essential in aiding the inflammatory response

contraindications: reasons, usually medical, whereby medications should not be given to a patient

cyclo-oxygenase pathway: a metabolic pathway that results in the formation of prostaglandins

cytochrome P450: a group of enzymes that help metabolize drugs

cytotoxic: toxic to cells, used to describe a class of chemotherapy drugs

D

decongestant: a drug used to unblock the upper respiratory tract

distribution: the distribution of drugs after absorption to their target sites

DNA: deoxyribonucleic acid, the genetic material of a cell

dopamine: neurotransmitter implicated in movement

E

elimination: removal of drugs and their metabolites from the body

enteric coating: protective coating that ensures a medicine is released after leaving the stomach

extrinsic pathway: blood clotting mechanism that is initiated by external damage to vessel

F

first pass: effect caused by metabolism of a drug by the liver resulting in only part of the drug reaching the circulation

G

gamma-aminobutyric acid (GABA): neurotransmitter associated with a dampening effect on brain activity

243

glucocorticoids: hormones secreted by the adrenal cortex

H

half-life: time taken for a drug to lose 50% of its plasma concentration in the body

histamine: substance that causes widespread vasodilation and increased permeability of blood vessels

I

ingestion: taking into the body

intramuscular (IM): injection into a muscle

intravenous (IV): injection directly into a vein

intrinsic pathway: blood clotting mechanism initiated without any external damage needed to vessel

L

laxative: drug given to promote defecation

lipid: a naturally occurring molecule that stores energy; examples are fats and cholesterol

M

malignant: a cancerous growth, or relating to cancer

metabolism: processing of a parent drug compound by enzymes in the liver

metastasis: cancer that has spread from its primary site

mycobacteria: rod-shaped acid-fast bacteria implicated in tuberculosis

N

neurokinin receptors: receptors for antiemetic drugs

neuroleptics: antipsychotic drugs

P

phantom limb pain: sensation of pain that is still reported by a patient after the removal of a limb/body part

plasma protein: proteins carried in the plasma with a range of physiological functions; target sites for drug binding

plasminogen: inactive plasma protein

potassium: major intracellular cation

prostacyclin: prostaglandin implicated in making platelets less sticky

proteolytic enzymes: enzymes that break down proteins within the cell membrane

prothrombin: inactive plasma protein involved in blood clotting

proton pump inhibitor (PPI): drug that stops production of hydrochloric acid in the stomach

R

renin: a hormone secreted by the kidney to help raise blood pressure

S

salicylates: group of drugs including aspirin which are acidic and given as analgesics

sepsis: overwhelming infection of the blood

serotonin: neurotransmitter implicated in alterations of mood

steady state: this is the point reached when the amount of drug being absorbed is the same as the amount being excreted

subcutaneous (SC): injection given into tissue just beneath the skin

systemic vasodilation: widening of the blood vessels throughout the body, including arteries and veins usually by smooth muscle relaxation; often leads to a reduction in blood pressure

T

T-lymphocyte: a type of white cell associated with the immune response and production of antibodies

therapeutic range: the range of plasma drug concentration in which medicine has its best effect

therapeutic index: reflects the relative safety of a drug; compares the amount of a drug required to induce a therapeutic response to the amount that would cause a toxic effect

thromboxane: implicated in platelet adherence

topically: the application of a drug directly to skin and mucous membranes

Answers

Chapter 1

Case study ① Mrs Asamoah

The following areas of assessment would help you identify factors influencing the absorption and distribution of the medication which Mrs Asamoah is taking:

- Assess Mrs Asamoah's mobility
- Assess the drug formulation: does she require liquids instead of tablets?
- Assess her age in relationship to plasma protein loss
- Assess if she is dehydrated
- Assess her nutritional status and when she takes her medicines in relationship to meals
- Is she taking any OTC medication?
- Check the BNF for any interactions between drugs that may affect absorption and distribution

Case study ② Mr Mambety

The following factors may influence Mr Mambety's ability to metabolize and excrete drugs during his post-operative recovery:

- The effects of alcohol on liver
- The effects of smoking on the systems of the body
- The effects of surgery on the movement of the intestine
- Fluid balance
- Urinary output

Case study ③ Ben Brown

You should consider the following when assisting Ben to take his medications appropriately:

- Ask about Ben's indigestion and what brings it on
- Elicit how much Gaviscon Ben is taking daily and when he takes the doses

- Explain to Ben that he needs to take his erythromycin 4 times per day and this must be evenly spaced
- Suggest he takes his erythromycin at set times, e.g. 8am, 12 noon, 4pm and 8pm
- Advise him that his Gaviscon should be taken regularly for the course of erythromycin at 10am, 2pm, 6pm and 10pm
- Explain that taking the drugs too close together would mean that the antibiotic may not be absorbed properly and will have a reduced effect
- Draw up a chart for him to tick when he has taken his medication and he should do this for the complete course of antibiotics
- Enlist the help of his family and carers where appropriate

Multiple-choice questions

1 a
2 a
3 d
4 c
5 b
6 b
7 d
8 b
9 d
10 a

Chapter 2

Case study ① Marek Brodzki

Your responsibilities regarding the antibiotics are:

- This may be a mild allergy
- Needs to be closely monitored
- No treatment necessary, although may give antihistamines
- Report rash to doctor
- The rash may become a more severe reaction

Your responsibilities regarding recording the incident are:

- Record extent of the rash, when first noticed: is it becoming worse, how irritant is it?
- Marek to tell health care professionals of any suggestion of antibiotic reaction

Your responsibilities regarding prevention of a reoccurrence are:

- Marek should inform health care staff if other members of the family have reactions
- Ensure it is documented on the patient's prescription chart and notes if he has an allergy
- Marek to carry information with him if he suspects a severe reaction (e.g. bracelet or medical card)

Case study ② Sue Kent

According to the BNF:

- Ibuprofen increases the actions of warfarin
- Sue may take some drugs like a COX2 inhibitor

Case study ③ Ethel Bassett

Discussion on the interaction between normal ageing and responses to drug therapy in older people may include:

- Age-related changes that increase risk for adverse drug events
  - chronic disease
  - polypharmacy
  - physiological and adaptive responses
- Determinants of physiological response to medications
  - race
  - ethnicity
  - genetic background
- Acute and chronic conditions may alter
  - pharmacokinetics (what the body does to the drug)
  - pharmacodynamics (what the drug does to the body)
- Age-related changes

- decrease in body water (as much as 15%) and increase in body fat
- increased concentration of water-soluble drugs
- more prolonged effects of fat-soluble drugs
- hepatic blood flow may be decreased by as much as 50% in individuals over 65 years
- increased toxicity with normal doses of 'first-pass effect' drugs
- less drug would be detoxified immediately by the liver
- decreases in serum albumin
- leads to altered binding capacity
- may cause increased serum levels of the 'free' or unbound proportion of protein-bound drugs
- may result in toxic levels of highly protein-bound drugs because more unbound drug is available to produce its effects
- considerable individual variation in the degree of decline of renal function
- Causes of changes in pharmacodynamics in the older person
  - decreased number of receptors
  - decreased receptor binding
  - altered cellular response to the drug–receptor interaction

Case study ④ Safiso

Discussion on the interaction between ageing and pharmacokinetics in a young person may include:

- Slower GI but faster IM absorption in infancy
- More body water vs. lipid in early life
- Limited protein binding in infants
- Larger liver/body weight ratio in infants
- Immature enzymes in neonates
- Larger brain/body weight ratio and higher blood–brain barrier permeability in younger children
- Immature renal function in infants

Multiple-choice questions

1 b
2 c
3 b
4 d

5   a
6   c
7   c
8   d
9   b
10 a

7   12.5mL
8   15mL
9   10 minutes
10 750mg

Chapter 3

Case study ① James Jones

Your task centres on:

- Doing the calculation: $60 \times 16 = 960$mg per day
- Divided into 4 doses = 960 / 4 = 240mg per dose
- This requires skills in multiplication and division, as well as application of a formula and a weight calculation
- Getting this right is important so James can receive the correct amount of drug for his body size, as too much risks overdose and too little would not achieve a therapeutic effect

Case study ② Helen Taylor

Your task centres on:

- Doing the calculation: the bottle contains 200mL at 2mg per mL, so:
- 300 / 2 × 1 = 150mL is needed
- 200mL × 150mL leaves 50mL over
- For the delivery: 150 / 60 = 2.5mL per minute
- This requires skills in multiplication, subtraction and division, as well as the application of a formula and a time calculation
- It is important to get this calculation correct, as there is a time schedule to adhere to for delivery of the dose; too fast a delivery may cause side-effects

Calculations

1   2000mcg
2   0.6g
3   1200mg
4   5000mcg
5   2 tablets
6   2 tablets

Chapter 4

Case study ① Dawn Mason

The mode of action of the two drugs:

- Actions on prostaglandins and nociceptors
- Talk about the cyclo-oxygenase pathway
- Opiates block calcium channels in pain pathways
- Opiates open potassium channels
- Opiates bind with receptors

The importance of stepping down from opiates to NSAIDS would involve:

- Give NSAIDs before taking Dawn off opiates
- Discuss analgesic ladder

The maintenance required to achieve a steady plasma concentration would involve:

- Make sure Dawn is taking regular doses so a steady state is achieved
- Ensure you evaluate Dawn's level of pain so that you know a steady level of analgesia has been maintained
- Discuss side-effects

You would explain the information by:

- Using understandable terms, diagrams or models and check the health care assistant's understanding

Case study ② Alex Smith

The mode of action of paracetamol and NSAIDS would involve:

- Actions of the drugs on the cyclo-oxygenase pathway 2 (COX2) and cyclo-oxygenase pathway 3 (COX3)

The need for regulator dosing to achieve therapeutic plasma concentrations would involve:

- Ensuring you evaluate Alex's level of pain so that you know a steady level of analgesia has been maintained
- Making sure Alex is taking regular doses so a steady state is achieved
- Discussing side-effects

You would pass on the information by:

- Checking Alex's and his parents' knowledge, plan information session, writing and agreeing learning outcomes, using understandable terms, using diagrams or models, and checking their understanding

Case study ③ Mr Nozic

The nursing observations you would be making on Mr Nozic during his immediate post-operative care might include:

- Return of sensation – you must make sure that the numb area is protected from pressure and injury until sensation returns. You must inform Mr Nozic that it takes 1.5 to 4 hours for feeling (sensation) to return to the area of his body that is numb and that he should tell the ward staff about any concerns or worries he may have. Mr Nozic should be informed that as sensation returns he may experience some tingling in the skin as the spinal anaesthetic wears off. At this point, he may become aware of some pain from the operation site and that he should ask for more pain relief before the pain becomes too severe. As the spinal anaesthetic wears off, ensure that Mr Nozic understands that he needs to ask for help when he first gets out of bed
- Low blood pressure – as the spinal anaesthetic takes effect, it can lower the blood pressure and make Mr Nozic feel faint or sick. This can be controlled with intravenous fluids and by giving drugs to raise his blood pressure if required
- Itching – this can occur as a side-effect of using morphine-like drugs in combination with local

anaesthetic drugs in spinal anaesthesia. If Mr Nozic experiences itching it can be treated, so long as you tell him to inform you when it occurs

- Difficulty passing water (urinary retention) – Mr Nozic may find it difficult to empty his bladder normally for as long as the spinal anaesthetic lasts. His bladder function should return to normal after the spinal anaesthetic wears off. He may require a catheter to be placed in his bladder temporarily, either while the spinal anaesthetic wears off or as part of the surgical procedure
- Headache – there are many causes of headache, including the anaesthetic, the operation, dehydration and anxiety. Most headaches lessen in intensity within a few hours and can be treated with pain-relieving medicines. Severe headache can occur after a spinal anaesthetic. If this happens to Mr Nozic, you should ask the anaesthetist to visit him. He may need special treatment for the headache
- Fluids and diet – tell Mr Nozic that he can normally drink fluids within an hour of the operation and may also be able to eat a light diet
- Nerve damage – this is a rare complication of spinal anaesthesia. Temporary loss of sensation, pins and needles and sometimes muscle weakness may last for a few days or even weeks but almost always the patient makes a full recovery over time. Permanent nerve damage is even rarer and has about the same chance of occurring as major complications of general anaesthesia.

Case study ④ Ruby Mtumba

Discuss the World Health Organization three-step 'analgesic ladder'.

Treatment should be started at the bottom of the ladder and the ladder ascended in accordance with the response to medication by this patient. Advise that ascending the ladder is the goal, though in some patients this is prevented by increasing side-effects.

Discussion of the WHO's analgesic ladder in order to explain how this lady's pain should have been pharmacologically managed may include:

- Paracetamol – at the foot of the ladder you should have discussed paracetamol as being sufficient for pain control of mild-to-moderate pain. Paracetamol is an effective analgesic, with no gastrointestinal side-effects, and is available in an array of formulations. Care should be taken to avoid overdosing, because this may cause liver damage
- NSAIDs – these have three actions: pain relief, a reduction in inflammation and bringing the patient's temperature down. They are particularly useful in conditions where the pain is accompanied by inflammation, such as rheumatoid arthritis. Some NSAIDs, such as naproxen, are associated with gastrointestinal problems, including stomach ulcers. Newer NSAIDs (COX-2 inhibitors, or coxibs) appear to have fewer gastrointestinal side-effects in some people and therefore are another option. It must be remembered that all NSAIDs and coxibs have the potential to cause renal dysfunction and should be used with caution in patients with cardiac disease
- Weak opioids – these include drugs such as codeine and dihydrocodeine. They are effective analgesics, but may cause drowsiness, constipation and other side-effects
- Strong opioids – these are on the top step of the ladder. Opioids may be important as part of the patient's overall pain management strategy. Strong opioids may be considered when other options have failed to control a patient's pain. It may be necessary to try different opioids before the best balance of efficacy and adverse effects is achieved for a particular patient. The treatment of chronic non-malignant pain, in particular, requires many factors (such as causative disease, previous analgesic history and extent of disability) to be considered before choosing whether to start a strong opioid and with which opioid to start treatment

Case Study ⑤ Jonti Williams

Options for analgesia:

- Use pain ladder – start with paracetamol
- Consider NSAIDs as an adjunct

- Opioids may not be an option due to poor effect in neuropathic pain and the potential interactions with gabapentin
- Increasing the dose of gabapentin may be considered so long as Jonti does not begin to exhibit side-effects related to the increased dose

Calculations

1 1.5mL
2 40mL
3 3 tablets: 20mg + 20mg + 10mg
4 3 capsules
5 0.8mL
6 12.5mL
7 8 tablets
8 0.4mL
9 0.7mL
10 0.75mL

Multiple-choice questions

1 a
2 d
3 b
4 d
5 c
6 b
7 a
8 c
9 d
10 c

Chapter 5

Case study ① Cynthia Day

Clarithromycin is:

- Bacteriostatic at low levels
- Bactericidal at high levels
- Inhibits protein synthesis
- Prescribed in penicillin allergy

The possible reasons why this drug has been chosen are:

- Active against most gram-positive bacteria
- Active against many penicillin-resistant bacteria

Answers

- Useful in treating respiratory tract infections
- Safe and least toxic of antibiotics

The clinical observations which would need to be made on Mrs Day include:

- Trend of pyrexia
- Cardiovascular status
- Nutritional and fluid status – promoting absorption, distribution and elimination of the drug
- Respiratory function and sputum examination (effect of drug)
- GI disturbances – side-effects of drug
- Skin rashes and pruritus – side-effects of drug

Case study ② Ella Jackson

Discussion of the difference between bacteria and viruses should include:

- Types of bacteria
- Difference between gram-negative and gram-positive bacteria
- Difference between our cells and bacterial cells

Discussion of mechanism of actions of antibiotics would include:

- How antibiotics work in different ways to destroy bacteria
- The difference between a bacteria and a virus

Alternative medications to relieve Ella's symptoms might include:

- The use antipyretics for pain relief

Case study ③ Scott Mosier

The nursing interventions for this patient with TB would include:

- Monitoring him for hepatic side-effects such as yellow eyes and skin, loss of appetite, dark urine and unusual tiredness. (Anti-tuberculosis agents, such as isoniazid and rifampicin, cause hepatic impairment)

- Monitoring him for neurological side-effects such as numbness and tingling of the extremities. (Anti-tuberculosis agents, such as isoniazid, cause peripheral neuropathy and depletion of vitamin B_6.) Give B_6 as required
- Monitoring for side-effects specific to various anti-tuberculosis drugs:
  - difficulty in voiding (pyrazinamide)
  - fever, yellowing of skin, weakness and dark urine (isoniazid, rifampicin)
  - GI system disturbances (rifampicin)
  - numbness and tingling of extremities (isoniazid)
  - red discoloration of body fluids (rifampicin)
- Collecting sputum specimens as directed by Trust. (This will determine the effectiveness of the medicine.) Instruct the patient in the proper technique needed to collect a sputum specimen
- Ensuring you follow the policies and procedures in order to establish infection control measures based on the extent of the condition. These measures help to prevent further spread of infection. Instruct patient in infectious control measures, such as frequent hand-washing, covering the mouth when coughing or sneezing, and proper disposal of soiled tissues
- Ensuring adequate rest, nutrition, hydration and relaxation. Teach the patient to incorporate health-enhancing activities, such as adequate rest and sleep, intake of essential vitamins and nutrients, and intake of 6–8 glasses of water per day
- Monitoring the patient's ability and motivation to be concordant with his medicines. It is important that the treatment continues for the full length of therapy to eliminate all *M. tuberculosis* organisms. Therefore, explain to the patient the importance of complying with the entire therapeutic plan, including:
  - taking all medications as directed by the physician
  - not discontinuing medication until instructed
  - wearing a medical alert bracelet
  - keeping all appointments for follow-up care

Case study ④ Lorenzo Chopra

Gentamicin is a member of the aminoglycoside family of antibiotics. Aminoglycosides act by disrupting protein synthesis at the bacterial ribosome.

You should make the following observations of the patient's condition:

- Monitor for signs of renal toxicity including unusual appearance of urine (dark, cloudy) intake and output ratio, and the presence of oedema
- Monitor for evidence of ototoxicity, including headache, dizziness or vertigo, nausea or vomiting with motion, ataxia, nystagmus, tinnitus, roaring noises, sensation of fullness of ears, and hearing impairment
- Monitor peak and trough drug levels. (Aminoglycosides have a narrow therapeutic range)
- Observe for symptoms of neurotoxicity or neuromuscular blockade such as muscle twitching, numbness, seizures, weakness or difficulty breathing
- Observe for signs and symptoms of bacterial overgrowth due to drug's effect to 'kill' all bacteria, even normal flora that can lead to superinfection. However, gentamycin only has a low incidence of provoking *Clostridium difficile* infections

Case Study ⑤ Josie

Opening capsules and ingesting the drug in another way changes the absorption properties of the drug, meaning less or potentially none of it reaching the systemic circulation. Advice should always be sought from a pharmacist as to whether or not this is a viable option for the prescribed drug and the nurse should never make this decision for themselves, or advise parents to do so. Doing so would also mean that the drug was given in a way not specified in the product literature supplied by the manufacturer upon gaining its marketing authorization (license), thus making the administration unlicensed.

The advice of the prescriber should be sought to determine whether it is acceptable to delay starting the course of the antibiotic until the liquid format becomes available. Again, nurses should not make this decision themselves.

As a 13-year-old with learning difficulties, Josie may not be able to provide valid informed consent to treatment and her parents should be involved at every stage. It may be necessary to determine if Josie has capacity to consent using the Fraser Guidelines to see if she is 'Gillick competent' and can make her own decisions. It may be necessary to act in her best interests and this is where involvement of the parent and the medical team becomes necessary.

Calculations

1 16mL
2 1.7mL
3 40mL
4 2 tablets
5 4.5mL
6 56 tablets
7 10mL
8 2mL
9 7.5mL
10 20mL

Multiple-choice questions

1 c
2 a
3 c
4 b
5 d
6 d
7 a
8 c
9 c
10 d

Chapter 6

Case study ① Radu Beligan

Action of steroids on the body:

- Steroids affect COX2 pathway

Side-effects of steroids may include:

- Increases blood glucose
- A fall in protein production
- Affects fat distribution in the body
- Sodium is retained
- Calcium is removed from bone

- Secondary diabetes
- Secondary hypertension
- Low blood calcium
- Lowered wound healing
- Lowered ability to fight infection

Other information that may be given to Mr Beligan would include:

- Need to carry card
- Do not suddenly stop taking medication
- Keep good stock of drug
- Inform his doctor and dentist

Case study ② Louise Mason

Discussion of the mode of action of ibuprofen, steroids and methotrexate may include:

- Discussion about prostaglandin synthesis
- Discussion about COX2 pathway
- Discussion about arachidonic acid formation
- Discussion about DNA in a cell and how methotrexate works on this

Discussion regarding maintaining drug therapy between stopping one drug and commencing another could include:

- Explaining steroids are only needed until the methotrexate begins to work

Discussion of the possible side-effects of steroids may include:

- Explaining the side-effects of steroids including high blood pressure, secondary diabetes, poor wound healing, masking of infection
- Checking Louise's parents' knowledge, plan session, writing/agreeing learning outcomes, using understandable terms, using diagrams or models, and checking their understanding

Case study ③ Darinda Novak

Discussion on what information the patient will require regarding side-effects of methotrexate may include:

- Feeling sick, upset stomach or diarrhoea. These problems frequently occur when the patient first starts the treatment and normally settle but may persist. The patient should be encouraged to report these problems. The symptoms can be helped in a number of ways:
  - they may be advised to increase the amount of the folic acid supplement they take
  - they may be advised to take an anti-emetic
  - their doctor may wish to change their treatment to methotrexate by injection once a week
- Effects on bone marrow or liver. Inform the patient that the blood tests to be performed during their therapy will help to monitor these potential problems. The patient should be told to report regularly catching infections, bruising or bleeding easily, and should be reassured that the doctor or nurse monitoring the treatment will contact the patient if there are any problems with the blood test results. Occasionally changes in the patient's blood may mean they have to stop the methotrexate
- Mouth ulcers, sore throat or sore mouth. If the patient experiences mouth ulcers, or a sore throat or mouth, they will need to speak to their doctor, nurse or pharmacist. It may be necessary for them to have a blood test to check how their body is coping, as these are signs that the bone marrow may be becoming depressed. In many cases, if blood tests are normal, the patient may then be given some medication to treat these problems
- Infections. As we have indicated, methotrexate may reduce the patient's ability to fight infections. It is important that the patient reports if they think they have an infection (for example, a wound that fails to heal promptly, pain or burning when passing water, or a chest infection)
- Rashes. If the patient gets a new rash or severe itching anywhere on their body, they should seek advice from their doctor, nurse or pharmacist
- Shortness of breath (breathlessness). Methotrexate can very occasionally cause inflammation of the lungs. This breathlessness can come on gradually or over a few days. The patient may also have a dry cough. If they feel breathless when resting and they don't have a heavy cold

(runny nose and temperature), they should be told to stop the methotrexate and contact their doctor or nurse. It is important that they see their doctor so that they can be examined, in case they have severe inflammation of the lungs

- Whites of the eyes become yellow or the patient develops severe itching of the skin. If this occurs, the patient should stop treatment and seek advice from their doctor or nurse, as these are sometimes signs of liver problems
- New unexplained bleeding or bruising. This sometimes means that the patient's blood cells are affected by the methotrexate. In this case, they can stop the methotrexate and seek advice from their doctor or nurse

Case study ④ *Phyllis Johnson*

Discussion of the inflammatory process and the medicine celecoxib describing the difference between cyclo-oxygenase 1 and 2 inhibitors should include:

- Cyclo-oxygenase (COX) is an enzyme that is responsible for the formation of what are known as prostanoids. The three main groups of prostanoids – prostaglandins, prostacyclins and thromboxanes – are each involved in the inflammatory response
- It is now clear that there are two different COX enzymes, COX1 and COX2. Cyclo-oxygenase-1 (COX1) is known to be present in most tissues. In the gastrointestinal tract, COX1 maintains the normal lining of the stomach. The enzyme is also involved in kidney and platelet function. Cyclo-oxygenase-2 (COX2) is primarily present at sites of inflammation. While both COX1 and COX2 convert arachidonic acid to prostaglandins, resulting in pain and inflammation, their other functions make inhibition of COX1 undesirable while inhibition of COX2 is considered desirable
- NSAIDS commonly prescribed to treat arthritis work by inhibiting prostaglandins. Traditional NSAIDs such as ibuprofen and naproxen, however, can cause gastrointestinal problems including gastric ulceration

- Traditional NSAIDs are considered 'non-selective' because they inhibit both COX1 and COX2. The inhibition of COX2 by traditional NSAIDs accounts for the anti-inflammatory effect of the drugs, while the inhibition of COX1 can lead to NSAID toxicity and associated side-effects such as ulcers, prolonged bleeding time and kidney problems

Calculations

1　6 tablets
2　5 tablets
3　The nearest accurate dose is 3.4mL
4　2 tablets
5　The nearest accurate dose is 4.3mL
6　2 tablets
7　450mg in each dose
8　The nearest accurate dose is 0.75mL
9　3.2mL
10　0.5mL

Multiple-choice questions

1　d
2　a
3　c
4　a
5　b
6　c
7　d
8　c
9　b
10　a

Chapter 7

Case study ① *Olek Krupa*

The advice that you would give Mr Krupa with regard to taking warfarin ought to include:

- Importance of carrying an anticoagulant card highlighting dosage
- Essential to make and keep blood check appointment
- To inform any doctor, nurse or dentist that he is receiving anticoagulant therapy

- To take tablets as prescribed
- To avoid alcohol, drugs containing aspirin and any other OTC medications
- To make an appointment with the GP or anticoagulant clinic if he notices any bleeding, bruising or indigestion
- To adjust lifestyle to avoid unnecessary trauma – for example, to be careful when using sharp gardening or domestic implements

Case study ② Mr Patel

Discussion around differences between the modes of action of warfarin and enoxaparin might include:

- Warfarin is a vitamin K antagonist, which means that it reduces the manufacture of a number of plasma clotting factors (II, VII, IX and X)
- Enoxaparin binds to and accelerates the activity of antithrombin III. By activating antithrombin III, enoxaparin preferentially potentiates the inhibition of coagulation factors Xa and IIa. Factor Xa catalyses the conversion of prothrombin to thrombin, so enoxaparin's inhibition of this process results in decreased thrombin and ultimately the prevention of fibrin clot formation

Discussion around Mr Patel's warfarin therapy before, during and after his procedure should include:

- He will stop his warfarin therapy 5–6 days prior to his procedure
- Bridging anticoagulation with enoxaparin is commenced 3 days prior to his surgery. The last dose of this should be given 24 hours before his surgery
- After surgery, bridging is resumed no earlier than 24 hours after surgery; at the same time, warfarin is restarted. Bridging is continued, typically for 4–6 days, until the anticoagulant effect of warfarin has resumed and the blood is sufficiently thinned again

Case study ③ Bo Wong

Discussion around teaching this lady how to give herself enoxaparin may include:

- Telling her to wash and dry hands thoroughly before giving the injection
- Telling her to sit or lie in a comfortable position, so that she can see her abdomen
- Choose an area on her abdomen at least 2 inches away from her naval
- Remove the needle cap
- Hold the syringe in her dominant hand
- With the other hand she should pinch her skin to make a mound and then insert the full length of the needle straight down – at a 90 degree angle into the mound of skin
- Press the plunger with the thumb until the syringe is empty
- Pull the needle straight out and let go of the skin mound
- Point the needle away from herself and others and press down on the plunger to activate the needle shield
- Place the used syringe in the sharps container

Calculations

1 5mL
2 4 tablets
3 0.525mL
4 0.9mL
5 3 tablets
   5mg + 1mg + 1mg = 7mg
   or
   1mg + 3mg + 3mg = 7mg
6 5mL per hour
7 0.1mL
8 500 units/mL in 40mL = 20,000 units
   20,000 units from 5000 units/mL = 4mL
   4mL of heparin and 36mL of saline = 40mL of solution
9 0.9mL
10 a) 0.25mL; b) 0.25mL; c) 0.5mL

Multiple-choice questions

1 c
2 a
3 a
4 d
5 c
6 b

7 a
8 c
9 c
10 d

Chapter 8

Case study ① *Joseph Olita*

Discussion around action of corticosteroid and bronchodilator may include:

- Reference to bronchodilators
- Reference to adrenoreceptors and stimulation of such receptors
- Reference to steroids and arachidonic acid
- Mention local side-effects like sore or dry throat
- Mention possibility of thrush formation

Discussion around inhaler technique may include:

- Talking Joseph through the inhaler technique outlined earlier in the chapter

You would inform Joseph by:

- Checking his knowledge, planning the session, writing/agreeing learning outcomes, using understandable terms, using diagrams/models

Case study ② *Elizabeth Jones*

Discussion around the action of corticosteroid salbutamol on the airways might include:

- Reference to bronchodilators
- Reference to adrenoreceptors and stimulation of such receptors
- Reference to steroids and arachidonic acid
- Mention local side-effects like sore or dry throat
- Mention possible thrush formation

Discussion to assuage Elizabeth's concerns may include:

- Checking her knowledge, planning the session, writing/agreeing learning outcomes, using understandable terms, using diagrams/models

Case study ③ *Faustina Olamba*

The candidiasis is probably caused by an inhaled corticosteroid. Her inhaler technique should be checked. It should be ascertained whether or not she has a spacer device and if not one should be provided. If she is using a spacer, it needs to be cleaned regularly. Faustina should also be taught good oral hygiene, especially immediately after taking her inhaled corticosteroid.

Calculations

1   56 tablets
2   50mcg
3   4
4   2mL
5   42 tablets
6   17 days
7   0.5mL
8   2
9   £490.23
10 £51.48

Multiple-choice questions

1   b
2   d
3   a
4   c
5   c
6   b
7   d
8   b
9   a
10 d

Chapter 9

Case study ① *Hannah*

Guidelines for the management of diabetes during surgery in the BNF are quite comprehensive and you should sit with Hannah and go through them with her, reassuring her and reinforcing that diabetes management during surgery is something the nurse, surgeons and anaesthetist are familiar with. Reinforce that as soon as she is able after surgery and tell her when she will be able to eat and drink and restore her normal insulin management. Access the following BNF source and familiarize yourself with the management: https://bnf.nice.org.uk/treatment-summary/diabetes-surgery-and-medical-illness.html

Case study ② Olly Phillips

Assessment of Olly's understanding in discussion with his mother should be undertaken before starting his teaching around managing his insulin. You need to consider the following points:

- Can Olly test his blood glucose and match this to his insulin needs?
- Can Olly draw up the dose accurately?
- Can he remember to give the dose at the correct time or will he need reminders or aids to do this?

Demonstrate to Olly how to give the injection and then allow him to do so under your supervision. Remember to include his mother at all times but acknowledge Olly's desire to become more independent. Ensure regular reviews in the near future to monitor his progress.

Calculations

1 63
2 0.25mL
3 0.04mL
4 60 doses
5 4 doses
6 6 tablets
7 1 tablet
8 1 × 15mg and 1 × 30mg = 2 tablets
9 0.28mL
10 16 full days

Multiple-choice questions

1 a
2 c
3 d
4 c
5 d
6 b

7 b
8 d
9 a
10 b

Chapter 10
Case study ① Tom McBrayer

Angiotensin-converting enzyme inhibitors work by blocking the effects of angiotensin II. They do this by preventing angiotensin I converting to angiotensin II. As angiotensin II is a powerful vasoconstrictor, ACE inhibitors open up blood vessels resulting in a lowering of blood pressure. You may also note that:

- Their mechanism of action not only helps to reduce blood pressure but also protects the kidneys of people with diabetes and hypertension
- Although ACE inhibitors are very effective in the treatment of blood pressure, the initial taking of this medication can cause a sudden fall in blood pressure, and so patients are advised to monitor their blood pressure initially
- ACE inhibitors do, however, have a side-effect of a dry irritating cough (especially at night) which can affect sleep

Case study ② Kevin Todd

Digoxin should be supplied with a patient information leaflet giving lots of information regarding the effects of digoxin on the heart rate and how to monitor it. Kevin should be reassured that digoxin is a medication that has been around for a long time and is well understood and commonly used for this condition. Taking time to explain to Kevin about his atrial fibrillation and the risks of not taking the medication is very important. This can allow him to make an informed choice about what medication is prescribed and help him adhere to the medication regime. Kevin should be taught how to take his own pulse as a measure of his heart rate before taking his digoxin each day. He should be made aware that if his heart rate drops below 60 beats per minute, he should omit his digoxin dose that day, and if it is regularly below 60 beats per minute each day, he should go to see his GP regarding the dose of his digoxin.

Case study ③ *Chuck Andrews*

- Need for medication. It is important to explain that although the surgery has corrected the blockage that caused the MI, he is still at risk of further episodes due to the diagnosis of coronary artery disease and this is the reason for ongoing medication. The medication will reduce his risk of suffering further cardiovascular events
- Action of medication. The medications he is on will have the following actions: 1) lessen his risk of suffering s further coronary event; 2) they will reduce his risks of other events such as embolism or stroke. An explanation of how the drug works should be given in simple layman's terms that Chuck is likely to understand, and jargon should be avoided
- Checking understanding. Ask Chuck to repeat back to you what his understanding is of the information you have given him and check that he knows when and how to take the medications he is prescribed
- Adherence. If Chuck understands what the medication is for, how it will help him and what might happen if he does not take his medication, he will feel fully informed to make his own choices. Patients who feel part of the prescribing process around medication and who have a good understanding are more likely to adhere to their medication regime. Asking him to articulate how he will take the medication and checking it with the prescriber's instructions are also important

Calculations

1. 2mL
2. 13mL
3. 26mL per hour
4. 3 tablets
5. 4mL of digoxin solution and 96mL of infusion fluid and 50mL per hour
6. 42 tablets
7. 16 weeks
8. 2mL
9. 6 sprays
10. 42 tablets

Multiple-choice questions

1. b
2. c
3. a
4. c
5. d
6. d
7. b
8. c
9. a
10. b

Chapter 11

Case study ① *Eric Vardey*

Discussion around the mode of action of levodopa and what the main side-effects of this medicine are might include:

- Levodopa remains the first-line treatment for Parkinson's disease
- Levodopa is a drug that can cross the blood–brain barrier and then be converted by the central nervous system into dopamine
- It is nearly always combined with another substance that stops peripheral enzymes breaking down dopamine. Examples of medicines that are combined or given with levodopa are carbidopa and benserazide
- When given levodopa, patients' response rates are good. However, this improvement is often only short-lived and as time goes by the levodopa becomes less effective
- Short-term side-effects quite often improve over a period of time. The person may feel sick, have no appetite and suffer a slight drop in blood pressure. This decrease in blood pressure could have a more serious effect if the patient is having anti-hypertensive therapy. A small number of patients may develop delusions and hallucinations as the brain is given extra dopamine, which is thought to mimic the high levels found in patients with schizophrenia

- Dyskinesia is when the individual develops a series of involuntary movements, causing acute embarrassment as they usually affect the face and limbs. If the dose is lowered, the dyskinesia does stop, but is replaced by the rigidity it had improved. This is a fine line that the patient and doctor walk in order to accept the consequences of both illness and treatment
- The 'on-off' effect – this is where, quite suddenly, the drug therapy seems to stop working. This can be quite distressing for the patient and can sometimes occur when they are in the middle of doing something. The reason for this fluctuation is not fully understood, but patients should be made aware of these side-effects when commencing treatment

Case study ② Younis Khan

- Phenytoin interacts with many other medications, yet it is still an effective medication for the control of epilepsy and has been started by the consultant for a reason

Let us look at how it interacts with the other medication on Younis' list:

- Insulin glargine – no listed interactions, so it is safe to co-administer
- Fluvastatin – interaction with lipid-regulating drugs, specifically fluvastatin and colesevelam. Consider changing lipid regulator to another that does not interact, such as atorvastatin
- Aspirin – phenytoin does interact with some anticoagulants but not aspirin, so it is safe to co-administer

All of the drugs Younis is taking are necessary for his chronic conditions. He should be regularly reviewed, and his medication monitored by the prescribing professional.

Calculations

1 42 tablets
2 8mL
3 5mL
4 10mL

5 1.25mL
6 0.5mL
7 91 tablets
8 12.5mL
9 375mcg
10 15mL

Multiple-choice questions

1 b
2 a
3 c
4 c
5 a
6 b
7 d
8 b
9 a
10 c

Chapter 12

Case study ① Debbie Butcher

Explain how SSRIs work as follows:

- Checking Debbie's knowledge, planning the session, using understandable terms, using diagrams/models, and checking her understanding of what you have told her
- Discussing the monoamine theory of depression
- Discussing what serotonin is and what is implicated with regard to mood
- Explaining what happens normally at a synapse
- Explaining how SSRIs affect the re-uptake of serotonin

Case study ② Anil Kahn

Discussion around the action of atypical drugs would including the following:

- Drugs block the dopaminergic pathways in the brain
- Most typical antipsychotic medications act on D_2 receptors
- Most atypical antipsychotic medications act on D_1 and D_4 receptors

Discussion around the difference between atypical and typical antipsychotics could include:

- Typical drugs are associated with more side-effects
- Atypical drugs are better at dealing with negative symptoms of schizophrenia
- Patients can gain weight and suffer secondary diabetes if on atypical drugs

Case study ③ Rona McKenzie

Discussion should centre on the need to treat the anxiety symptoms of the episode and identify the specific triggers for the anxiety state:

- Continuous treatment with SSRIs is not appropriate
- Benzodiazepines are not recommended for this type of anxiety
- Beta blockers to manage the anxiety symptoms would be the best pharmacological intervention
- Relaxation or talking therapies may help

Case study ④ Lisa Ryman

Areas to consider include:

- Lisa is likely to have anxiety-related episodes throughout her life and benzodiazepines should only be used in times of crisis and for a very short time
- Benzodiazepine use is related to poorer outcomes in panic disorder; refer to BNF guidance and NICE recommendations when explaining this to Lisa and her mother
- Suggest non-pharmacological strategies to deal with the anxiety
- Refer to experienced prescriber in autism spectrum disorder and anxiety if condition persists for consideration of SSRI

Calculations

1 2 tablets
2 3 tablets
3 4 tablets
4 2.5 tablets
5 0.4mL
6 0.25mL
7 2.5mL
8 1mL
9 4mL
10 2.5mL

Multiple-choice questions

1 d
2 c
3 d
4 a
5 d
6 b
7 a
8 c
9 b
10 c

Chapter 13

Case study ① Elizabeth Green

You may have included aspects of the following:

- Cyclophosphamide is an example of an alkylating agent
- Works directly on the DNA and prevents the cell division process
- Alkylating drugs are effective during all phases of the cell cycle
- Doxorubicin, which is a commonly used anthracycline chemotherapy agent
- Anthracyclines work by interacting with DNA and inhibiting production and function
- Fluorouracil is an antimetabolite which acts to disrupt normal cellular division

Case study ② Student nurse

You would probably offer the following information:

- Aprepitant is used to control nausea and vomiting in patients undergoing cytotoxic therapy
- It is an NK1 receptor antagonist and has its action in the chemotactic trigger zone and the vomiting centres of the brain

- It is useful in the acute and delayed onset of emesis in cytotoxic therapy
- It is important to consider the drug interactions of this drug, especially with warfarin

Calculations

1 3mg
2 46mg
3 0.7mg or 700mcg
4 2.5 hours
5 20 tablets
6 285mg
7 £4.21
8 15 doses
9 6 boxes
10 £1790.88

Multiple-choice questions

1 d
2 d
3 a
4 b
5 b
6 c
7 a
8 b
9 c
10 d

Chapter 14

Case study ① Kubi Garise

Strategies to improve Mrs Garise's compliance may include:

- Linking medication-taking with brushing teeth in the morning and evening
- Taking medications at coffee or tea breaks
- Taking medications at the same time as a favourite programme
- Involving others in ensuring medicines are taken
- Placing notes or reminders around the house
- Wearing an alarm watch that goes off when tablets are due

- Keeping a diary of when tablets have been taken
- Using a pill organizing box

Case study ② Ella Jenkins

Discussion around the importance of compliance with the patient may include:

- Checking the mother's knowledge, planning the session, using understandable terms, using diagrams/models, and checking her understanding
- Ascertaining if Mrs Jenkins appreciates the importance of Ella taking her medicine
- Ascertaining if Mrs Jenkins understands the consequences of Ella not taking her medicine

Improving Ella's compliance with taking her medication:

- Consider looking at the formulation – can the drug be given as a syrup which has a flavour Ella likes?

Case study ③ Oliver Paresi

Discussion should centre on the following points:

- His wife could help him with his medication but she needs to be informed of the following:
  - the indication for each medication
  - the time each dose should be taken
  - the side-effects to look out for
  - the risk of not giving the medication
  - safe storage
- Memory aids for Oliver to help him remember, special packaging from the pharmacy or use of reminder alarms

Calculations

1 2 tablets
2 2,500g
3 0.12mL
4 1,250,000mcg
5 2.5mL
6 2.5mL
7 200mL per hour
8 100,000mg

9 25g

10 300g

Multiple-choice questions

1 a

2 c

3 b

4 d

5 b

6 a

7 d

8 c

9 d

10 b

Chapter 15

Case study ① *Mr Ajani*

- The patient medicines administration chart is not a prescription but a direction to administer medication. It must be signed by a registered prescriber and authorizes the delegation to administer medication on the prescriber's behalf
- Check that the prescription chart is signed and dated by the authorized prescriber
- In exceptional circumstances, where medication (not including controlled drugs) has been previously prescribed and the prescriber is unable to issue a new prescription, but where changes to the dose are considered necessary, information technology (such as fax, text message or email) may be used but must confirm any change to the original prescription

Case study ② *Mrs Simpson*

The nurse must have completed and passed an accredited non-medical prescribing course to gain notation on her NMC registration as a V300 prescriber.

The fact the nurse is a prescriber and can issue the prescription provides Mrs Simpson with more rapid access to medication. This allows for service improvement and greater patient satisfaction and can promote improved patient–professional relationships. Even though Mrs Simpson could, in theory, buy paracetamol over the counter, you should bear the following in mind:

- her ability to go shopping
- the limited number of tablets she would be able to buy in a pharmacy
- the fact that Mrs Simpson is eligible for free prescriptions

Case study ③ *District nurse*

The patient will be well known to the district nurse if she visits regularly. Did the district nurse refer to the patient's notes when preparing for the visit? Was there a photographic identifier on the notes? Did the nurse greet the patient by name, and if so did the patient respond? All of these things are possible, so it would be important as a student nurse to ask the district nurse how she was sure she had the correct patient. Had you been asked to do the dressing and did not know the patient, it would have been appropriate to carry out an identity check.

Case study ④ *Josep Bosko*

The discussion should include:

- What are the licensed alternatives? There may be another similar medication in liquid form
- Prescribe an unlicensed alternative
- Prescribe a specially formulated liquid alternative
- Prescribe by another route. Are there suppository or patch formats?

Case Study ⑤ *Max Jones*

It is important to establish whether or not Max has capacity to consent to medication treatment. Although he is of a legal age to consent, his main disability may mean he lacks capacity. This means the person administering the medication should assess for capacity under the Mental Capacity Act 2005.

- Can Max understand the information regarding the need for medication?
- Can he retain this information?
- Can he use it to make a decision about whether he wants to take the medication or not?

Ascertaining the above will help to determine capacity and if it is found that Max lacks capacity, then best interests and necessity should take precedence. As his epilepsy is severe, it will be necessary to give medication to prevent or reduce seizure activity and this is in the best interests of Max. If Max regularly refuses to take this essential medication, then it is permissible to administer it covertly.

Multiple-choice questions

1 b
2 a

3 d
4 a
5 c
6 c
7 b
8 a
9 d
10 b

Index

Index

70138111R00166